AGING
Volume 15

Clinical Aspects of Alzheimer's Disease and Senile Dementia

Aging Series

Aging
Volume 15

Clinical Aspects of Alzheimer's Disease and Senile Dementia

Editors

Nancy E. Miller, Ph.D.
Gene D. Cohen, M.D.

Center for Studies of the Mental Health of the Aging
National Institute of Mental Health
Rockville, Maryland

Raven Press ▪ New York

Raven Press, 1140 Avenue of the Americas, New York, New York 10036

Raven Press, New York 1981

Made in the United States of America

Library of Congress Cataloging in Publication Data

Main entry under title:

Clinical aspects of Alzheimer's disease and senile
 dementia.

 (Aging; v. 15)
 "Derived from the proceedings of the Second International Conference on Alzheimer's Disease and Senile Dementia . . . held on the campus of the National Institutes of Health in Bethesda, Maryland."
 Includes bibliographies and index.
 1. Presenile dementia—Congresses. 2. Senile dementia—Congresses. I. Miller, Nancy E. II. Cohen, Gene D. III. Series. [DNLM: 1. Dementia, Presenile—Congresses. 2. Dementia, Senile—Congresses. W1 AG342E v. 15 / WM 220 C641 1978]
RC522.C57   618.97′68983   80–39741
ISBN 0–89004–326–4

Preface

Over the past decade, as the elderly have become the fastest growing segment of the population, Alzheimer's disease/senile dementia has emerged as one of this country's major mental health problems. Current estimates suggest that there are approximately one million severely demented persons and another three million mildly to moderately demented persons in the United States. This illness has deleterious effects on cognition, personality, and affect, and empirical evidence also suggests that the length of survival of severely demented individuals is only one-third to one-half that of age-matched controls. Although the economic and emotional burdens of caring for patients with this late-onset brain disorder are great, there have been few systematic efforts to integrate findings from the scientific research literature to yield practical suggestions for direct approaches to clinical care. The aims of this volume are to highlight critical aspects of the theoretic and empirical literature relating to clinical assessment, treatment, and care of the patient with Alzheimer's disease/senile dementia; to translate these research findings, where possible, into direct indications for patient care; and to direct attention to areas of investigation with high potential for practical application and theoretical significance.

Our introductory chapter provides a synopsis of the significant themes and major substantive issues that appear throughout the volume and highlights the most promising directions for future research in the field. The volume is organizationally divided into three major sections. The first section consolidates what is known about the nosology, diagnosis, and behavioral correlates of Alzheimer's disease/senile dementia, with special reference to recent developments in the psychiatric nomenclature as documented in DSM-III and to the often puzzling association between sociocultural variables and manifest symptomatology. In this section, new advances and current practice in neurologic and psychiatric assessment are specified, useful psychometric evaluative procedures are described, and the nature of the cognitive deficit itself, as revealed in experimental studies of memory, perception, and information processing, is more clearly outlined.

The second section includes comprehensive reviews of the efficacy, safety, and reliability of the major treatment and management modalities in current use with elderly dementing patients. It includes an overview of pharmacologic and somatic agents used in treating the effects of cognitive impairment in Alzheimer's disease and a review of useful therapeutic approaches to its affective concomitants. The state-of-the-art in behavioral techniques, and psychodynamic approaches to management and understanding are discussed, together with the effect of the environment on care of the patient.

The concluding section describes the role of the service delivery system, focusing on models of ambulatory care and community treatment as well as on innovative approaches to institutional care. In addition to formal institutional service delivery networks, the nature and value of the informal support network in helping to maintain the older person with dementia in the community is examined. The often neglected special difficulties associated with minority status are also addressed.

The final chapter reviews significant issues and trends in the formulation of social policy and public planning and assesses the economic and social impact of Alzheimer's disease/senile dementia on the fabric of American life.

The contributors represent internationally recognized authorities in the field and present new practical information, evaluate recent progress, highlight gaps in the structure of current knowledge, and outline high-yield areas for future research. The discussion sections interspersed throughout the text convey to the reader the sense of movement and excitement that characterizes this field today; they demonstrate the sense of hopefulness and lively controversy which is the mark of a newly developing system of scientific inquiry.

Although much remains to be learned about the cognitive pathologies of later life, they can no longer be regarded as invincible. This book comprises a rich and valuable resource for psychiatrists, neurologists, internists, family physicians, psychologists, behavioral scientists, social workers, graduate students, and all members of the health care team who share an interest in understanding and treating the older individual with Alzheimer's disease and his family.

Nancy E. Miller
Gene D. Cohen
Rockville, Maryland

Acknowledgments

This volume is derived from the proceedings of the Second International Conference on Alzheimer's Disease and Senile Dementia, jointly hosted by the National Institute of Mental Health, the National Institute on Aging, and the National Institute of Neurological and Communicative Disorders and Stroke and held on the campus of the National Institutes of Health in Bethesda, Maryland. The proceedings of the First Conference[1] focused on basic research in the etiology, pathophysiology, nosology, and epidemiology of this brain disorder. The emphasis of this Second Conference is on current clinical research and practice in the assessment, differential diagnosis, care, and treatment of the Alzheimer's patient within a practical and multidisciplinary framework.

---

[1] Katzman, R., Terry, R. D., and Bick, K. L., editors (1978): *Alzheimer's Disease: Senile Dementia and Related Disorders* (Aging, Vol. 7). Raven Press, New York.

Contents

Introduction

Introductory Statements

Clinical Description and Evaluation of Alzheimer's Disease and Senile Dementia

Contributors

Tom Airie
Department of Psychiatry
University of Nottingham Medical School
Nottingham, England

Odin W. Anderson
Center of Health Administration Studies
University of Chicago Graduate School of
  Business
Chicago, Illinois 60637

Klaus Bergmann
The Maudsley Hospital
London SE5 8AZ, England

Elaine M. Brody
Department of Human Services
Philadelphia Geriatric Center
Philadelphia, Pennsylvania 19141

Jacob Brody
Epidemiology, Demography and Biometry
  Program
National Institute on Aging
Bethesda, Maryland 20205

Paula J. Clayton
Department of Psychiatry
Washington University School of Medicine
St. Louis, Missouri 63110

Donna Cohen
Department of Psychiatry and Behavioral
  Sciences
University of Washington School of
  Medicine
Seattle, Washington 98195

Gene D. Cohen
Center for Studies of the Mental Health
  of the Aging
National Institute of Mental Health
Rockville, Maryland 20857

John M. Davis
Department of Psychiatry
University of Chicago
and
Illinois State Psychiatric Institute
Chicago, Illinois 60612

Maurice Dysken
University of Chicago School of Medicine
and
Illinois State Psychiatric Institute
Chicago, Illinois 60612

Carl Eisdorfer
Department of Psychiatry and Behavioral
  Sciences
University of Washington School of
  Medicine
Seattle, Washington 98195

Leon J. Epstein
Department of Psychiatry
Langley Porter Neuropsychiatric Institute
University of California School of
  Medicine
San Francisco, California 94143

William E. Fann
Department of Psychiatry
Baylor College of Medicine
and
Psychiatry Service
Veterans Administration
Texas Medical Center
Houston, Texas 77211

John A. Farell
St. Elizabeths Hospital
Washington, D.C. 20032

Donald S. Fredrickson
National Institutes of Health
Bethesda, Maryland 20205

xi

H. Harris Funkenstein
Department of Neurology
Peter Bent Brigham Hospital
and
Harvard Medical School
Boston, Massachusetts 02115

Charles M. Gaitz
Gerontology Research Section
Texas Research Institute of Mental
  Sciences
Houston, Texas 77025

Samuel Gershon
Department of Psychiatry
Wayne State University
Detroit, Michigan 48207

Ralph Goldman
Veterans Administration Central Office
Washington, D.C. 20420

Lars Gustafson
Psykiatriska Kliniken
Lunds Universitet
S-221 85 Lund, Sweden

Barry J. Gurland
Center for Geriatrics and Gerontology
Faculty of Medicine
College of Physicians and Surgeons
Columbia University
New York, New York 10032

Robert Hicks (deceased)
Section on Geriatric Psychiatry
Department of Medicine
University of Texas Medical School
Houston, Texas 77030

Gerald L. Klerman
Alcohol, Drug Abuse and Mental Health
  Administration
Rockville, Maryland 20857

M. Powell Lawton
Behavioral Research Division
Philadelphia Geriatric Center
Philadelphia, Pennsylvania 19141

Zbigniew J. Lipowski
Department of Psychiatry
Dartmouth Medical School
Hanover, New Hampshire 03755

Ronald Martin
Department of Psychiatry
Washington University School of Medicine
St. Louis, Missouri 63110

Harold Merskey
Department of Psychiatry
University of Western Ontario Psychiatric
  Hospital
London, Ontario N6A 4H1, Canada

Edgar Miller
Department of Clinical Psychology
University of Cambridge
Addenbrooke's Hospital
Cambridge CB2 1EL, England

Nancy E. Miller
Clinical Research Program
Center for Studies of the Mental Health
  of the Aging
National Institute of Mental Health
Rockville, Maryland 20857

Robert Nathan
Department of Mental Health Sciences
Division of Liaison Psychiatry and
  Psychosomatic Medicine
Hahnemann Medical College
Philadelphia, Pennsylvania 19102

Herbert Pardes
National Institute of Mental Health
Rockville, Maryland 20857

Eric Pfeiffer
Suncoast Gerontology Center
University of Southern Florida Medical
  School
Tampa, Florida 33612

Caroline Preston
Department of Psychiatry and Behavioral
  Sciences
University of Washington School of
  Medicine
Seattle, Washington 98105

Robert L. Ringler
National Institute on Aging
Bethesda, Maryland 20205

Sir Martin Roth
Department of Psychiatry
University of Cambridge
Addenbrooke's Hospital
Cambridge CB2 2QQ, England

Bruce Schoenberg
Neuroepidemiology Section
National Institute of Neurological and
*   Communicative Disorders and Stroke*
Bethesda, Maryland 20205

Ken Solomon
Department of Psychiatry
University of Maryland School of
*   Medicine*
Baltimore, Maryland 21201

Sheldon S. Tobin
School of Social Service Administration
University of Chicago
Chicago, Illinois 60637

Donald B. Tower
National Institute of Neurological and
*   Communicative Disorders and Stroke*
Bethesda, Maryland 20205

Ramón Valle
School of Social Work
San Diego State University
San Diego, California 92115

Adrian Verwoerdt
Department of Psychiatry
Duke University School of Medicine
Durham, North Carolina 27706

H. Shan Wang
Department of Psychiatry
Duke University Medical Center
Durham, North Carolina 27706

Jack Weinberg
Department of Psychiatry
Abraham Lincoln School of Medicine
University of Illinois
and
Illinois State Psychiatric Institute
Chicago, Illinois 60612

Charles E. Wells
Departments of Psychiatry and Neurology
Vanderbilt University School of Medicine
Nashville, Tennessee 37240

Jeanine C. Wheless
Department of Psychiatry
Baylor College of Medicine
Texas Medical Center
Houston, Texas 77211

Mark Wisen
Department of Neurology
University of Indiana
Bloomington, Indiana 47401

Richard Jedd Wyatt
Unit on Geriatric Psychiatry
and
Laboratory of Clinical
*   Psychopharmacology*
Division of Special Mental Health
*   Research*
National Institute of Mental Health
St. Elizabeths Hospital
Washington, D.C. 20032

*Clinical Aspects of Alzheimer's Disease and
Senile Dementia,* (Aging, Vol. 15), edited by
Nancy E. Miller and Gene D. Cohen.
Raven Press, New York 1981.

Introductory Statement: A View from the Alcohol, Drug Abuse, and Mental Health Administration

Gerald L. Klerman

Alcohol, Drug Abuse, and Mental Health Administration, Rockville, Maryland 20857

The clinical aspects of Alzheimer's disease and senile dementia—the disorders of later life—is an area of great concern across a range of categorical programs. The Alcohol, Drug Abuse, and Mental Health Administration (ADAMHA) is pleased to join the National Institute on Aging and the National Institute of Neurological and Communicative Disorders and Stroke in discussing this important area.

NIH and ADAMHA together fund approximately 90% of the nation's research in the biomedical, behavioral, and psychosocial aspects of health and illness.

Each of the three component Institutes of ADAMHA—the National Institute of Mental Health, the National Institute on Alcoholism and Alcohol Abuse, and the National Institute of Drug Abuse—has a particular and vital interest in the problems of aging.

The National Institute of Mental Health, with its Center for studies of the Mental Health of the Aging, has had the lead in the development of this conference. Such collaboration represents a dynamic aspect of the American research establishment, both in intramural and extramural programs. We have discovered various means of working together on large scale problems that cut across the categorical Institutes, while at the same time developing research focused on a particular manifestation of the problem.

This is the second joint conference called to deal with the problems of the dementias. That a distinguished group of investigators has again been brought together for these discussions indicates once again the capacity of the Public Health Service and of the scientific community to mobilize research efforts and knowledge for the further understanding of large-scale health problems.

It is our experience that through the valuable combination of basic and clinical research, public health problems can and do lend themselves to amelioration. Our continuing commitment to a balance between basic and clinical research stands as a fundamental principle of all our scientific endeavors, and particularly in the field of aging.

In the past the National Institute of Mental Health and the other Institutes of our agency may have emphasized the psychosocial and behavioral aspects of Alzheimer's disease, senile dementia, and other disorders. However, in recent years, the Institutes have supported increased activity in the neurosciences, including genetics, neurochemistry, and neuropharmacology. The boundaries between the biomedical and the behavioral sciences are increasingly becoming blurred; the distinctions between the purely behavioral and the biomedical approaches to a problem such as aging are more difficult to maintain. In this and other areas, as much cooperation is now required among the various scientific disciplines as has been required in the cooperation of several distinct Institutes in developing this series of conferences.

There have been notable advances in the basic neurosciences, especially in the understanding of the structure and functioning of the central nervous system, and in the psychological sciences, particularly as to the regulation of mood as occurs in depression among the aged, and the processes of memory and of cognition in aging. The clinical distinction between the pseudo-dementias of the depressions and the true dementias remains a major research problem to be addressed by the field.

I look forward to participating in these scientific deliberations and urge the three Institutes to plan other collaborative endeavors in this and other areas.

*Clinical Aspects of Alzheimer's Disease and
Senile Dementia,* (Aging, Vol. 15), edited by
Nancy E. Miller and Gene D. Cohen.
Raven Press, New York 1981.

Introductory Statement: A View from National Institutes of Health

Donald S. Fredrickson

National Institutes of Health, Bethesda, Maryland 20205

This volume represents the continuation of an exploration of the state of knowledge about Alzheimer's disease and senile dementia that was initiated in 1977 by the same sponsors. Its emphasis on the clinical aspects of these problems will, once again, be rooted in the findings of research and focus on what is known, but at the same time and perhaps in a more forcible way, bring us face to face with what is not known.

Joint sponsorship of these proceedings by the concerned Institutes—in this case crossing major organizational lines—exemplifies the kind of collaboration that enhances the efforts of each participating unit in dealing with different aspects of a common endeavor.

The dementias and their devastating human consequences constitute a significant public health problem of great economic dimensions. They primarily affect older people, a group that now constitutes 11% of the population and is responsible for 30% of the health care costs in this country. Brain deterioration represents perhaps the most critical aspect of aging, leading to loss of independence, withdrawal from active life, and often to institutionalization. It is one of the major reasons for admission to nursing homes—an extremely costly element in the nation's health bill.

It is predicted by the year 2000 there will be 32 million people over 65 years of age or 12% of our nation's population, and the number of the very old—those 75 and above—will be anywhere from 12 million to 18 million, depending on trends in mortality rates. So we are concerned here with a very substantial number of people and a huge economic burden.

If we can prevent or reverse some of the consequences of Alzheimer's disease and senile dementia, if we can improve diagnosis and clinical management, and if we can avoid or postpone institutionalization for even a small segment of the older population, we will be making a tremendous contribution to reducing the burden of medical care costs for the American people. Even more important, we will have made life better for all.

In the spring of 1978, the National Institutes of Health, together with the health-related agencies of the Department of Health, Education, and Welfare, began an intensive effort to develop a set of research principles to guide in the planning process by which the varied and substantial resources of the Department can be brought to bear on the nation's health needs.

This series of papers embodies precisely the intent of the planning principles—a commitment to fundamental research, and a recognition of the need not only to acquire new knowledge, but also to validate and apply it.

From such considerations, the National Institutes of Health has adopted research and research training in Alzheimer's disease and the dementias of aging as a special initiative. These Institutes are involved. The National Institute on Aging conducts research on basic science and clinical aspects of regional brain metabolism, neurochemistry and pharmacology. The major research effort of the National Institute of Neurological and Communicative Disorders and Stroke is to define etiology and pathogenesis and, in attempting to accomplish this, the Institute conducts clinical research projects, therapeutic trials, and epidemiologic studies. The possible role of a latent or slow virus in chronic dementia is being explored by the National Institute of Allergy and Infectious Diseases.

The total NIH financial commitment to Alzheimer's diesease and the dementias of aging increased from less than 7.5 million in fiscal 1979 to almost 11 million dollars in 1980 and the upward trend will be continued. These efforts, in coordination with those of ADAMHA, our sister agency, and of the scientific community at large, should certainly lead to more effective treatment and, I believe, the prevention of some of the dementias.

*Clinical Aspects of Alzheimer's Disease and
Senile Dementia,* (Aging, Vol. 15), edited by
Nancy E. Miller and Gene D. Cohen.
Raven Press, New York 1981.

Introductory Statement: Mental Health Perspectives

Herbert Pardes

National Institute of Mental Health, Rockville, Maryland 20857

With recent advances in the absolute number and relative proportion of older persons in the general population, growing attention has been focused by federal agencies on the devastating and disabling effects of those brain disorders that are associated with advancing chronological age. Among these disorders, senile dementia of the Alzheimer's type has been estimated to affect more elderly persons than any other brain disease, with 4 to 15% of the population over 65 being affected. Although the aged are disproportionately subject to mental and emotional problems, it is the individuals over 75 years of age, who are most vulnerable to the development of mental disorder, who also comprise the fastest growing segment of the elderly population.

The National Institute of Mental Health (NIMH), a component part of the Alcohol, Drug Abuse, and Mental Health Administration in the Public Health Service, is responsible for implementing the nation's major program in research and training for enhancing mental health and for understanding, treating, and preventing mental illness. In view of the great need for more fundamental information about how individuals function and fail to function, both emotionally and cognitively, in middle and later life, NIMH has actively embarked on a program of support to stimulate researchers to study these problems.

At NIMH, the Center for Studies of the Mental Health of the Aging (CSMHA) is the focal point for work in aging and the late life dementias. The major role of the Center is to stimulate, coordinate, and support research, training, and technical assistance efforts relating to aging and mental health. The Center, under the leadership of Dr. Gene D. Cohen, supports a wide-ranging, multidisciplinary set of studies that have both theoretical and applied implications. These include studies of the etiology, diagnosis, natural history, course, and prevention of mental disorders in later life, with special emphasis on the spectrum of dementias, affective disorders, and the interface between physical disease and psychiatric illness. The Center's interests range from support of studies applying advances in computerized axial tomography to problems in differential diagnosis, to systematic investigations of the role of the family in sustaining the psychological integrity of the patient with Alzheimer's diesease who is living in the community.

Other sections of NIMH also regard the mental health of the aging as a high priority area, and collaborate with CSMHA in the support and stimulation of innovative research. Psychopharmacology, for example, represents a rapidly advancing field of research, which has the potential for uncovering new clues in the etiology and basic mechanisms of the disease process itself. Studies are underway at the Psychopharmacology Branch at NIMH to measure the effects, for example, of naturally occurring substances such as small brain peptides on memory in senile dementia. The possible effects of increasing cholinergic activity on mental deficits associated with Alzheimer's disease are also being investigated, as are the effects of vasodilators, ergot alkyloids, and a variety of other psychotropic compounds.

The CSMHA also collaborates with the Biometry and Epidemiology Branch in fostering investigations that examine the distribution of late life dementias in the general population. Epidemiologic studies are urgently needed to define the prevalence, incidence, and risk factors associated with this disorder since available estimates of the incidence and prevalence of senile dementia are based on a patchwork of noncomparable studies. The absence of appropriate epidemiologic data therefore continues to be a major hinderance to the effective planning of appropriate health and mental health services for the elderly. In the context of its major Epidemiologic Catchment Area initiative, the Center for Epidemiologic Studies, in collaboration with the CSMHA and the National Institute on Aging, plans to oversample the elderly living in both institutions, and in the community, in various geographic regions of the United States. There is also interest in evaluating the interplay of genetic and environmental factors on the expression of symptomatology in dementing illnesses. One recent epidemiologic investigation supported by NIMH revealed that relatives of probands with histologically confirmed Alzheimer's disease manifested excessive morbidity from Alzheimer's disease, Down's syndrome, and hematologic malignancies. These findings raise the specter of a common genetic deficit in the development of Alzheimer's diesease, Down's syndrome, and various malignancies, and point the way to possible etiologic mechanisms.

Other portions of the Institute also play important roles in advancing investigations of the psychopathology of later life. As one of its many foci, the Clinical Research Branch, for example, supports studies on the nature, specificity, and efficacy of psychological interventions on various types of mental illness, including conditions of altered brain function, and the Mental Health Services Development Branch assists in the formulation of innovative approaches to mental health service delivery, including a focus on elderly persons with brain impairment.

As a scientific research institute, NIMH is rather unique in its mandate to provide support not only for research training, but also for services, and for the clinical training of mental health professionals. Critical to the advancement of understanding, prevention, and treatment of these late life disorders is the presence of an adequate pool of high caliber professionals, both researchers and clinicians, who are knowledgeable regarding the diagnostic and therapeutic dilemmas presented by the dementias of late onset. Programs sponsored by both the Center for Studies of the Mental Health of the Aging and the Division of Manpower and Training are currently underway in an effort to increase the number of geriatric specialists in the core mental health disciplines.

At the intramural level, a new research unit in Geriatric Psychiatry has been set up under the direction of Dr. Richard Jedd Wyatt. The unit has shown impressive progress in studies of neuroplasticity and in pharmacological research. This group has also been involved in the development of new and sensitive methods for measuring aluminum, a neurotoxin, and in research on slow viruses, in collaboration with the National Institute of Neurological and Communicative Disorders and Stroke. Extramurally, the relationship of hypertensive disease to dementia is being examined as part of a long-term clinical trial supported jointly by the National Heart, Lung, and Blood Institute, the National Institute on Aging, and the National Institute of Mental Health.

A major area of NIMH's interest is in the development of improved models for integration of mental health with health services. Full access to mental health services for those needing care constitutes a high priority Institute goal. Underserved populations, especially elderly persons with cognitive disorders, who have received only minimal treatment in the past, will be especially represented in this initiative. From another angle, the treatment and care of the chronically mentally ill, including individuals with senile dementia of the Alzheimer's type, is of special concern both to NIMH and throughout the Department of Health and Human Services. This attention would include a focus on those patients with psychopathology addressed in the Mental Health Systems Act, as well as those encompassed in the newly developed National Plan for the Chronically Mentally Ill. In addition to the broad scope of these activities, and to an expanding HHS interest in the quality of long-term care, there is the proposed federal initiative specifically focused on Alzheimer's disease and the dementias of aging, which will bring together the combined resources of the National Institute of Mental Health, the National Institute on Aging, the National Institute of Neurological and Communicative Disorders and Stroke, and the National Institute of Allergy and Infectious Diseases.

In conclusion, although the etiology of these dementias, in most cases, remain unknown, although their diagnosis remains problemmatic, and their effects on the family—in disrupting human ties, in causing the loss of productive members of society, and resulting in profound social and emotional hardships—are great, much effort, thought, and fresh initiative is being brought to bear on this devastating public health problem, on the part of the National Institute of Mental Health, and its sister agencies and Institutes, across the span of the Public Health Service. The opportunities for finding new solutions for this crippling disorder have never been brighter.

*Clinical Aspects of Alzheimer's Disease and
Senile Dementia,* (Aging, Vol. 15), edited by
Nancy E. Miller and Gene D. Cohen.
Raven Press, New York 1981.

Introductory Statement:
Neurological Perspectives

Donald B. Tower

*National Institute of Neurological and Communicative Disorders and Stroke, National
Institutes of Health, Bethesda, Maryland 20205*

At the first conference of Alzheimer's disease–senile dementia, I pointed out a number of neurobiological aspects that represent intriguing and urgent research challenges (7). In particular there is the very special relevance to the overall problem of aging of the human nervous system, with the likelihood that aging of most of the body is a function of the "health" of the nervous system. Thus, we of the National Institute of Neurological and Communicative Disorders and Stroke (NINCDS) recognize a close identification with the many problems confronting the National Institute of Aging (NIA), and indeed we are engaged in a continuing dialogue with our colleagues in the NIA over this and many other program concerns.

In this volume we begin consideration of the clinical aspects of the dementias, where the interests and responsibilities of the NINCDS clearly overlap those of the National Institute of Mental Health (NIMH). Since the inception of these two institutes more than 25 years ago, we have tended to divide research responsibilities between the neurosciences (NINCDS) and the behavioral sciences (NIMH). As Dr. Klerman has already indicated, these distinctions are hardly tenable today. The borders have become blurred as those in behavioral studies are confronted with biochemical circuitry, modulatory peptides and hormones, and neuropharmacological agents that have specific correlations with behavioral phenomena. At the same time neuroscientists are forsaking the simpler neuronal networks and electrophysiology for the problems of central processing, adaptation, plasticity, and all those complex integrative functions that comprise behavior. Nowhere is the confluence of the two streams of research more critical than in the problems posed by the human dementias.

Among the clinical problems presented by the dementias, we at the NINCDS view at least three as particularly important. First, there is the sheer magnitude of the problem in terms of numbers of patients—an aspect discussed at some length in the first conference (6). Secondly, there is the currently perplexing variety of dementias encountered in clinical neurological and psychiatric practice.

There is the dementia that develops in Huntington's disease—a genetically determined autosomal dominant disorder characterized by massive destruction

9

of neurons in the striatum and consequent involvement of cerebrocortical neurons (1). There is the population focus of Parkinson-dementia among the native Charmorros on Guam—a disorder in which the parkinsonism can be effectively managed with L-DOPA and its congeners without affecting the relentless course of the dementia, and in which there are neuropathological changes characteristic not only of Parkinson's disease but also of Alzheimer's disease (5). There is the slow-virus group of disorders—the transmissible spongioform encephalopathies, like Kuru and Creutzfeldt-Jakob disease, in which dementia is the final expression of the destruction of neurons in many gray matter areas, together with pronounced astroglial changes (4). And there is the Alzheimer-senile dementia group of disorders under specific consideration here.

This is not an exhaustive list, but even these examples illustrate some of the epidemiological, etiological, and clinical dilemmas. And these are too often complicated by vascular, nutritional, visual, and auditory disorders that plague the aging population. Moreover, many such patients commonly go to the neurologist, although they have major behavioral components that warrant sharing with the psychiatrist—or vice versa. We hope that new research approaches like positron emission transverse tomography (PETT) will be instrumental in unravelling some of the unknowns in these peculiarly human disorders. What CT scans have done for the demonstration of morphology and pathology in the living human brain, the PETT scans will do for metabolism and function (3). For the first time, we are promised an opportunity to probe harmlessly in the living patient's brain the mysteries of such peculiarly human disorders as the dementias.

Finally, the dementias confront all of us with major catastrophes in patient care and services. In this respect each of the examples just cited are all too familiar to the neurologist, the psychiatrist, and the gerontologist. During the public hearings recently held by the Congressionally mandated National Commission on Huntington's Disease, those of us who attended such hearings heard over and over again the destruction wreaked on families, their financial disasters, and the often fruitless search for medical help and institutional care that the havoc of the Huntington's disease dementia creates (2). And Huntington's disease is by no means unique in these respects. Thus, the needs for research that will provide the clinician with preventive, screening, counselling, and therapeutic measures are obvious. But until these measures become realities, we must deal with the dementias by providing regional, comprehensive centers for care and services as well as providing effective solutions to the financial and institutional care problems.

Thus, from the NINCDS perspective we emphasize three points: the continuum of research from basic mechanisms and animal models in the laboratory to the clinical problems at the patient's bedside; the essential pooling of research talents and resources by the concerned institutes—NINCDS, NIA and NIMH; and the imperatives for all of us in DHHS to address the acutely desperate needs in the areas of patient care and services.

This conference-workshop must develop advice and recommendations for planning clinical research, management, and services, and for the allocation of necessary resources. The problems are important and immense; the challenges are extraordinary. I cannot emphasize too strongly that for our older citizens especially, the health of the nervous system is *the* critical factor in the quality of their lives.

REFERENCES

1. Chase, T. N., Wexler, N., and Barbeau, A. (eds.) (1980): *Second International Huntington's Disease Symposium.* Raven Press, New York.
2. Commission for the Control of Huntington's Disease and Its Consequences (1977): *Report, Vol. I: Overview* (DHEW Publication (NIH) 78–1501) U.S. Dept. Of Health, Education, and Welfare-PHS-NIH, Bethesda, Maryland.
3. Fox, J. L. (1978): Methods map brain functions chemically. *Chem. Engineer. News,* 56:20–22.
4. Gajdusek, D. C., and Gibbs, C. J., Jr. (1975): Slow virus infections of the nervous system and the laboratories of slow, latent and temperate virus infections. In: *The Nervous System, Vol. 2: The Clinical Neurosciences,* edited by T. N. Chase and D. B. Tower, pp. 113–135. Raven Press, New York.
5. Hirano, A., Malamud, N., and Kurland, L. T. (1961): Parkinsonism-dementia complex, an endemic disease on the island of Guam. II. Pathological features. *Brain,* 84:662–679.
6. Katzman, R., Terry, R. D., and Bick, K. L. (eds.) (1978): *Alzheimer's Disease: Senile Dementia and Related Disorders.* Raven Press, New York.
7. Tower, D. B. (1978): Alzheimer's disease-senile dementia and related disorders: Neurobiological status. In: *Alzheimer's Disease: Senile Dementia and Related Disorders,* edited by R. Katzman, R. D. Terry and K. L. Bick, pp. 1–4. Raven Press, New York.

*Clinical Aspects of Alzheimer's Disease and
Senile Dementia,* (Aging, Vol. 15), edited by
Nancy E. Miller and Gene D. Cohen.
Raven Press, New York 1981.

Introductory Statement:
Aging Perspectives

Robert L. Ringler

National Institute on Aging, National Institutes of Health, Bethesda, Maryland 20205

In the United States, the elderly constitute one of the fastest growing segments of the population. The 24.4 million persons over 65 make up just over 11% of the population (8), and we expect that this figure will jump to the range of 17 to 21% by 2030 (2). More striking than this is the rate at which the elderly population is growing compared with the population at large. Between 1970 and 1977, the number of persons 65 and over increased by 18%, whereas the general population increased by only 5% (1).

As a response to the dramatic increase in the total number of elderly, the U.S. Congress passed the Research on Aging Act early in 1974, thereby creating a National Institute on Aging (NIA) to conduct and support biomedical, behavioral, and social research to improve the quality of life in the later years.

Health care professionals are also beginning to appreciate the significance of the changing age structure. Faced with a growing number of elderly patients, physicians are becoming more aware of the dangers of accepting negative stereotypes of old age and more concerned with providing effective treatment for the special needs and problems of the aged.

Despite many advances and many positive changes in attitudes toward the elderly, however, research on the chronic dementias of aging has been comparatively neglected. The belief that these disorders are both inevitable and intractable continues to prevail.

The NIA supports the position that the dementias are not concomitant with old age; rather, they represent pathological disease states that should be subject to investigation, skilled diagnosis and treatment, and, given further research, preventive activities.

In keeping with the Institute's goal to enhance the quality of life in the later years, the NIA considers research toward an understanding of senile dementia to be a major priority. Approximately 1 million people in the United States over age 65 suffer severe dementia with global intellectual deterioration and inability to carry out the normal tasks of daily living. An additional 2 to 3 million are mildly or moderately affected. Of these, it is estimated that between 500,000 and 1.5 million persons suffer from senile dementia of the Alzheimer's type—so called because clinical presentation, postmortem pathology, electron microscopy, and histochemical studies all support the concept that senile dementia and Alzheimer's disease are indistinguishable with the exception of age of onset (4).

In an effort to serve as a catalyst for research in this area, the NIA joined with the National Institute of Neurological and Communicative Disorders and Stroke (NINCDS) and the National Institute of Mental Health (NIMH) in sponsoring the first conference of this series (5). Since that time, the NIA has instituted a neuroscience program both extramurally and intramurally.

Last year, the extramural neuroscience element—which supports research at universities, medical centers, and other research institutions—funded several significant research projects dealing with senile dementia and with age-related changes in the central nervous system. One NIA-supported study in animal models is already yielding data suggesting that the brain may be able to compensate for some forms of cell loss (6). Since many older persons suffer death of neurons, which is also one of the hallmarks of senile dementia, this is an area deserving of further research. In other studies of major import, scientists are developing a better understanding of structural and neurochemical changes that accompany senile dementia in human research subjects.

Also, in this past year, Dr. Stanley I. Rapoport, who is well-known for his work on the blood-brain barrier, became the first director of the Laboratory of Neurosciences at NIA's intramural research facility in Baltimore. The importance of continued research on the barrier can hardly be exaggerated, particularly in light of our interest in the etiology of senile dementia. The barrier normally provides selective nutrition for the brain, excludes antibodies from the brain that could kill cells or alter function, and may play a role in viral passage.

One collaborative project currently being planned involves using positron emission transverse tomography to study cerebral metabolism in humans, specifically, the uptake of an analog of glucose. Using this noninvasive technique, NIA investigators can measure functional changes in the brain activity of persons with Alzheimer's disease or senile dementia, as well as persons who are aging normally.

Many of the participants at the first conference of this series noted that the baseline data necessary for scientific study of senile dementia are not available. Under the direction of Dr. Jacob Brody, the NIA has now established an Epidemiology, Demography, and Biometry Program to develop information on the incidence and prevalence of senile dementia and other diseases that afflict the old. Currently, most older people escape all medical and statistical attention; as a result, health planning is often based on incomplete information.

To develop valid and reliable quantitative instruments and measures of dementia, and to determine the magnitude of the problem, Dr. Brody is collaborating with clinical and laboratory scientists and epidemiologists at NIMH, NINCDS, and NIA, as well as internationally renowned investigators such as Sir Martin Roth of Great Britain.

The NIA Epidemiology, Demography, and Biometry Program is also collaborating with epidemiologists at the NINCDS in supplementing the NIMH population or catchment area studies of community mental illness being directed by Jerome Myers of Yale University.[1] The goal is to determine the number of older people with senile dementia who have remained in the community.

Dr. Brody also hopes to join NINCDS in its study of amyotrophic lateral sclerosis-parkinsonism dementia complex in Guam. Neurofibrillary change, which is a common histological feature of senile dementia of the Alzheimer's type, is also seen extensively in the brains of those suffering from the severely debilitating and progressive dementia, which is essentially indigenous to the Chamorro population of Guam.

On the clinical side, NIA supports the position that health care professionals must rule out the possibility of a treatable disorder before establishing a diagnosis of Alzheimer's disease/senile dementia. Although there are numerous references in the medical literature to the physiological and psychological disorders that can mimic senile dementia, the NIA initiated a special effort to develop guidelines for the diagnosis and treatment of mental impairment in the elderly (7). It is tentatively estimated that such disorders may account for as much as 30% of those cases diagnosed as irreversible, with untold institutional costs.

At the same time, we look forward to the development of clinical programs designed to test treatment modalities for the so-called irreversible disorders. These disorders are by no means hopeless ones.

Before closing, I would like to highlight a very positive development of this past year. Until recently, the victims of Alzheimer's disease/senile dementia and their families have had to cope as best they could. When suddenly faced with a diagnosis of Alzheimer's disease—often after years of going from one physician to another—they were given little hope or information. When trying to care for the affected person at home, the family was given minimal support. In addressing this group last year, Dr. Robert N. Butler advocated the founding of an organization to aid the families of persons with Alzheimer's disease in facing the personal and financial crisis this often entails, as well as the disruption of family life (3). Several such groups have now formed to assist the family and increase public awareness of the need for research support for the dementias.[2]

Much has been accomplished since the meeting a year and a half ago, but there is still a need to increase our fundamental knowledge of the chronic dementias through basic, clinical, behavioral, and epidemiologic research; and to apply that knowledge to improved health care. The National Institute on Aging sincerely believes that joint efforts such as this meeting represent one approach to the attainment of the overall goal of ameliorating or preventing the dementias of aging.

---

[1] Myers, J., The Epidemiologic Catchment Area Program. (National Institute of Mental Health grant U01-MH-34224.)

[2] In October 1979, seven self-help groups dealing with Alzheimer's disease and related disorders in Boston, New York, Pittsburgh, Minneapolis, Columbus, Seattle, and San Francisco united to form the Alzheimer's Disease and Related Disorders Association (292 Madison Avenue, New York, New York 10017).

REFERENCES

1. Brotman, H. B. (1978): The aging of America: A demographic profile. *Natl. J.,* 10:1622–1627.
2. Bureau of the Census (1978): *Demographic Aspects of Aging and the Older Population in the United States.* (Special Studies Series P-23, No. 59). U.S. Government Printing Office, Washington, D.C.
3. Butler, R. N. (1978): Alzheimer's disease—senile dementia and related disorders: The role of NIA. In: *Aging: Vol. 7: Alzheimer's Disease: Senile Dementia and Related Disorders,* edited by R. Katzman, R. D. Terry, and K. L. Bick, pp. 5–9. Raven Press, New York.
4. Gruenberg, E. M. (1978): *Patterns of Disease Among the Aged.* National Institute on Aging, Bethesda, Maryland (HEW Publication No. NIH 78-1410).
5. Katzman, R., Terry, R. D., and Bick, K. L. (eds.) (1978): *Aging, Vol. 7: Alzheimer's Disease: Senile Dementia and Related Disorders.* Raven Press, New York.
6. Scheff, S. W., Bernardo, L. S., and Cotman, C. W. (1978): Decrease in adrenergic axon sprouting in senescent rat. *Science,* 202:775–778.
7. A Task Force Sponsored by the National Institute on Aging. (1980): Senility reconsidered: Treatment possibilities for mental impairment in the elderly. *JAMA,* 244:259–263.
8. U.S. Senate Special Committee on Aging (1979): *Developments in Aging: 1978.* U.S. Government Printing Office, Washington, D.C.

Clinical Aspects of Alzheimer's Disease and Senile Dementia, (Aging, Vol. 15), edited by Nancy E. Miller and Gene D. Cohen. Raven Press, New York 1981.

Clinical Aspects of Alzheimer's Disease and Senile Dementia: Synopsis and Future Perspectives in Assessment, Treatment, and Service Delivery

Nancy E. Miller and Gene D. Cohen

Center for Studies of the Mental Health of Aging, National Institute of Mental Health, Rockville, Maryland 20857

Senile dementia of the Alzheimer's type is a disorder of growing medical importance, and one of immense social and economic impact. It is a chronic, progressive, deteriorative neuropsychiatric brain disease accompanied by profound and devastating effects on memory, cognition, and ability for self care. Historically, senile dementia has been assumed to be an inevitable result of normal advancing chronological age. Current scientific trends, however, suggest that this serious and irreversible impairment of brain function represents an insidious disease process that is separate and distinct from normal aging: The majority of older persons do not develop this disorder within their lifespans, and it is estimated that only 5 to 7% of the population at age 65 have moderate to severe dementia of the Alzheimer's type. However, the incidence of Alzheimer's disease is strongly age-related, and the risk of developing this disorder increases as one grows older. Given the steadily rising proportion of the population that is elderly, and given conservative estimates that one out of every five Americans will be past 65 within the next half century, the public health implication and the social and economic impact of the problem is obvious and overwhelming.

This volume presents a practical, theoretical, and multidisciplinary approach to contemporary clinical knowledge in the assessment and treatment of Alzheimer's disease, senile dementia, and related conditions.

The scope of the volume ranges from a comprehensive focus on questions of nomenclature and differential diagnosis to an inquiry into intrapsychic, affective, and cognitive concomitants of the disorder. It includes analyses of the safety and efficacy of a variety of behavioral, pharmacologic, and other somatic treatment regimens, offers multiple perspectives on models of care and service delivery, and considers the emotional, social, and economic costs of developing this disease at the family, community, and societal levels.

The volume is written for those with an interest in any number of aspects of the chronic dementing conditions of late life, with the expectation that an understanding of one's own area of expertise may be significantly enhanced by a fresh awareness of the multiple factors impinging on the care and well-being of the elderly individual with senile dementia of the Alzheimer's type.

The volume constitutes the second set of proceedings to emerge from a series of conferences on Alzheimer's disease and senile dementia, jointly sponsored by the National Institute of Mental Health, the National Institute on Aging, and the National Institute of Neurological and Communicative Disorders and Stroke. The initial publication, entitled *Alzheimer's Disease: Senile Dementia and Related Disorders* (Katzman, R., Terry, R. D. and Bick, K. L., eds., Raven Press, New York, 1978), which presents an extensive scientific overview of the field, focuses largely on basic etiological and pathophysiological studies of the dementing disorders of later life. The present volume, in contrast, tackles the clinically oriented problems of diagnosis and management, which in many respects are more difficult to study, in that they are less amenable to precision in scientific investigation, and must take into account not only factors on the molecular, cellular, and neurophysiological levels, but must also consider more molar aspects of the problem on the organismic and societal levels as well.

As the initial volume suggests, considerable progress has been made over the course of the past decade in delineating new etiological models of dementia and in studying possible metabolic, neurochemical, genetic, immunological, and viral abberations associated with dementing conditions of later life. Yet, as the contents of this volume reveal, although much has been learned, the extent of our ignorance is still staggering, and current challenges to clinical investigators could not be more stimulating or provocative.

In the process of reviewing the chapters included in this volume, which were prepared by authors representing widely divergent theoretical perspectives and differing experimental approaches to clinical knowledge, a number of themes or consistently expressed problems began to repeatedly manifest themselves with significant consistency and clarity. Because in many instances these concerns appear so obvious, basic, and deceptively simple, they are especially prone to neglect by the serious investigator. Yet, many of these items constitute important variables, which are often difficult to address empirically because they represent a complex series of confounded factors, frought with methodological pitfalls and colored in many instances by emotional preconceptions and closely cherished beliefs. In the course of briefly reviewing the major issues addressed in this volume, these special themes will be highlighted and described.

A number of these themes present themselves at the most basic clinical levels of knowledge. For example, serious questions continue to be raised regarding nomenclature and how this disease, or spectrum of diseases, should be classified—what it should be called, and what the nature of the clinical criteria should be for positive identification of the disorder in the living patient. Since there is no chemical, radiologic, or psychometric examination or indicator that is specific for Alzheimer's disease, the diagnosis can only be reliably made postmortem on the basis of histopathologic data or clinically by a process of excluding potentially treatable dementias. Accordingly, reliable data regarding the prevalence of the disorder are difficult to obtain, and much of the reported literature is problematic because of great variability in the methods of classification and diagnostic procedures used in identifying the disorder. Almost without exception, both authors and discussants in this book underscore and reiterate the serious difficulties that accrue in research as the result of the lack of a uniform, well-defined nosology for classifying the dementias of later life.

The opening chapters review this problem in detail. Zbigniew J. Liposki provides a historical perspective on the language of psychopathology related to brain disorders and describes the ambiguous and overlapping terminology that has been used to characterize these states in the past. He depicts the more rudimentary efforts to classify organic mental disorders that have taken place over the span of centuries, and brings us up to date with an analysis of the more recent development of the classification of mental disorders in American psychiatry. This includes conceptualizations used in the American Psychiatric Association's second edition of the *Diagnostic and Statistical Manual of Mental Disorders* (DSM-II) published in 1968, and continues through the significantly revised and recently published third edition of this manual, DSM-III. The chapter broadly discusses the place of senile dementia and Alzheimer's disease in the context of, and in relation to, other organic mental disorders, and describes the distinctions specified in DSM-III among classifications of delirium, dementia, amnestic syndromes, organic hallucinosis, as well as among the organic delusional syndromes, organic affective syndromes, and organic personality disorders. Lipowski underscores a second theme that is also expressed repeatedly, from various theoretical perspectives, and across disciplines throughout this volume. This regards the critical importance of psychological and social factors as essential components coloring the manifestation of the illness and the fresh appreciation that symptomatology in all organic/mental disorders is multifactorial in origin.

In further delineating aspects of nomenclature, Paula Clayton and Ronald Martin focus on the historical development of the senile and vascular dementias as specific nosological entities, and outline the rationale in DSM-III for encompassing senile dementia of the Alzheimer's type under the classification of "primary degenerative dementia." They also describe the rationale for selection of the term "multi-infarct" dementia to describe stepwise deterioration of intellectual function in the face of focal neurological signs and a fluctuating course of disease. The current DSM-III classification has eliminated the distinction between "psychotic" and "nonpsychotic" aspects of organic mental disorder, and has incorporated the recognition that mental, neurologic, and pathologic findings appear to be indistinguishable in Alzheimer's disease regardless of whether onset is in the senium or the presenium. The DSM-III incorporates a new multiaxial approach to diagnosis, which yields a far more complex and comprehensive picture of the patient: In the context of this classification system, the first axis reflects the primary disorder, the second includes personality description, the third lists associated medical disorders, the fourth indicates the presence of recent life stress, and the fifth describes highest level of adaptive ability in everyday life during the past year. The authors of both nomenclature papers were active members of the Section on Organic Brain Disorders in the Committee on Nomenclature and Statistics of the American Psychiatric Association, and they therefore can provide the reader with a bird's-eye view of the developing conceptualization and logic behind the most recent shifts in nosology descriptive of the organic mental disorders. The new classification has been clinically tested and has been reviewed, rewritten, and changed in response to criticisms and suggestions from the field. Only far more extensive use over time, however, will confirm the validity and utility of these new adjustments.

It is clear that different nosological schemes often reflect different aims of classification and different unstated assumptions underlying their purpose and development, and that such classifications may manifest different strengths and weaknesses, depending on the context in which they are used. In keeping with this, the lively discussion following these papers highlights two somewhat divergent approaches to nomenclature, the more circumscribed and phenomenological approach to classification of organic mental disorders, as exemplified in the 9th edition of the *International Classification of Diseases,* ICD-9, as formulated by the World Health Organization, and the broader, operationally descriptive American view as exemplified in DSM-III. The discussants from Great Britain cogently note, for example, that although the International classification (ICD-9) ranks dementing states by operationally defined grades of severity, the DSM-III has not incorporated a formalized system for indicating severity in its classification of organic mental disorders. Some degree of discomfort is also expressed regarding the new American system of labeling symptomatic affective and schizophreniform psychoses, occurring concomitantly with organic states, as "organic affective syndromes," "organic personality syndromes," or "organic delusional syndromes." The British contend that such a nosological schema fosters the unproven assumption that it is the underlying organic states themselves that are both necessary and sufficient causes for manifestation of the concomitant behavioral symptomatology. It is their view that since the causal association between these is unknown, and the clinician may simply be dealing with the conjunction of two relatively discrete and independent groups of phenomena, it would do well to describe these states on the basis of further empirical research rather than deciding them at the outset by "arbitrary" diagnostic rules. However, views on this point differ, and although some worry that widening the scope of definition of the psychoorganic syndromes may result in the blurring of conceptual parameters of diagnosis, others feel that, on the contrary, by including diagnoses such as hallucinosis, organic delusional syndrome, organic affective disorders, and organic personality disorders, fresh research on the borderland of disorders spanning the range between organic and functional psychopathology will be significantly enhanced. It is hoped that the new classification will stimulate the formulation of testable hypotheses, loosen entrenched conceptions about organicity, and encourage a fresh look at these unresolved issues. Such lively controversy is likely to remain in this area for some time to come, and represents a healthy indication that scientists continue to ponder and struggle with complex questions of classifying behavioral symptomatology in the face of definitive brain disease. If the new formulation advanced in DSM-III serves to provoke more discussion, fresh conceptualization, and the uncovering of new etiologic clues, the result is likely to be a rapidly advancing field, a more secure knowledge base, and a richer understanding of the nature and possible treatment of these multifactorial brain disorders.

That the situation grows increasingly complex is indicated in the following chapter on "The Borderlands of Dementia." Here, Barry Gurland suggests that not only do serious questions remain regarding the optimal methods to be used in classifying the brain disorders of later life, but also that even more basic are those questions pertaining to the nature of the actual criteria used in identifying the presence of senile brain disease of the Alzheimer's type. Depending on the manner in which the diagnosis is formulated, the effect of socio-cultural variables on rates of disease appear to differ. A number of studies undertaken in both the United States and Great Britain, for example, suggest that when dementia is measured by psychological indicators such as mental status questionnaires or rating scales, rates and severity of dementia appear to vary with socio-cultural factors. On the other hand, the association between dementia and social class appears to be weaker when diagnosis formulated by a clinician is the indicator, rather than when a psychological instrument acts in this capacity. This discrepancy raises the specter of the differential validity of various techniques commonly employed in the assessment of brain disorder in older persons. Much remains to be learned about precisely what it is that is being measured in each type of evaluation, and what the systematic effects are of the numerous intervening variables that color expression of symptoms and manifest behavior. Since biologic or behavioral markers pathognomic of the disease have not yet been found, there is as yet no real agreement regarding the most favorable approach to positive identification of the disease. Results from empirical studies continue to be inconsistent, and it remains unclear whether clinical diagnosis, say in the hands of a psychiatrist or neurologist, is more reliable than other techniques, such as tests and rating scales, for the classification of dementing psychopathology. Accordingly, many of the significant discrepancies in prevalence rates of dementia reported in different community surveys may be partially due to differences in the methods and criteria used for diagnoses. Furthermore, there may be an overabundance of brains in the advanced stages of dementia that come to autopsy, as well as a social class bias in the collection of brain tissue, such that sociocultural differences in prevalence could easily be missed in those studies based only on postmortem examinations.

Gurland also raises fundamental issues regarding the whole nature of the brain-behavior relationship in dementia. He notes that although severity of cognitive deficit is typically correlated with severity of changes in the neurophysiological substrate, there appear to be many exceptions to this rule, with some subjects showing gross brain pathology but minimal performance decrements, and others showing mild structural changes in brain accompanied by massive behavioral incompetence. It is not clear to what extent performance on mental status examinations is influenced by both dementia and sociocultural characteristics, and whether the relationship between test performance and brain deterioration in the dementing process is more common in certain sociocultural groups. These issues arouse continuing controversy regarding the relationship between structure and function, between the nature, degree, and extent of damage to the neurophysiologic substrate and the resulting variety and severity of manifest cognitive and behavioral deficit. They raise questions regarding the functional plasticity and modifiability of neural systems, the role of nature and nurture, the effects of learning, of cortical redundancy, and of the reserve capacity of the brain.

Gurland speculates about mechanisms that may underlie an association between cortical reserve capacity, brain insults, sociocultural characteristics, and prevalence rates of a dementing process, and suggests that premorbid personal, intellectual, and adaptive factors may have a profound influence on the behavioral sequelae associated with altered brain function in later life. Social class and education may, for example, be associated with the preservation of social skills and personal habits that enable the older person with dementia to survive in the community for far longer periods of time.

As the animated panel discussion following Gurland's paper suggests, current knowledge regarding the specificity of brain-behavior relations in dementing conditions and the role of auxiliary sociocultural variables and character traits remains an open question. As such, it constitutes a critically important research challenge for the future.

H. S. Wang, in "Neuropsychiatric Procedures for the Assesment of Alzheimer's Disease," underscores the view of both Drs. Gurland and Lipowski in suggesting that Alzheimer's disease is a complicated disorder that is influenced by a broad variety of physical, psychological, and social factors. In the course of formulating a diagnosis and establishing a treatment plan during the neuropsychiatric evaluation, Wang suggests that it is important to take many different levels of function into account. The evaluation should include measures of memory and cognition, assessment of functional and structural brain impairment, a review of behavioral manifestations affecting the individual's capacity for self-care, as well as quality of the patient's interpersonal relations and ajustment. In keeping with former authors, Wang stresses that often there is not a one-to-one correlation between brain impairment, behavioral or affective dysfunction, and capacity for self-care, such that many levels of analysis are necessary in order for a comprehensive, realistic treatment appraisal to be formulated.

The chapter reviews the validity, efficacy, and comparative cost of neuropsychiatric measures and procedures currently available for evaluation of various aspects of Alzheimer's disease, including an overview of relevant history taking, and the psychiatric and neurological examination. A concise description of the efficacy of various laboratory procedures is provided, including plain skull X-ray films, pneumoencephalography, cerebral angiography, radioisotope brain scans, cisternography, electroencephalography, cerebral blood flow, brain biopsy, computerized axial tomography, and positron emission transverse tomography.

In the following paper, Edgar Miller considers the goals of psychological assessment in Alzheimer's disease, which include the measurement of cognitive and perceptual change from premorbid levels, the formulation of a differential diagnosis, and the rendering of decisions about management and placement. In his report, Miller considers each of these subjects in turn, reviewing what is known on a systematic basis and highlighting areas in need of further work.

Since the success of any systematic study of dementing conditions depends most importantly on the reliability or accuracy of the formulated diagnoses, Miller approaches the recurrent problem of differential diagnosis from a rigorously empirical perspective, asking methodological questions that few clinical investigators working in the field have taken seriously into account. The chapter addresses basic issues concerning diagnostic validity, problems relating to direct and indirect contamination effects, questions regarding the homogeneity of subject samples, shifts in base rates of disease, and how and where cutoff points should be set in order to optimize overall levels of correct classification. For example, it is clear that opinions and value judgments often enter the classification process in unspecified ways, and that differential costs and benefits accrue, depending on the nature of the goal to be ascertained. Thus, as Miller states, "It could be argued that since depression is a treatable condition, it is a much more serious error to misdiagnose a depressed patient as demented, than the reverse. Would you set the cutoff score to minimize this type of error, even at the expense of a greater risk of falsely classifying a dement as depressed?"

In addition to questioning the adequacy of test norms for assessing the elderly, and especially the effects of changes in cohort characteristics over time on age-rated normative data, the author also underscores the great need for cross-validation in assessment research, as well as the need for more and better multiple test forms in order to control for practice effects.

In addition, the chapter reviews the utility of a wide variety of psychometric instruments including tests of IQ, memory, verbal learning, design copying, language, and orientation, as well as traditional neuropsychological measures, rating scales, and mental status examinations. Automated procedures, such as matching to sample techniques and the use of direct observational methods, are also discussed.

Although psychological tests are often quite useful in determining differential diagnoses, they generally are less successful in measuring cognitive decline from premorbid levels. Only rarely is reliable premorbid information available to the clinician, and even when factors such as education and occupation are controlled for, it is suggested that there is still considerable fluctuation in intelligence levels within categories. Moreover, in many instances, even if differences are found at a group level, it is not always possible to reliably and accurately interpret data obtained from the individual case.

These methodological parameters are more fully considered in the following report on the "Nature of the Cognitive Deficit in Dementia." Here the author is not so much concerned with issues facing the clinician in the diagnostic setting as with providing a comprehensive synopsis of the experimental research literature on the nature of cognitive and perceptual impairment in demential disorders. Since dementia is associated with diffuse and wide ranging pathological changes in the brain, it is not surprising that a broad spectrum of functional and behavioral deficits has been identified by experimental investigators. Since so many behavioral capacities are eroded by senile dementia of the Alzheimer's type, Miller emphasizes the need not only for more descriptive research but also for research based on explanatory theoretical models, which can be confined to a single behavioral system. In the area of cognitive research especially, there have been few systematic attempts to explain a particular problem in depth. Rather, the knowledge base is meager, with many of the areas studied representing fragmented efforts, which have not built on findings reported by others. The need, therefore, is great for investigators to make sustained career commitments to research in this area. Many experimental studies of cognition in dementia suffer from major methodological flaws, especially stemming from problems in the selection of subjects. Again, the theme is reiterated that study samples are poorly described, that criteria used in selection vary markedly, and that results, accordingly, are often noncomparable and inconsistent.

Miller discusses what is known about cognition in dementia, and presents the available evidence regarding distractibility, disturbances of attention, utilization of acoustic coding in short-term memory, performance on tests of iconic memory, long-term storage, free recall, memory for remote events, acquisition and retrieval, etc., but concludes that, overall, many aspects of intellectual function memory in dementia remain unexplored. In addition, although senile dementia of the Alzheimer's type is a slowly progressive disease, there are no empirical reports in the literature following the development of cognitive impairment across different stages of the course of disease. Moreover, there have been extremely few studies of such functions as perception, information processing, visuospatial abilities, and thinking in dementia. For example, although clinical impression suggests that there appears to be an increased incidence of sensory impairment in dementia, both visual and auditory abnormalities have been minimally investigated. Similarly, although some reports indicate that naming difficulties in senile dementia of the Alzheimer's type differ from those occurring in more usual types of dysphasia, there have been few investigations of narrative speech in this disorder. Rather than simply exploring the presence or absence of a particular deficit, however, Miller advises investigators to attempt to approach experimental research in this area from a clinical management perspective. Given that the etiological factors in this disorder remain unknown, the predominant problem presented by the patient with dementia is one of management—that is, how can the clinician diminish the importance of cognitive deterioration and ensure that the individual retains his functional capacities for as long as possible? Accordingly, the experimental question then shifts from trying to define the deficits to attempting to establish under what circumstances these are either maximized or minimized. For example, how well do older patients with dementia retain information under different conditions of acquisition?

Some innovative and beginning approaches to these questions are explored in the following section, which focuses on somatic, behavioral, and environmental treatment and management parameters in the dementing states of later life. Although many of the attributes and subtleties of the cognitive impairment accompanying dementia remain to be systematically described, on a gross and descriptive level, the clinical hallmark of dementia consists of symptoms of progressive deterioration of intellect and memory. In keeping with Edgar Miller's suggestion regarding investigations that attempt to establish under what conditions the severity of dementia impairment can be ameliorated or minimized, there have been a host of studies undertaken that have made the attempt to identify a chemical agent capable of reducing, halting, or reversing the intellectual decline associated with dementia.

In the following chapters, Drs. Funkenstein, Hicks, Dysken, and Davis review the substantial literature on the major classes of drugs that have been used in an effort to improve cognitive function in elderly patients. Some of the agents touched on in this chapter include classes of cerebral vasodilators, central nervous system stimulants, anabolic substances, RNA-like compounds, anticoagulants, vitamins, chelating agents, and cholinomimetic substances. After reviewing the available evidence, the authors conclude that although no drug has demonstrated any clear degree of efficacy in reversing the cognitive failure of dementia, some of the drugs reported on may be useful in certain types of patients. In many of the studies, however, reports of improvements may actually be secondary to changes in mood state rather than a result of enhanced cognitive function. Pharmacological research on the dementias of later life is no less affected by methodological pitfalls than are other substantive research areas. Such studies, for example, often exhibit a lack of precision in describing the character of the experimental sample and the nature of the outcome measures used. In addition, in many of the drug studies, terms used to describe beneficial outcomes often indicate an affective rather than a cognitive locus of action, with the investigators stating in their conclusions that the patients are "brighter," "less irritable," or "more socializable," etc. Investigators often fail to separate gains due to mood enhancement from primary effects on intellectual function, and do not use psychometric instruments capable of reliably measuring cognition. Moreover, few of these studies actually control for the effects of medication on affective status and motivation levels. Research in this area is progressing rapidly, however, and many promising leads are still in the experimental stages of development.

Although truly effective pharmacologic treatments for intellectual deterioration in dementia have not yet been formulated, significantly greater success has been achieved in ameliorating those psychopathologic affective states that are often seen to develop concomitantly with dementing processes in later life.

Often, the affective and interpersonal symptoms accompanying senile dementia such as depression, anxiety, agitation, irritability, withdrawal, paranoia, etc. can accelerate deterioration. Yet, as Fann and Wheles reveal in their chapter, many of the symptoms of these concomitant conditions are treatable, and adaptive behavior is generally seen to improve when the affective symptoms are effectively identified and managed. This chapter yields practical suggestions for pharmacological management of the affective components of senile dementia, and reviews relevant studies of drug trials with antipsychotics, anxiolytics, anticoagulants, MAO-inhibitors, ergot alkaloids, vasodilators, central nervous system stimulants, cholinergic agents, hormones, enzymes, vitamins, nootropic drugs, etc. The studies reviewed vary significantly in their degree of methodological rigor, ranging from open studies with no placebo control groups, to double-blind, placebo-controlled, crossover designs. Even in the latter studies, however, many of the reports manifest methodological shortcomings, which continue to make it difficult to assess the accuracy of their contributions. The frequent presence, for example, of simultaneous physical and psychiatric disorder in older demented persons and the consequent effects of polypharmacy often make it difficult to differentiate the intended effects of the experimental drug from side effects, placebo effects, etc. Furthermore, in various of the studies of anti-anxiety, antidepressant, and antipsychotic agents, the homogeneity of the experimental group is not always assured, and oftentimes, deteriorated subjects at the endpoint of dementia are used for study. Furthermore, sample sizes are frequently too small and the trial period for the experimental agent is often too short. On the whole, however, the authors conclude that enough reliable evidence is available to suggest that much can be done to ameliorate coexistent anxiety, depression, agitation, and paranoia, and that when used appropriately, psychopharmacological treatment can significantly relieve emotional distress in the dementing conditions of later life.

Both the authors and the panel discussants highlight the fact that because older persons have reduced tolerance to psychotropic medication, they require lower doses to reach a desired therapeutic effect. Older patients may manifest frequent and severe side effects at essentially therapeutic doses. Side effects include drug-induced Parkinsonism, tardive dyskinesia, for example, or the exacerbation of psychotic symptoms associated with anticholinergic toxicity. There appears to be reliable consensus among both researchers and clinicians regarding recommendations to limit the use of agents with potent anticholinergic side effects in older persons. In treating depression, for example, the use of antidepressants that have minimal anticholinergic activity is strongly advised, and it is suggested that agents such as the monoamine oxidase inhibitors be given greater consideration with this population than they have had in the past. Not much evidence from double-blind studies is available regarding the differential effects of antipsychotics and antidepressants in elderly persons with dementia, and the question of using electroconvulsive therapy (ECT) in the management of the affectively depressed older person with organic brain disease has been even less adequately explored. It is speculated that ECT may be an extremely effective method for the treatment of depression in cases of senile dementia, but further studies are urgently needed. Fuller consideration of specific practical issues such as the somatic treatment of choice in cases with mixed symptomatology, the nature of drug side effects in the elderly, specific contraindications, dosage schedules, drug-interaction effects, and problems resulting from longer term trials of medication can all be found in the discussion sections following each of the chapters on somatic approaches to treatment.

The question of affective response to illness is explored from a different perspective in Adrian Verwoerdt's innovative chapter on the use of individual psychotherapy with senile dementia patients. This chapter was specifically invited in an effort to counter the strong sense of nihilism so often manifested by clinicians and staff about older persons with brain disorder. Such attitudes are often, at least partially, the result of the staff's own feelings of helplessness and despair, which often stem from unrealistic expectations and goals. Although intellectual function and capacity for self-care may be severely limited in older persons with Alzheimer's disease, the capacity for affective responsivity is often preserved until the end stages of disease.

Verwoerdt suggests that a psychodynamic approach to treatment of the demented patient is both feasible and appropriate when incorporated as an integral part of a comprehensive treatment plan. Such an approach can serve to deepen the clinician's understanding of the conflicting emotions, fears, and intrapsychic mechanisms that color the patient's subjective world, that substantially affect his adaptation to neuronal impairment, and that impinge on the therapist's own subjective motivation to become involved on a sustained basis in the treatment process. The chapter is rich in clinical examples and filled with a wealth of practical information regarding treatment on the clinical level. It is based on the recognition that no matter what symptoms the patient presents, there is always something the practitioner can do to give relief. The aim of treatment, which the author suggests must be continued indefinitely throughout the course of the disease, is to facilitate optimal functioning as long as possible, by maintaining and utilizing residual skills, enhancing mastery and adaptive coping, and by relieving concomitant emotional distress. Verwoerdt reiterates the importance, stressed throughout this volume, of adopting a patient approach to long-term management, rather than treating the individual with expectations derived from a short-term, acute approach to care.

The chapter describes a variety of psychological defensive techniques aimed at mastery and control, at conservation of energy, and at retreat from threat, which are commonly manifested by elderly patients with brain impairment. The behavioral patterns commonly associated with these techniques, and the implications of these for the individual's adjustment and clinical management, are presented.

The chapter also traces common obstacles to the therapist-patient relationship and describes the dementia patient's penchant for primary process thinking, his impaired capacity for abstraction, and his common use of paleologic thought, analogies, displacement, and condensation. As a result of these deficits in cognition, Verwoerdt suggests that the use of a nondirective interviewing style is contraindicated with dementia patients. Instead, an approach providing the patient with consistency, predictability, cognitive structure, and the opportunity for closure is substantially more useful.

Patients with Alzheimer's dementia often present with acute traumatic anxiety and/or with feelings of depletion, abandonment, helplessness, and shame. Depressive loneliness is extremely common in these individuals, and as Fann and Wheles note, tends to exacerbate the severity of symptomatology. The author describes the practical management of a variety of defensive operations and discusses various clinical approaches to problems of combativeness, apathetic withdrawal, paranoia, mania, hypochondriasis, dependency, regression, etc. Although the goal of treatment is aimed at reducing helplessness and encouraging a sense of self-control, Verwoerdt poignantly and aptly reminds us that "self-care has appeal only to the extent that there is something to live for."

This chapter speaks knowledgeably about those emotional phenomena and personality changes that, although difficult to classify and quantify, appear to exert a powerful effect on the expression of behavior in persons with progressive senescent brain impairment. Although systematic research in this area has been sparse, every clinician working on the front lines with demented patients is aware of their presence and in some way must come to terms with them. As the discussion section following the chapters on nomenclature indicates, consensus is far from unanimous in regard to how these symptoms should best be classified. Whether the associated symptoms of dementia are described from a psychoanalytic perspective, or from a behavioral framework, whether or not one assumes that a close correspondence exists between brain structure and specificity of behavioral impairment, whether the symptoms are classified as integral parts of the organic spectrum of disease, or as independent syndromes, their presence needs to be acknowledged and understood, carefully diagnosed, and appropriately treated. At this point there is little to indicate, on an empirical basis, the parameters of these affective symptoms or syndromes, their frequency of occurrence, their differential responsiveness to various treatment modalities, or their long-term prognostic significance. It is evident that much difficult work remains to be done.

The need for more research is also emphasized in the chapter on behavioral therapies by Carl Eisdorfer, Donna Cohen, and Carolyn Preston. The authors reinforce previously reiterated views, suggesting that behavior is multidetermined, that therapeutic nihilism is deleterious, and that much of the literature examining efficacy of treatment strategies continues to focus on acute methods of curative treatment, rather than on the management and maintenance of function in chronic disease.

Eisdorfer et al. focus on what is known about a broad variety of treatment approaches with elderly persons with dementia, which include different operant techniques, cognitive interventions, and psychosocial treatments. The efficacy of efforts to change a variety of maladaptive behaviors such as muteness or screaming, for example, or bowel and bladder incontinence, poor personal hygiene, obsessional rituals, self-injurious behavior, etc. are explored, and techniques to increase social interaction, enhance cognitive skills, improve ability for self-care, and prevent deterioration are also presented. Included among these approaches are techniques such as reality orientation, remotivation, resocialization, activity therapy, and group, milieu, and family therapies.

Questions concerning the effects of relocation stress, and the fostering of dependency and learned helplessness are taken into account, as are descriptions of covert treatment goals, such as staff assumptions regarding the importance of "conforming" behavior on the part of the patient. The chapter reviews a broad scope of treatment literature and contains descriptions of practical and successful approaches to problems in patient care. It also highlights the minimal amount of outcome research that has been done in this area.

These sentiments are echoed by M. Powell Lawton in his description of the ecological context in which persons with dementia live. Lawton suggests that as an individual's base of behavioral competence erodes, the effect of the environment assumes increasing importance in determining well-being.

He hypothesizes that although brain-impaired aged are more vulnerable to noxious environments, on the other hand, small environmental improvements may produce disproportionate effects in "low competent" individuals. Accordingly, to the extent that the environment surrounding the demented individual is either deprived or stressful, behavior and affective outcomes will be more negative than necessary. Behavioral mapping of the daily activities of demented elderly persons in institutionalized settings reveals a low diversity of spatial experience, significant impoverishment of social behavior, and high frequencies of isolated and passive activity, such as sleeping or sitting.

Since the institutional milieu of demented patients verges on sensory deprivation, Lawton suggests that it would be useful to emphasize diversity within the circumscribed treatment area, and to attempt to produce greater variation in the types of behavior demanded of individuals with dementia. On the other hand, Lawton notes that despite the intention that treatment-environment improvements should enhance or increase sensory stimulation, orientation, self-maintenance, and social behavior, only limited empirical evidence is available to suggest that any of these aids are, in fact, effective. Edgar Miller's remark—in the chapter on the nature of the cognitive deficit—indicated that there exist apparent perceptual abnormalities in individuals with dementia, but that little is known about these; similarly, more needs to be evaluated regarding the effects of sensory deprivation and sensory overload, stimulus complexity, and novel experience on demented patients. Although it is often asserted that persons of lower cognitive competence require simpler environmental stimulus fields, if adaptive behavior is to result, again, there is little systematic evidence on this point.

As Gurland, Miller, Verwoerdt, Eisdorfer, and Lawton have all suggested, more needs to be known about the possibility of modifying behavior, and the available plasticity of response in these patients. Moverover, if demented persons do manifest an improvement in behavioral activity as the result of a specific environmental intervention, what are the implications of this for management, housing, and approaches to institutional care? Should those with senile dementia, for example, be clustered in a single location, or housed in areas where fully mentally competent persons reside? Lawton suggests that the literature is equivocal on this point, and notes that although some studies suggest the importance to demented patients of the presence of mentally competent persons, if social interaction is to take place at all, oftentimes strong objections to this are raised by both relatives and staff.

In addition to questions regarding how the progressive chronic brain disorders of later life are to be classified, diagnosed, treated, and managed, there is a real need to better understand how effectively, in what contexts and settings, and at what cost these clinical and social services are delivered to patients and their families.

In their chapter on community treatment for aged persons with altered brain function, Robert L. Kahn and Sheldon F. Tobin provide a historical perspective regarding the effectiveness of mental health models for treating older persons with altered brain function in their own community. They suggest that the provision of community mental health services to the aged has declined precipitously and consistently since the end of World War II, such that, at present, most community service programs have policies of screening out older persons with Alzheimer's disease and senile dementia. With the pressures toward deinstitutionalization, the emptying of state mental hospitals, the failure of community mental health centers to treat major mental disorders of the aged, and the effects of recent health care legislation, there has emerged a "new custodialism," exemplified by the accumulation of masses of older persons with brain disorders in nursing homes. With few exceptions, services for the elderly in the community today remain fragmented and uncoordinated, with limited integration between psychiatric, medical, and social service networks.

Outside of the nursing home, the focus is not on long-term assistance in helping to maintain chronically ill patients in their natural communities so much as on expensive, technology-intensive care, oriented toward treatment of acute medical illness. The authors cogently describe the deleterious effects of custodialism, and of the provision of overintensive, overprotective services on the functional capacity of the elderly patient with brain impairment. They note that such individuals commonly develop what is described as "excess disability," in that they manifest greater functional disability than warranted by their health status. As a result of institutionalization, a "social breakdown syndrome" occurs, in which the individual is torn from his or her moorings in the community, and added impairment is superimposed on that due to intrinsic properties of the pathology. Once social supports collapse, as when the old person is admitted to an institution for a prolonged period, they are often difficult to reconstruct.

In order to circumvent this, a series of basic principles of community mental health care of the aged is delineated, which includes an emphasis on (a) early identification and prompt treatment, and a focus on minimal dislocation by providing home evaluation and treatment in the community, if possible, and strictly time-limited hospitalization, close to home, if not; (b) building a relationship of trust and commitment with a community catchment area by providing integrated service alternatives, which include such services as assessment units, home care, day care programs, holiday relief for families, time-limited hospitalization and continuity of care—such that the same personnel are responsible for the patient in different settings and times, etc. A number of progressive and effective European and American models of community care are described that have successfully integrated these principles of minimal intervention.

When interpreting findings from the literature in this area, it is often useful to note the manner in which results are colored by particular value judgments and unspecified covert assumptions. In some studies, for example, presumably benign outcomes are limited to relatively trivial criteria of effectiveness. Additionally, therapeutic strategies often do not distinguish primary pathological behavior patterns from those patterns arising as a result of institutionalization itself. Moreover, as noted by Eisdorfer et al., there is often confusion in distinguishing between basic goals, such as the slowing of intellectual deterioration in the patient, and more limited goals, such as the value of having compliant patients, who cause few management problems for the staff. In many instances, the achievement of the latter may contradict the attainment of the former. Investigators often fail to acknowledge that very difficult and complex calculations of value, of costs and benefits, need to be made in these situations, and that sometimes the best solution for the family member may not constitute the best solution for the patient. Often, for example, relief to relatives and the best interests of the patient do not coincide. A delicate balance must be struck between providing for community care that fosters survival of the older person in the community for long periods and one that, at the same time, does not strain community tolerance and the family burden. The authors indicate that institutional care, by itself, can be either custodial, with negative effects, or therapeutic, by being brief and time-limited.

Elaine Brody presents a contrasting perspective regarding the value of long-term care institutions, noting that for many persons with brain dysfunction, these provide an important, appropriate, and necessary component of care. She skillfully describes how the current climate favoring deinstitutionalization places community care for institutions in a false position of competition, rather than of mutual and interactive support. She notes the need for community care services to be expanded enormously, and concomitantly, the need for "deinstitutionalizing" the institution.

The chapter exhaustively reviews the legislative and economic factors giving impetus to the growth of institutional facilities on the United States over the past 30 years, and lists the rates of institutionalization of the over-65 population in different countries. Although data specifically focused on long-term care rates of Alzheimer's disease are inadequate, it is estimated that the current 5% figure in the United States—as a proportion of the institutionalized aged—represents a serious underestimate.

In line with the theme repeated by Eisdorfer, by Verwoerdt, by Fann, Kahn, Miller, etc., Brody also indicates that an acute care model has been imposed inappropriately on long-term care. She stresses the importance and desirability of a social-health model to replace a model based on acute and episodic care. Brody notes that risks of being admitted to an institution are multiply determined, and are significantly related to age, sex, race, and health status, such that individuals most likely to be institutionalized are over 80, white, female, and preponderantly from lower socioeconomic groups. Although the primary precipitant to institutionalization is poor health, the critical factor as to who is institutionalized involves the availability of adequate social support systems, especially family. Although at present fewer institutionalized persons are married and have children than age-matched controls living in the community, this situation may alter significantly, concomitant with the shifts in demography, social values, and life styles that are taking place in America today. In years to come, a clearly increasing burden of care will be placed on the institution and formal support system as a result of the rapid growth of the very old, and of those individuals at highest risk for dementia and institutionalization. In addition, as a result of women's changing life styles, their substantial increase in labor force participation will make them less available to give the overwhelming preponderance of home health services that they provide at present. Moreover, given the continuation of present trends of high rates of divorce and remarriage, complex and multiple, and often strained, filial loyalties may ensue.

Finally, the specter of people in advanced old age being cared for by aging children who have their own age-related problems, chronic disabilities, interpersonal losses, retirement, and lowered income to face is growing more common.

Senile dementia is one of the most socially disruptive diseases, placing severe burden on family members who, in most cases, have little recourse from community services. The burden on the family in terms of emotional strain, interference with employment and daily life, the effects on children, etc. is considerable. Accordingly, there is a significant need to reassess the whole question of burden, and the differential response to it, on the part of available health and social services.

In reference to this, the discussion section highlights the new and rapidly emerging community phenomenon of Alzheimer self-help groups, with information describing the origin and development of these local support networks into a national organization. These groups emerged partially as an answer to the extraordinarily stressful and complex effects an individual with Alzheimer's disease has on his own family members, with spouses often traveling in desperation from one medical center to another, searching for a cure or for definite answers, and refusing to institutionalize the patient. With the advent of these groups, physicians diagnosing the disorder now have a place to direct the family that will assist them in their emotional adjustment, ease the stress of living with chronic illness, and supply behavioral methods to spouses and relatives to assist them in maintaining the patient at home. The rapid development of these groups indicates the presence of a profound need on the part of relatives and family members, and accentuates the importance of involving the patient's family in the formulation and development of a realistic treatment plan.

Ray Valle's chapter looks into these issues one step further, describing what is known about natural support systems, not only generally, but also specifically, as they are differentially constituted in different sociocultural and ethnic groups. In the decades to come, partially as a result of improved life expectancy, there will be far greater numbers of minority elderly, yet there continues to be a serious dearth of information regarding the prevalence of dementia in these groups. Little is known regarding the role ethnocultural factors play, for example, in determining the expression of symptomatology and patterns of coping in the dementing illnesses of later life. Valle suggests that various minority groups experience greater exposure to high-risk occupations and toxic substances, and speculates that different subcultures may have different dietary habits or immune system deficits that could affect the development of illness or the nature of the symptom picture in dementia. Minority groups typically occupy the lowest rung of the economic ladder, manifest lower life expectancies and higher morbidity rates, and are more vulnerable to developing such conditions as diabetes, hypertension, lung disease, and heart disease than are individuals in the majority culture. Accordingly, these ethnic and cultural groups are placed in "multiple jeopardy," often presenting to the physician at more advanced and severe stages of disease, while at the same time underutilizing available health resources. Valle outlines the different forms of natural support networks that constitute endogenous caregiving systems, and suggests that clinicians and community-based systems of care often fail to adequately take the strengths and contributions of these family supports into account. He underscores the very great need for reliable data on variables relating to altered brain function in later life as manifested in different sociocultural, racial, and ethnic groups.

In summing up these multiple trends for the volume, and looking toward the future, Odin W. Anderson, in the concluding chapter, questions the benign assumption that the solutions to formulating and implementing public policy in the area of senile dementia will soon become self-evident. Anderson wonders, given the demographics of the situation, and the ponderous behavioral problems regarding self-care, "whether we as a society will be capable of managing the increasing pressure of the sick aged gracefully." In agreement with Brody, Anderson notes that the nuclear family is geared not to the home but to the work-a-day world, and, as more and more women are employed, the social system and the family unit are becoming seriously overloaded. All data, he suggests, point in the same direction, that of facing exceedingly difficult answers in the years to come. Anderson echoes again what others have reiterated in previous chapters: Health legislation has not been developed to optimally benefit the demented elderly. Medicare, for example, was designed primarily for short-term, acute episodes of illness, but long-term chronic illnesses constitute not an episode, but a way of life until death, with a constant and increasing drain on health resources. Although institutional care accounts for about 70% of all personal health services for the aged, little is known empirically about the cost of home care services, and knowledge of the interrelationships between family structures, delivery of home services, and care of the demented is exceedingly meager. Senile dementia is a disease process that places an enormous strain on the family, that often arouses nihilistic expectations and approaches to treatment on the part of the helping services, and one that is often obscured in the political process. Anderson bemoans the erosion of the ethic of service and duty, and espouses an emphasis on peace and comfort, and the shifting of attitudes toward chronic, rather than acute, models of care. He cautions, however, that there are no neat, social engineering solutions and reminds us, as Kahn and Tobin did so eloquently before, that all social objectives demand tradeoffs.

Although this overview touches on some of the highlights of the chapters to come, it can in no way convey the richness, detail, and complexity of the papers themselves. Each one of them is well worth reading in its entirety.

The volume reveals the complexities and the tragic effects of this disorder on patients, on their families, and on the community at large, on the one hand, yet amply spells out multiple areas in which substantial opportunities for innovation and discovery in research exist. It is our hope that in coming decades many of these questions will be answered by systematic research, if not for our parents' sake, then for our own and our children's sake. The chapters, as a group, suggest that a unitary model of illness and treatment is insufficient, that multiple perspectives on different levels are necessary, ranging from understanding at the molecular and cellular level, to consideration of the human organism in its entirety, including assessment of the nature, intrapsychic dynamics, premorbid intelligence, and sociocultural variables, as well as the patient's interface with family and society.

A variety of themes and concerns specific to the clinician weave their way through the chapters of this volume, reiterating over and over again such matters as the continuing controversy over the best method of classifying Alzheimer's disease and related disorders, distress over the high rates of error and lack of precision in characterizing current approaches to diagnosis, and the absence of reliable rates of disease incidence and prevalence in different geographic areas, social classes, and cultural groups. Also highlighted, and judged worthy of considerably closer scrutiny, is the broad spectrum of affective and behavioral symptoms that often accompany the core deterioration of intellect, and that, though typically overlooked, are in many instances responsive to appropriate treatment. In addition, considerable interest is focused on the role of premorbid character, on sociocultural, and educational variables as factors coloring the symptom picture, either by compensating for, or exacerbating, cognitive incapacity; and related to this, of course, must be the continuing effort to better specify the relative closeness-of-fit in brain-behavior relationships in senile dementia of the Alzheimer's type. The nature of stage-specific changes in cognition, perception, and affect over the course of disease, and the compensating effects of sensory stimulation and environmental complexity on adaptation are also in need of further attention. Persistent themes on a more molar level involve questions regarding the differential social and economic costs of institutionalization versus maintenance in the community, the interface of service delivery structures with family networks, changing lifestyles and demographics on costs and patterns of care, and finally, the effects and ramifications of a basic shift in the philosophy of care delivery from acute intervention to chronic management.

The presence of the chapters in this volume suggest that important questions are being raised, that the field is at the threshold of developing a solid base of knowledge, and that interest in the dementias of late life—which has expanded so significantly in the course of the past decade—will continue, vigorous and unabated, for many years into the future.

Clinical Aspects of Alzheimer's Disease and Senile Dementia, (Aging, Vol. 15), edited by Nancy E. Miller and Gene D. Cohen. Raven Press, New York 1981.

Organic Mental Disorders: Their History and Classification with Special Reference to DSM-III

Z. J. Lipowski

Department of Psychiatry, Dartmouth Medical School, Hanover, New Hampshire 03755

Mental disorders causally related to cerebral disease in the elderly have emerged as a major public health problem, one that is casting "a sombre shadow into the 21st century," as a recent editorial in the *British Medical Journal* (9) put it. The editorial speaks of "dementia—the quiet epidemic." The burden of dementia has personal, social, and economic dimensions. The disorder is defined in psychological or behavioral terms which specify its chief clinical manifestations. It is necessary to emphasize this semantic point at the outset so as to avoid confusing dementia, a term referring to a cluster of behavioral abnormalities, with senile dementia, denoting a form of brain disease. The core problem in dementia is a change in personality and behavior resulting in some degree of failure of adaptive social functioning. Underlying such change and adaptive failure is impairment of memory and information processing, especially of new and complex information inputs.

Dementia has been recognized since antiquity, as suggested by the following quotation from one of Juvenal's satires (18): "Worse by far than all bodily hurt is dementia: for he who has it no longer knows the names of his slaves or recognizes the friend with whom he has dined the night before, or those whom he has begotten and brought up. And by a cruel will he disinherits his own and makes over all his property to Phiale; well does she understand how to entice him with her halitus oris: not for nothing had she set herself up in a brothel years before."

Thus during the second century a perceptive poet noted some of the main symptoms of dementia: failing memory, impaired judgment, and defective impulse control. It is a task of science to systematize such casual observations of behavior, label them, and classify clusters of observed behavioral aberrations for the purpose of clear communication and diagnosis, and for the generation of testable etiological hypotheses. Woodger (29) points out that "science demands great linguistic austerity and discipline." By contrast, the language of psychopathology related to brain disorders offers an example of semantic muddle. It features ambiguous, overlapping, and inconsistently used terms which hamper communication, teaching, and research. For 3 years a task force of the American

Psychiatric Association was preparing the third edition of the *Diagnostic and Statistical Manual of Mental Disorders (DSM-III)* (12). Since the main clinical manifestations of Alzheimer's disease and senile dementia are behavioral, these diseases have been traditionally classed among mental disorders. This classification, however, encompasses a whole range of behavioral abnormalities encountered in all age groups. It seems logical, therefore, to discuss the place of senile dementia and Alzheimer's disease in the context of, and in relation to, other mental disorders, especially those referred to as "organic." A psychiatric classification reflects current knowledge and assumptions about etiology. The mere fact that only some mental disorders are classified as "organic" implies an etiological hypothesis. "Organic" in this context connotes that disorders so labeled are believed to result from cerebral damage, metabolic derangement, or both. This does not imply, however, that psychological and social factors play no role in their causation and treatment. On the contrary, if these factors were omitted, one would be substituting the brain for the person, hardly a satisfactory solution.

DSM-III reflects not only current opinions but also history. Our present conceptions of organic mental disorders and the terms we use become more meaningful when viewed in a historical perspective. It is germane, therefore, to start with a broad outline of their evolution.

HISTORICAL DEVELOPMENT OF THE CONCEPT OF ORGANIC MENTAL DISORDERS

Mental disorders due to brain disease, primary and secondary to systemic disease, were known during antiquity. Hippocrates (17) described phrenitis (or delirium), a mental disorder associated with physical, especially febrile, diseases. During the first century A.D., Celsus (7) introduced the terms "delirium" and "dementia." Delirium, or phrenesis, referred to acute mental disorder associated with fever. Celsus noted that phrenesis could be followed at times by "continuous dementia." Aretaeus of Cappadocia (1), active during the second century, classified diseases into acute and chronic, and distinguished among the chronic ones senile dementia, which started during old age and was marked by "a torpor of the senses and a stupefaction of the gnostic and intellectual faculties" (1). His contemporary Galen (15) viewed delirium as a condition secondary to many physical illnesses and due to disorder of the brain arising by "consensus" in diseases such as pneumonia. Phrenitis and lethargus were similar to delirium but were caused by primary brain disease.

Thus by the end of the second century the rudiments of a classification of organic mental disorders had been formulated. What followed was growing terminological confusion as the original terms acquired additional connotations and new terms were coined to compete with the ancient ones. The oldest terms, delirium and dementia, were at times used synonymously to denote insanity in general. On the whole, however, delirium was more likely to be used in its narrower and modern sense. Both of these terms turned up in the English medical literature in 1592, when Cosin (8) defined delirium as "that weakness of conceite and consideration which we call dotage: when a man, through age or infirmitie, falleth to be a childe againe in discretion" (8). Dementia signified for Cosin "a passion of the minde, bereaving it of the light of understanding." His contemporary Barrough (2) described concurrent impairment of memory and reason, and called it in Latin *fatuitas* or *stultitia* and in English "foolishness" or "doltishness." During the seventeenth century, Willis (28) gave an excellent description of delirium. He stated clearly that it meant the same as dementia and denoted "such an annoyance of the animal Function, as arising in the Fits of Fevers, Drunkenness, and sometimes in the Passions called Hysterical, induces Men to think, speak, or do absurd things . . . for a short time" (28). Willis also described a chronic mental disorder, one characterized by defects of memory, understanding, and judgment, and designated it "stupidity." It could be inherited or acquired during old age or as a result of head injury, drunkenness, epilepsy, and extreme sadness. "Stupidity" was usually incurable but could improve.

For Willis, as for Hippocrates, mental disorders were manifestations of brain disease (30). At the beginning of the eighteenth century, Stahl (26) proposed for the first time that some abnormal mental states are of a physical or organic origin, and others have a psychological causation. This distinction was generally ignored until Pinel (22) revived it in 1801. In his influential *Treatise on Insanity,* he wrote that "derangement of the understanding is generally considered as an effect of an organic lesion of the brain, consequently as incurable, a supposition that is, in a great number of instances, contrary to anatomical fact" (22). Pinel distinguished five classes of mental derangement, one of which he called "dementia," or "the abolition of the thinking faculty." It featured a rapid succession of unconnected ideas, volatile emotions, and wild eccentricity. This description resembles what we would call schizophrenia. Pinel used the term "idiotism" to refer to a mental disorder characterized by intellectual impairment. His student Esquirol (14) defined dementia as a cerebral affection marked by a weakening of the sensibility, understanding, and will. Reasoning, recent memory, attention, and capacity for abstraction were all impaired. Three varieties of dementia could be distinguished: acute, chronic, and senile. The acute form could be caused by fever or hemorrhage and was curable. Chronic dementia could be produced by masturbation, drunkenness, or excessive study, or might follow mania or epilepsy. It was rarely cured. Senile dementia resulted from the progress of age. It was heralded by general excitement and irritability, followed by defects of recent memory and other intellectual deficits. It could not be cured, but its progression might be slowed down by country air and moderate exercise. In general, the causes of dementia could be physical or moral. Esquirol's description of acute and chronic forms suggests that his concept of dementia encompassed what would now be called schizophrenia and atypical psychoses.

Pinel and Esquirol were immensely influential in France and beyond. Rush

(24), the author of the first American textbook of psychiatry, published in 1812, wrote: "Related to intellectual madness is that disease of the mind, which has received from Mr. Pinel the name DEMENCE. The subjects of it in Scotland are said to have 'a bee in their bonnets.' In the United States, we say they are 'flighty,' or 'hair-brained,' and, sometimes, a 'little cracked' " (24). Rush proposed to substitute "dissociation" for "dementia" because the core feature of the disorder was inability to associate perceptions and ideas coherently. Like Pinel, Rush reserved the term "idiotism," or "fatuity," to designate a mental disorder characterized by impaired reason and memory. "Fatuity could come on in old age," wrote Rush, "in consequence of the brain becoming so torpid, and insensible, as to be unable to transmit impressions made upon it to the mind" (24).

In 1837 an English psychiatrist, Prichard (23), developed Esquirol's concept of dementia further. He classified dementia as primary and secondary to other disorders of the brain, e.g., mania, apoplexy, or paralysis. He described four degrees, or stages, of dementia and thus outlined its natural history. The first stage was marked by impairment of recent memory with intact remote memories. The second stage involved loss of reason, the third incomprehension, and the fourth loss of instinctive action. All four stages could be readily observed in the gradual development of senile dementia. The latter was not a universal feature of old age but rather the result of harmful influences such as excessive striving for success, "intense and unremitted application to studies," and abuse of alcohol. In the later stages of dementia, the patient's personality became changed, his ability to reason abolished, and his mind totally disorganized.

Several French students of Esquirol focused on the general paralysis of the insane, a condition featuring pathological brain changes and mental disturbances. This observation encouraged the search for cerebral causes of other mental illnesses. This trend reached its extreme expression in Germany, where Griesinger (16) asserted in 1866 that "psychiatry and neuropathology are not merely two closely related fields; they are but one field in which only one language is spoken and the same laws rule" (16). One could hardly be more wrong in fewer words. Griesinger's reductionism threatened to lead the search for behavioral correlates of cerebral disorders to a dead end. Meanwhile, other French followers of Esquirol derived and detached from his concept of dementia the syndrome of "mental confusion." The latter provided a basis for classifying together many acute mental disorders, organic and psychogenic. Its essential features included impairment of thinking, perception, and spatiotemporal orientation, with or without a hallucinatory, dream-like or oneiric state. From the word "confusion" were derived terms still used today, e.g., acute confusional state, confusional insanity, episodic confusions. During the 1880s German and Russian writers introduced a related and equally influential concept: "clouding of consciousness." Bonhoeffer (6) made it the hallmark of the acute organic mental disorders or, as he called them, "exogenous reaction types." He asserted that any systemic disease causing acute brain dysfunction could give rise to one of five reaction types: delirium, epileptiform excitement, twilight state, hallucinosis, or amentia. Clouding of consciousness was the key feature of all of them except hallucinosis, which was characterized by recurrent or persistent hallucinations experienced during clear consciousness. Delirium was the commonest exogenous type. This syndrome was the first organic mental disorder to be described (19). In 1813 Sutton (27) coined the term "delirium tremens" for delirium following withdrawal from alcohol. Its flamboyant clinical features have inspired some writers to view it as the prototype of delirium in general and to refer to the hypoactive and lethargic variant as "acute confusional state."

Several terms are used currently in English medical literature to designate acute organic psychiatric syndromes, i.e., acute brain syndrome, delirium, acute confusional state, and toxic psychosis. Such usage of overlapping terms makes clear communication impossible.

The concept of chronic organic mental disorders followed a more tortuous course. Senile dementia became clearly distinguished by the 1830s. Esquirol's chronic dementia became purified, as it were, at the end of the nineteenth century when Kraepelin (13) detached from it the various clinical subtypes of dementia praecox or schizophrenia. He adopted the term "organic dementias" for psychoses due to diseases of the central nervous system, e.g., neurosyphilis or head trauma. In 1916 Bleuler (3) defined the so-called organic psychosyndrome, or a set of behavioral manifestations of chronic diffuse cerebral cortical damage. It featured impairment of memory, judgment, critical faculty, perceptual discrimination, attention, and orientation as well as labile emotionality and deficient impulse control. The patient's whole personality was changed: "Tenderness, consideration, tact, piety, esthetic sensibility, sense of duty, sense of right, feeling of sexual shame—all these may fail at any moment, even when they are present" (3), wrote Bleuler. He stressed that the various cognitive functions were not impaired uniformly and that the most highly developed and practiced abilities were remarkably resistant to deterioration. Bleuler observed that focal brain lesions gave rise to affective rather than cognitive disturbances.

Bleuler's formulation of the organic psychosyndrome was a landmark in the development of psychiatric nosology. What remained to be done was to evolve the concept of the focal organic psychosyndromes. Bleuler's son, Manfred Bleuler, stated that the focal psychosyndrome was first recognized after the epidemic of encephalitis during World War I and that it features disturbances of impulse control, drives, and mood, with preservation of intellectual functions (4). Manfred Bleuler classified organic mental disorders into three groups: (a) acute exogenous reaction type, which includes delirium, hallucinosis, simple confusion, and acute amnestic syndrome; (b) organic psychosyndrome due to diffuse chronic cerebral disease; and (c) organic psychosyndrome of chronic focal brain damage and endocrine disease. Speaking of the psychosyndrome due to diffuse pathology, Bleuler (5) wrote that "forty years ago our clinic called this syndrome 'psycho-organic syndrome'; this was at a time when it was not known that many other organically caused psychosyndromes existed." One year after these words were written, the first edition of the official manual containing the classification of mental disorders adopted by the American Psychiatric Association (DSM-I) was published (10). It adopted the elder Bleuler's concept of the organic psychosyndrome as a "basic" characteristic of *all* organic brain disorders. Thus an obsolete conception of a single and homogeneous organic psychosyndrome became embalmed in the official American classification and is still with us.

CRITIQUE OF CURRENT CLASSIFICATION (DSM-II)

The currently used second edition of the diagnostic Manual, or DSM-II (11), was published in 1968. It distinguishes a class of organic brain syndromes (OBS) due to or associated with impairment of brain tissue function and manifested by the "organic brain syndrome." The latter is defined as a "basic mental condition characteristically resulting from diffuse impairment of brain tissue function from whatever cause" (11).

Its component features include: (a) impairment of orientation; (b) impairment of memory; (c) impairment of all intellectual functions, e.g., comprehension, calculation, knowledge, learning; (d) impairment of judgment; and (e) lability or shallowness of affect.

This syndrome is nothing but a replica of Eugene Bleuler's "organic psychosyndrome." It leaves no room for psychopathological effects of focal brain lesions, endocrine diseases, or drugs and poisons, which may not give rise to the so-called basic syndrome yet may be logically viewed as "organic." The Manual distinguishes between psychotic and nonpsychotic organic brain syndromes, a distinction of doubtful value. It recommends as an option that one should distinguish acute and chronic (i.e., the reversible and irreversible brain syndromes) but offers no guidelines for how to do it. The so-called basic symptoms are stated to be present to some degree in acute and chronic syndromes. As a result of this classification, the literature is replete with references to "OBS" as if it was an invariable, all-or-none condition such as pregnancy. Reversibility of organic symptoms is not an all-or-none feature; rather, there are degrees of restitution to the premorbid state which reflect such factors as availability of treatment, time for the healing processes, influence of the social environment, and the patient's emotional state. Furthermore, the degree of reversibility of psychopathology does not necessarily parallel that of the underlying cerebral pathology. The concept of the chronic or irreversible brain syndrome encourages the deplorable tendency to view as hopelessly incurable any person to whom such label is attached.

PROPOSED REVISION

An alternative classification (20,21) of organic mental disorders has been proposed, one designed to reflect clinical observations more adequately. The proposed revision has been adopted, with some changes, in the current draft of DSM-III (12). As it now stands, this classification has the following features: First, the class "organic mental disorders" comprises seven descriptive psychopathological syndromes. To avoid confusion by introducing new terms, some of the ancient designations (e.g., delirium and dementia) were retained. Second, organic mental disorders as a class are defined as behavioral manifestations of transient or permanent cerebral dysfunction whose presence needs to be independently confirmed by laboratory evidence, physical examination, and/or the history of exposure to an organic factor (e.g., a drug or poison) known to produce behavioral symptoms of the type presented by the patient. Third, it is recommended that each patient be diagnosed and coded by the presenting organic brain syndrome as well as the organic etiological factor involved, e.g., dementia associated with brain tumor, delirium associated with pneumonia, hallucinosis associated with alcohol withdrawal. Fourth, the seven organic brain syndromes encompass a wide range of behavioral abnormalities which are believed to be caused by diffuse or focal cerebral damage and dysfunction as well as by cerebral effects of toxic agents. This formulation departs from the traditional view that cerebral disorders can give rise to only one psychiatric syndrome characterized by global impairment of intellectual or cognitive functions. It leaves open the possibility that affective and schizophrenia-like disorders may at times have organic etiology. Fifth, no distinction is made between acute and chronic and psychotic and nonpsychotic organic brain syndromes, respectively. It is assumed that reversibility is not a sound taxonomic principle, as it reflects prognostic judgment that one may not be able to make in a given case as well as the availability of effective treatment. For example, as long as no treatment for neurosyphilis existed, the associated mental disorders could be viewed as chronic, incurable, or irreversible. Sixth, each organic brain syndrome is defined by its psychopathological diagnostic criteria (12).

The seven proposed organic brain syndromes are as follows:

A. Those with relatively global cognitive impairment
   1. Delirium
   2. Dementia
B. Those with relatively selective cognitive abnormality
   1. Amnestic syndrome
   2. Organic hallucinosis
C. Those with predominantly affective or personality disturbances
   1. Organic delusional syndrome
   2. Organic affective syndrome
   3. Organic personality syndrome

It should be stressed that DSM-III is still in a draft stage and does not in any way represent an official or final classification. Diagnostic criteria for all of the organic syndromes have been formulated but remain subject to modification in the final draft. Pending possible further modifications, the seven syndromes are clinically defined as follows:

Delirium: A syndrome characterized by rapid onset of a fluctuating clinical picture involving disturbance of attention, memory, thinking, perception, orientation, psychomotor activity, and the sleep–wakefulness cycle.

Dementia: A syndrome featuring deterioration of previously acquired intellectual abilities sufficiently severe to interfere with social or occupational functioning, or both. Impairment of memory, abstract thinking, and judgment is evident in a fully developed case. Defective impulse control and personality change in the form of either accentuation or alteration of premorbid personality traits is usually present. The clinical course may be progressive, static, or partly or fully remitting. "Dementia" does not imply irreversibility.

Amnestic syndrome: The essential feature is retrograde and anterograde amnesia occurring as the only or the predominant clinical manifestation.

Organic hallucinosis: A syndrome characterized by persistent or recurrent hallucinations in a state of full wakefulness and alertness, and attributed to a clearly organic factor.

Organic delusional syndrome: The essential feature is the predominance of delusions in a state of full wakefulness and alertness. Other symptoms encountered in schizophrenic disorders may be present. These symptoms are attributable to a clearly defined organic factor, e.g., intoxication with amphetamines.

Organic affective syndrome: The essential feature is a clinical picture in which the predominant symptom is a mood disorder, depressive or manic, attributed to an organic factor, e.g., antihypertensive drugs or Cushing's syndrome. It does not meet the criteria for any other organic syndrome.

Organic personality syndrome: The essential feature is a marked change in personality involving primarily expression and control of emotions and impulses as well as social judgment. It does not meet the criteria for any other organic syndrome.

It should be emphasized that the proposed classification was not developed specifically for geriatric patients but for *all* age groups and *all* organic etiologic factors, be they primary intracranial diseases, metabolic encephalopathies, systemic infections, intoxications, etc. Some aspects of this classification have been criticized on the grounds that they blur the concept of the organic mental disorders. Such criticism ignores the purpose of classifying natural phenomena. As Sokal (25) points out, the main purpose of classification is to stimulate further research. The proposed classification of organic mental disorders loosens to some extent the encrusted rigidity of the conception of organicity which was developed more than 60 years ago. This should lead to new testable hypotheses on the role of cerebral disorders in the etiology of behavioral aberrations and thus to therapeutic advances.

By tradition, the section on Mental Disorders of the International Classification of Diseases and of the Diagnostic Manual has included the so-called senile and presenile dementias. Clayton and Martin discuss them in relation to DSM-III elsewhere in this volume.

REFERENCES

1. Aretaeus (1861): In: *The Extant Works of Aretaeus, the Cappadocian,* edited by F. Adams, p. 103.
2. Barrough, P. (1596): *The Method of Physick.* Field, London.
3. Bleuler, E. (1924): *Textbook of Psychiatry.* Macmillan, New York.
4. Bleuler, M. (1977): Personal communication.
5. Bleuler, M. (1951): *Br. Med. J.,* 2:1233–1238.
6. Bonhoeffer, K. (1912): In: *Handbuch der Psychiatrie,* edited by G. L. Aschaffenburg, pp. 1–60. Deuticke, Leipzig, Spez. Teil 3.
7. Celsus (1938): *De Medicina,* translated by W. G. Spencer. Heinemann, London.
8. Cosin (1963): Quoted in: *Three Hundred Years of Psychiatry, 1535–1860,* edited by R. Hunter and J. MacAlpine, pp. 43–44. Oxford University Press, London.
9. Dementia: the quiet epidemic (editorial). (1978): *Br. Med. J.,* 1:1–2.
10. *Diagnostic and Statistical Manual. Mental Disorders* (1952): American Psychiatric Association, Washington, D.C.
11. *Diagnostic and Statistical Manual of Mental Disorders,* ed. 2. (1968): American Psychiatric Association, Washington, D.C.
12. *Diagnostic and Statistical Manual of Mental Disorders,* DSM-III draft (1978): American Psychiatric Association, Washington, D.C.
13. Diefendorf, A. R. (1915): *Clinical Psychiatry.* (Abstracted and adapted from the seventh German edition of Kraepelin's "Lehrbuch der Psychiatrie.") Macmillan, New York.
14. Esquirol, J. E. D. (1965): *Mental Maladies.* Hafner, New York.
15. Galen (1937): Quoted in: *Historical Notes on Psychiatry,* by J. R. Whitwell. Blakiston, Philadelphia.
16. Griesinger, W. (1941): Quoted in: *A History of Medical Psychology,* by G. Zilboorg, p. 436. Norton, New York.
17. Hippocrates (1950): *The Medical Works of Hippocrates,* translated by J. Chadwick and W. N. Mann. Blackwell, Oxford.
18. Juvenal (1967): Quoted in: *Diseases in Antiquity,* edited by D. Brothwell and A. T. Scandison, p. 718. Thomas, Springfield, Ill.
19. Lipowski, Z. J. (1980): *Delirium: Acute Brain Failure in Man.* Thomas, Springfield, Ill. *(in press).*
20. Lipowski, Z. J. (1978): *Compr. Psychiatry,* 19:309–322.
21. Lipowski, Z. J. (1975): In: *Psychiatric Aspects of Neurologic Disease,* edited by D. F. Benson and S. Blumer. Grune & Stratton, New York.
22. Pinel, P. (1962): *A Treatise on Insanity.* Hafner, New York.
23. Prichard, J. C. (1837): *A Treatise on Insanity.* Haswell, Barrington, and Haswell, Philadelphia.
24. Rush, B. (1812): *Medical Inquiries and Observations Upon the Diseases of the Mind.* Kimber and Richardson, Philadelphia.
25. Sokal, R. R. (1974): *Science,* 185:1115–1123.
26. Stahl, G. E. (1941): Quoted in: *A History of Medical Psychology,* by G. Zilboorg, pp. 277–280. Norton, New York.
27. Sutton, T. (1813): *Tracts on Delirium Tremens, on Peritonitis and on Some Other Inflammatory Affections.* Underwood, London.
28. Willis, T. (1973): *The London Practice of Physick,* pp. 458–459. Milford House, Boston.
29. Woodger, J. H. (1952): *Biology & Language,* p. 8. Cambridge University Press, Cambridge.
30. Zilboorg, G. (1941): *A History of Medical Psychology.* Norton, New York.

Clinical Aspects of Alzheimer's Disease and Senile Dementia, (Aging, Vol. 15), edited by Nancy E. Miller and Gene D. Cohen. Raven Press, New York 1981.

Classification of Late Life Organic States and the DSM-III

Paula J. Clayton and Ronald Martin

Department of Psychiatry, Washington University School of Medicine, St. Louis, Missouri, 63110

Many recent books on aging have been marred by the lack of a uniform, well-defined nosology classifying the conditions under discussion. In an effort to bring clarity to a confusing field, the DSM-III Organic Mental Disorders Committee has made some rather major decisions about the psychiatric nomenclature associated with organic disorders and in particular the dementias. A brief review of the nosological history of dementia demonstrates why these changes were long overdue.

According to Menninger (19) the first definite syndrome description of a mental illness was of a senile deterioration, described in Prince Ptah-hotep around 3000 B.C. Although Hippocrates described psychiatric problems in his writings, he did not use the term dementia. Senile dementia was first used by Aretaeus "The Incomparable" of Cappadox early in the second century. Thereafter, there was continuous shuffling and reshuffling of symptoms and syndromes in various disease categories. Noted men such as Immanuel Kant and Philippe Pinel published their own classifications which included "dementia" but did not always use it in reference to the same entities.

After falling into disuse, the term senile dementia began to reappear in the classification during the late 1800s. It is found in the textbooks of Emil Kraepelin (1883) and Theodor Ziehen (1894), but not in Carl Wernicke's textbook (1900). Kraepelin revised and expanded his nosologic system in each new edition of his text. In his eighth and last edition, published in four volumes from 1909 to 1915, he had 17 groups of mental conditions, the seventh of which was "senile and presenile conditions." He was influenced, of course, by his now immortalized neuropathologist Alois Alzheimer, who in 1906 reported the case of a 51-year-old woman who developed delusions, then loss of memory and disorientation, and later depression and hallucinations. Her illness progressed over 5 years to a state of profound dementia and death (28). At autopsy Alzheimer found her brain to be atrophied. The cortex contained miliary lesions (senile plaques). Using silver impregnation he noted a curious clumping and distortion of the cortical neurofibrils. It is said that Kraepelin proposed that this dementia with a presenile onset and such neuropathologic findings be named Alzheimer's disease. This introduced the debatable convention into our nosology of dichotomizing the dementias into "presenile" and "senile."

American classification, for the most part, followed the European classification. During the late 1800s the term senile insanity was used and later changed to senile psychosis (equating psychosis with commitability). In 1917 the American Medico-psychological Association (which became the American Psychiatric Association in 1921) adopted an official classification which was largely Kraepelinian in principle. It contained 22 categories, including senile psychosis and psychosis with cerebral arteriosclerosis. This is the first reference to a vascular dementia we could find. Although physicians such as Adolf Meyer, Smith Ely Jelliffe, William A. White, and Ernest Southard proposed different classifications, the 1917 classification remained in use for over 15 years.

In 1933 the first edition of the *Standard Classified Nomenclature of Disease* was published. It contained a section on the classification of mental illness, and an official APA classification was developed in 1934 to correct its weaknesses. It was planned on an "etiologic basis" and extended the categories to 24 with 82 subdivisions. The eighth category was "psychoses with cerebral arteriosclerosis," the eleventh was "senile psychoses" with five subtypes, and the thirteenth was "psychoses due to other metabolic, etc., diseases," again with five subtypes, the third of which was Alzheimer's disease.

Based on his experiences in World War II, Menninger again revised the classification. He designed a classification which emphasized the "newer (Freudian) theories of personology and psychodynamics" (19). It was designed to facilitate discharging men from the armed services. It de-emphasized "psychosis" and considered most conditions "reactions." This de-emphasized disease entities and implied knowledge about etiology, but unfortunately paid little attention to the dementias. It was adopted by the U.S. Army in 1945, the Veterans Administration in 1946, the U.S. Navy in 1947, and in a revised form by the International Statistical Classification in 1948.

In 1952 the first edition of the *Diagnostic and Statistical Manual: Mental Disorders* (DSM-I) was published (2). Perhaps in response to Menninger's neglect of disorders associated with demonstrable organic etiology and/or structural change, this very expanded and detailed nomenclature introduced the terms "acute" and "chronic" brain syndromes. Circulatory disease became "acute brain syndrome associated with circulatory disturbance," or "chronic brain syndrome associated with cerebral arteriosclerosis." Dementia became "chronic brain syndrome associated with senile brain disease," "chronic brain syndrome associated with other disturbances of metabolism, growth, or nutrition" (includes presenile, glandular, pellagra, familial amaurosis), and "chronic brain syndrome associated with diseases of unknown or uncertain cause" (includes multiple sclerosis, Huntington's chorea, Pick's disease, and other diseases of a familial or hereditary nature). This nomenclature, as discussed by Lipowski *(this volume),* proved to be unsatisfactory as the terms acute and chronic denoted prognosis (regardless of reversibility) rather than underlying pathology. In addition, the term "acute" implied a sudden onset and/or brief duration which need not be related to reversibility. Sudden-onset syndromes (e.g., head trauma) may be irreversible whereas syndromes with an insidious onset (normal pressure hydrocephalus, thyroid deficiency) may be reversible. Why the term "brain syndrome" and the confusing dichotomy of "acute" and "chronic" was adopted by psychiatry is unclear.

The DSM-II (3), published in 1968, intended to correct some of the confusion of DSM-I. The concept of "acute" and "chronic" was retained as a qualifying phrase, and diseases were classified as "psychotic or nonpsychotic" organic brain syndrome. In DSM-II, senile dementia and presenile dementia reappear. For the first time Alzheimer's and Pick's disease are categorized together as presenile dementias. Also for the first time it was recognized that the presenile dementias present a clinical picture similar to those of senile onset but characteristically have an earlier onset. The DSM-II had an additional advantage. A great deal of work by Morton Kramer went into integrating it with the International Classification of Diseases (ICD-8) promoted by the World Health Organization and used by many countries. This was at least a step in the direction of a uniform international nomenclature (23,24).

The DSM-III was to appear 10 years after the DSM-II (4). Planning for it began in 1973, and the Committee on Organic Mental Disorders was formed. The first decision was to define everything as a disorder. Thus "organic brain syndrome" which was often used imprecisely as a wastebasket diagnosis was eliminated. The seven syndromes (as described by Lipowski, *this volume*) were developed, reviving classic descriptive terms that connote disease phenomena (17). The next decision was to classify together the dementias which are not associated with clinically identifiable specific neurologic disorders. Thus senile, presenile, and circulatory dementias occur in the same class as "primary degenerative dementias, senile and presenile onset, and multi-infarct dementia" (Table 1). This emphasizes their shared phenomenology.

Based on the bulk of the evidence currently available, it was concluded that the mental and neurologic status as well as the pathologic findings are virtually indistinguishable whether Alzheimer's disease had a presenile or a senile onset

TABLE 1. *Senile and presenile dementias*[a]

Code phenomenology in fifth digit as:
  0 = (uncomplicated)
  1 = with delirium
  2 = with delusional features
  3 = with depressive features

290.0x Primary degenerative dementia, senile onset A:33
290.1x Primary degenerative dementia, presenile onset A:33
290.4x Multi-infarct dementia A:35

[a] Draft of Axis I of DSM-III classification (January 1980).

(5,14,18). Genetically they also segregate in the same families. Constantinidis reportedly found both forms in the same families (14). In addition, a review of the 1963 Larsson et al. monograph, which is commonly cited as an argument for maintaining a dichotomy, showed that some of their secondary cases of senile dementia (in this case, in siblings) had an onset prior to age 65, yet were not classified as Alzheimer's disease (15). Probably this occurred because of the authors' definition of Alzheimer's disease, which contained *three* criteria: (a) the occurrence of *aphasic* disturbance; (b) rapid progression to profound mental deterioration; and (c) as a rule, a comparatively early onset (although they maintain that the disease may occur as late as during the seventh and eighth decade). They record 10 cases of "presenile psychosis," although in their discussion they comment that no cases of Alzheimer's or Pick's disease were found (probably because these cases had no aphasia). The age of onset of the "senile dementia" in the probands varied from 56 to 92 years. Similarly, in another report the same group of investigators again required that "aphasia" be present before the diagnosis of Alzheimer's was established (22). With this requirement the average age of onset of Alzheimer's disease in the probands was 61, with the age in decades ranging from 20 to 89 years. Thus they clearly used a symptom and not age as a differential diagnostic point, an idea not accepted by most investigators. Heston also found the two diseases in the same families and concluded that "while there may be widespread heterogeneity within the Alzheimer's disease–senile dementia [group], age of onset is not a rational criterion for delimiting subgroups" (11,12). Therefore the committee decided to accept them as variants of the same disease.

The DSM-III Committee had also decided not to retain any eponyms in Axes I and II, which are the sections that deal with mental disorders per se. Because of that, Alzheimer's disease was not used in the nosology, although it is referred to in the body of the text. On the basis of this, it was decided to name it "primary degenerative dementia" and to order the more frequent but less severe senile onset dementia first (290.0x) and to place presenile onset second (290.1x). The age of demarcation was set at the traditional 65. Note that the categories "primary degenerative dementia, presenile onset, or senile onset" do not differentiate between Alzheimer's and Pick's. In the case of the senile dementias, they almost invariably will be of Alzheimer's type. The presenile dementias could be Alzheimer's or Pick's, or even unspecified types (13), but this discrimination can be made reliably only on the basis of histopathologic data, information a clinician does not generally have at hand. When such neuropathologic data are at hand, the specific form of the progressive idiopathic dementia should be made on Axis III.

When a dementia secondary to some other known disease occurs (e.g., a brain tumor, Huntington's disease, or vitamin B_{12} deficiency), the specific disease should be noted on Axis III, and the presence of the dementia is noted by using a different number, 294.10, as described by Lipowski *(this volume)*.

The essential feature of primary degenerative dementia is the insidious onset of a dementia with a uniformly progressive deteriorating course for which all other specific causes have been excluded by history, neurological examination, and laboratory investigation. The fifth digit is 0 when it is uncomplicated, 1 when it appears with delirium, 2 when it has delusional features, especially paranoia, or 3 when it has depressive features. Depressive symptoms are common, especially early in the disease, but diminish as it progresses. In the early stages, only memory deficit is generally apparent. Often mild personality changes occur, e.g., apathy, lack of spontaneity, and a quiet withdrawal from social interactions. Individuals tend to remain neat, well-groomed, and, aside from occasional outbursts, cooperative and appropriate. In the middle stage, a variety of mental disturbances become more obvious and behavior may be disturbed. The individual may be querulous, slovenly, irritable, or agitated. In the late stages he is mute, inattentive, and uncooperative. The most common age of onset of progressive idiopathic dementia is during the seventies. Prior to modern medical advances the average longevity from age of onset to death was 5 years. Now, primarily as a result of the improved treatment of infectious diseases, the course has lengthened and may be as long as 12 years. With this increased longevity, the prevalence of dementia is increasing. It may be as high as 6% for men and women over the age of 65 in Western industrialized nations (8). Ten years ago it was estimated to be between 2 and 4%. The disorder is perhaps more common in women than men.

Another interesting question is whether Alzheimer's disease should be dichotomized into familial and sporadic types. Familial factors appear to be involved in at least some cases. There are pedigrees of families showing striking aggregation that suggest single gene transmission. When families of consecutively selected patients are studied, however, a lesser tendency for familial aggregation is seen. Overall, the risk to primary relatives is around four times the age-specific morbidity risk for the general population. There are recent findings regarding the unconventional virus transmission of the subacute spongiform dementias: Kuru and Creutzfeldt-Jakob disease suggest another line of investigation that must be considered before assuming genetic transmission. Gajdusek and co-workers transmitted a dementing illness (a spongiform encephalopathy) to primates from three Alzheimer's patients, two of whom were from families showing familial aggregation (20,25). They have not however, despite repeated attempts, transmitted illness from a typical sporadic case. Whether the so-called familial and sporadic cases represent two separate illnesses is as yet to be established.

The gross pathology in the majority of cases comprises cortical atrophy, widening of the sulci, and large ventricles. This may be (but not necessarily) demonstrated in the live patient by computerized axial tomography (7). Microscopically there are usually three characteristic histopathologic changes—senile plaques, neurofibrillary tangles, and granulovascular degeneration of the neuron.

Mild degrees of intellectual impairment may be common in elderly people. In the majority of the cases, however, this does not interfere with social functioning. In one study, by Roth and associates, those who had mild deterioration seldom went on to develop dementia, and most new cases of dementia were not predicted by early, mild deterioration (21). Therefore the diagnosis of progressive idiopathic dementia should be reserved for those cases in which there is clear evidence of progressive and significant deterioration in function. This means that those authors who stress the need for using "early cases" in testing drugs to arrest the progression of dementia (e.g., choline) may be encouraging researchers to include in their study population patients who do not have progressive idiopathic dementia at all and would not show progressive deterioration regardless of treatment (16). Thus only carefully controlled, blind studies should be considered in evaluating the efficacy of any potential treatment.

The diagnosis of a primary degenerative dementia is one of exclusion. An important differential diagnosis is with potentially treatable dementias, e.g., those associated with subdural hematomas, normal pressure hydrocephalus, brain tumors, substance intoxication, metabolic diseases, vitamin deficiencies, and other medical diseases, as well as other psychiatric syndromes, especially "major depressive disorders."

Individuals require complete medical and neurologic evaluation to exclude one of the treatable causes of dementia. A review of several studies of patients diagnosed as having chronic brain syndromes showed 15% to be amenable to treatment. In addition, a certain percentage were found not to be demented at all but suffering from depression or even schizophrenia. In other follow-up studies, some patients diagnosed as having a "chronic organic brain syndrome (OBS)" on psychiatric units were found to be depressed at follow-up (26,27).

Despite the fact that a sizable percentage of our older psychiatric patients have a dementing illness, it must be remembered that the majority of people retain their intellectual competence. A recent study of 70-year-olds found that their intellectual functioning was, for the most part, as good as that in younger individuals, despite the fact that more often they were living in social situations that should or could have influenced their basic physical and mental function (1).

In DSM-II the dementia associated with vascular disease was OBS, psychosis associated with cerebral arteriosclerosis. However, because the severity of the dementia seldom appeared to be pathologically related to the extent of cerebral arteriosclerosis, cerebral vascular dementia seemed to be a more descriptive term. With more consideration and consultation, it was decided to adopt the term "multi-infarct dementia," which the neurologists use for a more limited and more specific group of patients who at autopsy show multiple small and large infarcts of the brain (6,10). It was felt that rather than use the term "multi-infarct dementia," which we took to connote multiple simultaneous infarcts, we would adopt the term "repeated infarct dementia," which we thought was more descriptive of the essential pathologic findings (old and new infarcts). However, after the last meeting of the National Institute of Aging (June 1977), it was decided that we should not confuse the issue further by introducing another term, and we returned to the term "multi-infarct dementia." This dementia is distinguished from the others in that it often shows focal neurologic signs and symptoms and a stepwise deterioration in intellectual function that, early in the course, leaves some intellectual functions relatively intact (patchy deterioration). The onset is typically abrupt, and the course is fluctuating rather than uniformly progressive. The pattern of deficits is patchy depending on which regions of the brain have been destroyed. Thus certain cognitive functions will be unaffected, and others will be impaired. Examples of focal neurologic signs are weakness in limbs, reflex asymmetries, extensor planter responses, dysarthria, and small step gait. Generalized vascular disease is presumed present. Often hypertension exists, and there may be evidence of cardiac enlargement. Known predisposing factors include arterial hypertension, extracranial vascular disease, and valvular or other disease of the heart that may cause thromboemboli.

The prevalence is unknown, although it is surely much less common than progressive idiopathic dementia. The sex ratio is unknown, although if it is similar to the cases previously called arteriosclerotic it is more prevalent in men.

The differential diagnosis includes the same differential that might be postulated for progressive idiopathic dementia. It is to be distinguished from the more common situation where a single stroke causes relatively circumscribed change in the mental state, e.g., in aphasia following damage to the left hemisphere or an amnestic syndrome from infarction in the territory of the posterior cerebral arteries. It is rare for a single stroke to result in a permanent dementia. With multiple infarcts, however, the full syndrome of dementia can occur. Hachinski showed that by using an "ischemia score" patients with multi-infarct dementia could be differentiated from those who had similar "dementia scores" with primary degenerative dementia (9).

In a minority of cases of dementia there are elements typical of primary degenerative dementia as well as multi-infarct dementia. In these cases, both diagnoses are made. At autopsy many of these cases have pathologic findings characteristics of both types of dementia.

As Menninger so aptly noted, "There are many ways to organize miscellaneous data, and classification is one of the basic devices for bringing order out of chaos both in the universe and in our own thinking" (19). In 1949 the APA's official Committee on Nomenclature and Statistics was reviewing the new classification used by the Army and Veterans Administration system. In the minutes of the meeting there occurs the following quote: "Reports from the Army and Veterans representatives indicated that the new system of nomenclature had been found more satisfactory by both clinicians and statisticians. The dire prophecies of utter chaos previously expressed have failed to develop and after 3 years' experience with the new nomenclature both organizations have found their modifications superior to present APA nomenclature" (19). This sounds familiar.

We hope that this new nomenclature serves the clinician and the researcher better than the DSM-II that emerged on the heels of the above quoted consideration.

ACKNOWLEDGMENT

This paper was supported in part by USPHS grants MH-31302 and MH-25430.

REFERENCES

1. Andersson, E., Berg, S., Lawenius, M., and Svanborg, A. (1978): *Acta Psychiatr. Scand.,* 57:59–66.
2. *Diagnostic and Statistical Manual: Mental Disorders* (1952): American Psychiatric Association, Washington, D.C.
3. *Diagnostic and Statistical Manual of Mental Disorders (DSM-II)* (1968): Second Edition. American Psychiatric Association, Washington, D.C.
4. *Diagnostic and Statistical Manual of Mental Disorders (DSM-III)* (1980): Third Edition. American Psychiatric Association, Washington, D.C.
5. Fields, W. S. (1975): *Neurological and Sensory Disorders in the Elderly.* Stratton Intercontinental Medical Book Corp., New York.
6. Fisher, C. M. (1968): In: *Cerebral Vascular Diseases: Sixth Conference,* edited by J. F. Toole, R. G. Siekert, and J. P. Whisnant, pp. 232–236. Grune & Stratton, New York.
7. Freemon, F. R., Allen, J. H., Duncan, G. W., and Randle, G. P. (1978): *Arch. Neurol.,* 35:129–132.
8. Gruenberg, E. M., Hagnell, O., Ojesjo, L., et al. The rising prevalence of chronic brain syndrome in the elderly. Presented at the symposium "Society, Stress and Disease: Aging and Old Age," Stockholm, Sweden, June 14–19, 1976 *(in press).*
9. Hachinski, V. C., Iliff, L. D., Zilhka, E., Du Boulay, G. H., McAllister, V. L., Marshall, J., Russell, R. W. R., and Symon, L. (1975): *Arch. Neurol.,* 32:632–637.
10. Hachinski, V. C., Lassen, N. A., and Marshall, J. (1974): *Lancet,* 2:207–210.
11. Heston, L. L. (1977): *Science,* 196:322–323.
12. Heston, L. L. (1977): *Arch. Gen. Psychiatry,* 34:976–981.
13. Hughes, C. P., Myers, F. K., Smith, K., and Torack, R. M. (1973): *Neurology,* 23:344–351.
14. Katzman, R. (1976): *Arch. Neurol.,* 33:217–218.
15. Larsson, T., Sjogren, T., and Jacobson, G. (1963): *Acta Psychiatr. Scand.,* 39(Suppl.):167.
16. Levy, R. (1978): *Lancet,* 2:944–945.
17. Lipowski, Z. J. (1978): *Compr. Psychiatry,* 19:309–322.
18. Lishman, W. A. (1978): *Psychol. Med.,* 8:353–356.
19. Menninger, K. (1963): *The Vital Balance.* Viking Press, New York.
20. Roos, R. P., and Johnson, R. T. (1977): In: *Dementia,* 2nd ed., edited by C. E. Wells, pp. 93–112. Davis, Philadelphia.
21. Roth, M. (1976): *Psychiatr. Ann.,* 6:57–101.
22. Sjogren, T., Sjogren, H., and Lindgren, A. G. H. (1952): *Acta Psychiatr. Neurol.,* Suppl. 82.
23. Spitzer, R. L., and Wilson, P. T. (1975): In: *Comprehensive Textbook of Psychiatry/II,* Vol. 1, 2nd. ed., edited by A. M. Freedman, H. I. Kaplan, and B. J. Sadock, pp. 826–845. Williams & Wilkins, Baltimore.
24. Stengel, E. (1959): *Bull. WHO,* 21:601–603.
25. Traub, R., Gajdusek, D. C., and Gibbs, C. J. (1977): In: *Aging and Dementia,* edited by W. L. Smith and M. Kinsbourne, Chap. 5. Spectrum Publications, New York.
26. Wells, C. E. (1977): *Dementia,* 2nd ed. Davis, Philadelphia.
27. Wells, C. E. (1978): *Am. J. Psychiatry,* 135:1–12.
28. Wolstenholme, G. E. W., and O'Connor, M. (1970): *Alzheimer's Disease and Related Conditions,* Churchill, London.

DISCUSSION

Dr. Schoenberg: I would first like to emphasize two principles of particular concern to the epidemiologist that should be considered in the critical evaluation of any study dealing with the classification of human subjects.

The first principle concerns the accuracy of the diagnosis and the detailed characterization of the patients under study. This point was well summarized by a British statistician who many years ago wrote: "The government are very keen on amassing statistics— they collect them, add them, raise them to the *nth* power, take the cube root and prepare wonderful diagrams. But what you must never forget is that every one of those figures comes in the first instance from the . . . village watchman, who puts down what he damn pleases" (2).

Unfortunately we are now in a situation with no agreed-on minimal criteria either for diagnosis or for staging, and we must rely on our village watchmen recording whatever they please. It is critical that investigators studying the problem of senile dementia describe their study subjects in as much detail as possible so that one study may be compared with another. This is essential not only because of the many diseases presenting with dementia, but also because the patient with senile dementia is changing over time.

The second important principle concerns representation. Our knowledge of senile dementia is based on either clinical or pathologic experience. But, how representative is a particular group of study subjects? This problem pervades all branches of science, and is highlighted in a quote by an American philosopher, George Boas, who noted: "Some scientists will study two or three dozen pigeons in a laboratory and then write a book entitled *Pigeons.* They should call it *Some Pigeons I Have Known*" (1). In our investigations we must exercise great care in relating particular study subjects to all individuals with senile dementia.

Two specific questions are directed to Drs. Lipowski and Clayton: Classifications can have many uses and it is impossible to judge the value of a given system of nosology unless one is aware of the particular goals of the classification scheme. Diseases can be grouped by clinical features at onset, or at a certain time period following onset. They can be grouped according to clinical course, prognosis, pathologic findings, etiology, when that is known, and one could go on and on. Now, is it possible to devise a system of classification that will maximally address all possible uses and if not, what is the specific goal of your proposed classification scheme?

Dr. Bergmann: I would like to address myself to the contributions from Drs. Lipowsky and Clayton. The former has diagnosed the problems of DSM II, and set up a whole set of new problems when we get DSM III in the future.

The first question I asked was: Why did he ignore the W.H.O. Scientific Group reports on psychogeriatrics? These propose a nosology based on the International Classification of Diseases (ICD) commanding international agreement. They have the advantage of classifying dementing states by empirically defined grades of severity. This leads to Dr. Clayton's observation: She rightly points out that we do not know whether mild, moderate, or severe dementias are part of a continuum. Surely it is because we do not know the answer to this question that the dementias should be defined independently and followed up longitudinally.

In our Newcastle follow-up studies of borderline senile dementia, one-third of our subjects became evidently demented, one-third remained doubtful after 3 or 4 years, and the other group turned out to be intellectually and socioeconomically deprived. Why then prejudge this issue when proposals exist to label grades of severity purely on an operational basis?

Finally, my most serious worry about Dr. Lipowsky's statement must focus on the totally unjustified labeling of so-called symptomatic affective and schizophreniform psychoses that happen to be associated with bodily or localized cerebral disease. The assumption is made that organic factors provide both necessary and sufficient causes for these conditions. It does not allow for any flexibility in measuring the weight of a variety of factors that may be associated with psychoses in later life.

The reserpine-induced depression is called organic psychiatric disorder, but those people receiving this treatment who do not become depressed have no psychiatric classification at all. It is self-evident that not everyone with organic deficits develops a particular form of psychosis. So, I consider the inclusion of symptomatic functional psychosis an extremely dangerous practice discouraging further research and investigation.

Finally, I think that the abolition of paraphrenia as a diagnostic classification is unfortunate. I hope there is still time to reconsider these difficulties and to examine the report of the W.H.O. specialist group on psychogeriatrics. This, I think, represents at least the possibility of international agreement.

Sir Martin Roth: I would like to reinforce what Dr. Bergman has said. I reacted with a certain astonishment, I have to say, to the classification of organic syndromes in the DSM III. I find it difficult to understand the detailed logic behind it.

My remarks are concerned with the classification of the organic schizphreniform and affective syndromes and the organic delusional and personality syndromes. Why are these inadmissible in a group of psychiatric organic disorders? They are inadmissible because in amnestic syndromes, clouded and delirious states, and the chronic psycho-organic syndrome of dementia, the organic lesion is both sufficient and necessary. In every case of an amnestic syndrome there is a specific lesion in the limbic, hippocampus, mammillary bodies, thalamic dorso-medial nucleus, or related structures. A lesion will be found in 100% of cases.

This is not the state of affairs in relation to the new syndromes that are being recommended for inclusion among the organic psychiatric disorders. The nature of the relationship between the psychiatric syndrome and the organic lesion is obscure and uncertain. When schizophrenic-like diseases are associated with organic disease, the strength of the correlation and the causal relationship between them is unknown. It needs to be defined by further research. The problem cannot be decided by ad hoc and arbitrary diagnostic rules.

We may take the example of what is perhaps the most clearly established form of hallucinosis without psychiatric organic features. I refer to chronic alcoholic hallucinosis. The psychosis is dominated by auditory hallucinations of a rather characteristic content and the psychosis is late in onset and circumscribed, leaving the personality intact. Even in this well-studied phenomenon the organic factor (usually withdrawal from chronic intoxication) is neither necessary nor sufficient. Similar hallucinosis may be seen without any contribution from alcoholism or any other toxic or organic factor. On the other hand, among a large group of alcoholics comparable in all relevant respects, only a small minority will develop hallucinosis.

However, much more serious diagnostic and conceptual confusion is likely to arise if one looks at a wider range of somatic diseases that precede or coincide with, let us say, schizophrenic-like psychoses. The psychiatric disorder may have been preceded by influenza during the previous week, a minor operation a fortnight earlier, hepatitis 2 months ago, or a fracture entailing immobility 3 months previously. Is such a psychosis to be diagnosed as organic schizophreniform disorder?

If so, what evidence is there to justify such a practice, seeing that such psychoses respond to treatment in exactly the same manner as schizophrenic-like disorders without associated organic disease? Of course it has been known for a considerable time that there is some measure of overlap between schizophrenic, other delusional, and affective psychoses on the one hand and organic diseases on the other. The association is greater than could have been expected to occur by chance.

But this does not justify calling the relevant disorders organic, paranoid, affective, and other syndromes for the following reasons. The physical illness may subside but the psychiatric syndrome continues. This course of events is well known in the depressions that follow influenza or infectious hepatitis or the paranoid state in clear consciousness following surgery in old people. The opposite sequence may be observed. The physical disease continues, but the psychiatric disorder disappears. In the case of the paranoid and affective psychosis of old age, the psychiatric disorder may respond to the same pharmacological treatment as do the "functional" forms of these disorders despite the fact that the physical disease continues.

We therefore deal with the conjunction of two relatively independent groups of phenomena. The strength of the association between them can be determined only by further investigation. To place such conditions into the same class as dementia, delirium, and other typical organic syndromes appears to be misconceived. That these disorders present diagnostic problems is undeniable. But the solution for this in clinical practice is to enter the descriptive psychiatric diagnosis and associated physical diseases under separate headings.

I believe the same practice should be followed in relation to the group described by Dr. Lipowsky as "organic personality syndrome." There is a case for classifying patients with a frontal lobe syndrome following injury or some other form of cerebral damage with the organic disorders. But how is one to deal with the patient who exhibits a severe life-long personality disorder and also manifests a borderline EEG abnormality or perhaps a small nonepileptic focus or a history of a road traffic accident 3 years previously? Are these to be regarded as organic personality disorders, and if not, why not?

I would have refrained from taking up so much time if this were not such an important question. I believe that to widen the concept of psycho-organic syndromes in the manner suggested can only cause blurring of the concept and confusion in practice. There is a real problem in this area, but it should be solved in my view by (a) further scientific research and (b) separate diagnostic statements and descriptive and etiological terms in relevant cases without any prejudice about the strength of the association between them.

Dr. Lipowski: I will try to respond briefly to the comments of Sir Martin and Dr. Bergman, and will say a few words about the thinking behind the proposed new classification of organic mental disorders.

Both Dr. Bergman and Sir Martin criticize me for failing to separate delirium from dementia, although in fact both those syndromes are clearly distinguished and defined in both DSM III and in my paper. Explicit clinical diagnostic criteria for both delirium and dementia have been formulated in DSM III, and are more likely to sharpen rather than blunt the distinction between those syndromes. In addition, Dr. Bergman and Sir Martin raised objections to the inclusion of hallucinosis, organic delusional syndrome, organic affective syndrome, and organic personality disorder in DSM III. Such inclusion is certainly controversial and calls for an explanation. I believe that by including those syndromes in the DSM III Classification we will succeed in stimulating research on that whole borderland between the organic and the so-called functional psychopathology. Sir Martin clearly agrees that we have important research questions here but objects to what he views as our premature closure on the issue of causal relationships. Yet I believe that the nature and strength of such relationships will be definitively clarified as a consequence of research encouraged by our explicit inclusion of those disorders in the class of organic syndromes. To say that a mental disorder is organic does not, in my opinion, contradict current belief that all mental disorders are multifactorial in origin, although in a given disorder one factor may have more weight than others.

It appears that our disagreements boil down to different views on the functions of classification. I believe that a classification is not a collection of immutable platonic ideas of the classified phenomena, but simply reflects current knowledge and serves as a methodological tool, a stimulant for the formulation of testable hypotheses about causal relationships and for research that may help in the advancement of knowledge. It was really our purpose to formulate the classification in such a way as to loosen up some of the entrenched conceptions and conceptual rigidities, and to encourage a fresh look that is justified by clinical observations made in the past 50 years or so.

The new classification is far from being an arbitrary and idiosyncratic effort by one person only. On the contrary, it is a product of joint efforts by the Task Force preparing DSM III, a product discussed and critically reviewed by special sub-committees comprised of psychogeriatricians, of experts on drug abuse and alcoholism, and of other people concerned with organic mental disorders. I have personally solicited comments from many interested colleagues in this country and abroad, such as Dr. Lishman and Professor Manfred Bleuler. The outline of the new classification has been published twice and changes have been made in it in response to specific criticisms. On the whole, however, the classification has so far provoked few substantial criticisms or major objections. Let me stress that the whole process of formulating this classification has been thoroughly public and empirical, in that the new diagnostic categories are being tested in field trials in a wide range of psychiatric settings in this country. After all, a classification of organic mental disorders has to take into account not only the needs of psychogeriatricians but also of psychiatrists working with all the other age groups and in all types of therapeutic and diagnostic settings.

There is little doubt that some people will find the changes introduced by us extremely unpalatable and disturbing, as they fail to conform to some time-honored notions and preconceptions. Responses by informed critics will be seriously considered by the Task Force, whose job has not yet been finished. Some controversy is likely to remain, as we can't satisfy everybody. If our formulations provoke a discussion and even irritation of some critics, the result is likely to be the establishment of much-needed studies and, ultimately, improved knowledge and treatment of the so-called organic mental disorders.

Dr. Clayton: It was not our intent to devise a classification that was etiologic. That would be premature. Our classification was to be descriptive. We were simply trying to classify together those entities that had shared phenomena, that might predict outcome or course. In regard to the dementias being "senile" and "pre-senile," we left those descriptors of pre-senile and senile onset merely to tie in with the ICD eight and nine, which both include the terms pre-senile and senile onset. We have made concessions in order to make the two more comparable. I think the ICD nine is difficult to use too. I believe there is an ICD nine CM that is especially formulated for clinicians to use, with slightly different terms, so that no one classification can satisfy everyone.

With respect to multi-infarct dementia, you are absolutely right in pointing out that it has been over-used and over-diagnosed. As I indicated in my paper, this more specific type of cerebral dementia is much less common than the senile dementias. We used this term because we thought it might discourage the indiscriminant use of cerebro-vasodilators.

We did not have an opportunity to present the whole of DSM III as comprehensively as we would have liked, and that may have added to your confusion. For instance, there is a whole section on paranoia, and I would doubt that patients would be grouped into organic classifications if they had some kind of paranoid reaction. It should be recalled that there are five different axes, with the second including personality descriptors. The third is a medical axis, to note the presence of a physical, medical condition. Finally, the fourth is a stressor axis, and the fifth is a functioning axis. Both stress and adaptive ability can be taken into account on the new DSM III axis, which should add to the richness and comprehensiveness of information about the patient.

REFERENCES

1. Lawrence, J. G. (1978): *Johns Hopkins Magazine.* 29:4.
2. Stamp, J. (1929): *Some Economic Factors in Modern Life,* pp. 258–259. P. S. King and Son, London.

Clinical Aspects of Alzheimer's Disease and Senile Dementia, (Aging, Vol. 15), edited by Nancy E. Miller and Gene D. Cohen. Raven Press, New York 1981.

The Borderlands of Dementia: The Influence of Sociocultural Characteristics on Rates of Dementia Occurring in the Senium

Barry J. Gurland

Center for Geriatrics and Gerontology, Columbia University, New York, New York 10032; and Department of Geriatrics Research, New York State Psychiatric Institute

EPIDEMIOLOGY

Rates of Dementia as Measured by Psychological Indicators

It has long been recognized that rates and severity levels of dementia occurring in the senium, at least as measured by psychological tests, vary with sociocultural factors. In 1961 Kahn et al. (34) published a report on a study of a random sample of 605 elderly persons in long-term care institutions in New York City and pointed out that their measures of mental functioning were more closely related to educational level than to age. The main measure they used was the Mental Status Questionnaire (MSQ), which was significantly inversely correlated ($p < 0.001$) with the number of years of education (Table 1).

TABLE 1. *Relation of MSQ to education*

MSQ error score	No. of pts.	% Distribution by years of education			
		0–7	8	9+	Total
0	119	26	29	45	100
1	85	41	33	26	100
2	54	48	28	24	100
3	50	42	24	34	100
4	45	62	29	9	100
5	37	57	22	22	101
6	38	60	26	13	99
7	37	65	22	13	100
8	27	74	22	4	100
9	35	80	14	6	100
10	78	80	13	8	101

From ref. 1.
Correlation between MSQ and education = 0.33 ($p < 0.001$).

It is indicative of the puzzling nature of the sociocultural associations of dementia occurring in the senium that despite the lengthy period of time that has intervened since Kahn's finding this association is still attracting new interest and new speculation. In 1975 Pfeiffer (49) reported data from the application of the Short Portable Mental Status Questionnaire (SPMSQ) (almost identical to the instrument used by Kahn) to a random sample of 997 elderly persons in Durham County, North Carolina, and two nonrandom samples (141 and 102 persons, respectively) from a multipurpose clinic and long-term care institutions in the same region. Again the findings included a statistically significant correlation between SPMSQ scores and level of education (Fig. 1). This relationship held true for black and white subjects.

Still more recently, in 1978, Gurland et al., reporting data (24) from the United States–United Kingdom Cross-National Project, confirmed the association described above in a study of random samples of elderly persons living outside institutions in New York and London ($N = 445$ and 396, respectively). Subjects were over 65 years of age, randomly selected, and interviewed in their homes.

Data from the New York sample is presented in Table 2 to show the relationship between educational level and scores on an indicator scale of dementia, taking age into account. The dementia indicator scale is based on the MSQ; a criterion score (4 or more) is used to separate high from low scorers, with higher scores reflecting more errors in response. Educational levels are divided into those with 8 or fewer years of school and those with more. High scores on the dementia scale are overall 2.5 times more frequent in the low-education group (17%) than in the high-education group (7%). However, since age is related to education (Table 2, line a) and scores on the dementia scale (Table

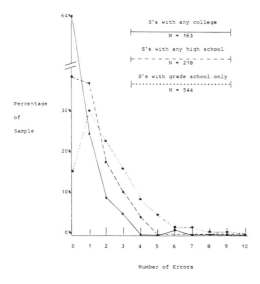

FIG. 1. Distribution of survey sample by educational attainment and number of errors on short portable MSQ. (From ref. 2.)

2, line c), the relationship between education and the dementia scale may be confounded by age and should be examined for each age group separately (Table 2, line b). Within each of the 5-year age groups from 65 to 79 and for those 80 and over, high scores on the dementia scale are more frequent in the lower than in the higher educational groups.

The major measure of mental functioning used in the above studies is the MSQ developed by Kahn and his colleagues (33), with or without minor modification. This is a widely used instrument consisting of a short set of questions (usually 10) on orientation, memory, and recent events. The number of errors scored on the MSQ is predictive of the clinical diagnosis of organic brain syndrome from any cause. In settings where the majority of organic brain syndromes are chronic and of the Alzheimer's type or related dementias, the MSQ is predictive of these clinical diagnoses and of mortality, discharge from hospital, institutionalization, nursing needs, and scores on other psychological test indicators of dementia, as well as more direct measures of brain pathology by, for example, electroencephalography (EEG) and postmortem examination (23).

Since there is a high correlation between educational level and social class, race, ethnic membership, or immigration status, it is not unexpected that each of these characteristics has been found to be related to the MSQ (24,49). It is not at all clear whether the other sociocultural relationships with the MSQ would hold up if it was possible to adequately control the effects of education. For example, the data from Pfeiffer show a higher rate of SPMSQ errors for blacks than for whites, and this is evident for each of three educational categories (grade school, high school, and college level). However, the quality of education is not the same for the two races, and the gross educational categories only partially control for the effects of education. Similarly, in the Cross-National Project data, higher scores on the MSQ (Dementia Scale) occur predominantly in the lower social classes, immigrant groups (including Europeans and Puerto

TABLE 2. *US–UK Cross-National Geriatric Community Study, New York: relationship between dementia scale score,[a] educational level, and age*

Parameter	Age 65–69		Age 70–74		Age 75–79		Age 80–98		
No. of patients	136		117		93		77		
Education[b]	*Low* 45	*High* 55	*Low* 53	*High* 47	*Low* 61	*High* 39	*Low* 77	*High* 33	(a)
Percent with high dementia[c]	11	3	8	2	19	14	32	21	(b)
	7		5		17		28		(c)

All results are expressed in percent.
[a] The Dementia Scale is modified from the MSQ.
[b] Low education = ≤ 8 years. High education = > 8 years.
[c] High dementia equals a score of 4 or more on the rational scale of dementia.

Ricans), and blacks. The extent to which the quality of education or other sociocultural factors could account for the subcultural differences in MSQ scores is difficult to determine, even though the differences remain when quantity of education is kept constant.

Relationship Between Performance and Brain Deterioration

There can be little doubt then that there is a relationship between MSQ scores (or many other psychological tests of memory and other cognitive functions) and sociocultural factors, but it is clear that the nature of this relationship is open to several interpretations. The simplest hypotheses available to explain this relationship are: (a) that the MSQ or other similar psychological tests are indicators of a dementing process (i.e., deterioration of the brain) and that the dementing process is more common in certain sociocultural groups, or (b) that performance on the MSQ or other similar psychological tests is influenced by dementia and sociocultural characteristics, e.g., education. The latter hypothesis allows that dementia rates may be constant between sociocultural groups even where the MSQ scores or other similar psychological test scores vary between the groups.

This possible discrepancy between the structural alteration of the brain by the dementing process and the performance level of the sufferer is a special case of a more general debate that has raged for almost half a century since Rothschild emphasized in 1937 (55) the disparity between the brain changes of senile dementia as noted at postmortem examination and the level of performance of the subject on psychological tests or in everyday activities before death. Some subjects had gross brain pathology but were little affected in their performance, whereas the converse also applied.

Other researchers have argued powerfully in favor of a close fit between brain change and behavior. Roth (54) reviewed the work of his own group and others showing that contrary to the emphasis given by Rothschild there is on the whole an orderly relationship between postmortem findings and premortem measures of performance. Roth asserts that previous studies which failed to show this orderliness were misled by the inclusion of cases of acute brain syndrome and pseudodementia among the group of persons judged to have had behavioral signs of dementia so that the absence of postmortem brain changes of dementia in this group is not surprising. Furthermore, he points out that these previous studies relied on a classification of dementia that treated it as an all-or-none phenomenon. In his own studies he took degrees of impaired performance and of brain changes into account. He found a strongly positive correlation between the amount of brain softening or the histological signs of dementia (neurofibrillary tangles and senile plaques) on the one hand and psychological tests of memory and orientation and informant reports of level of function in everyday activities on the other hand. The correlation between postmortem brain changes and performance levels was of the order of 0.77 ($p < 0.001$), although among the subjects who were markedly demented there was no significant correlation between the degree of dementia and number of senile plaques.

Tomlinson (61) estimates that on the basis of quantitative changes alone (i.e., senile morphology and cerebral softening), 70% of dements are markedly different from nondemented subjects in old age, but he goes on to postulate that as yet unquantified elements such as neuronal loss may account for those cases of dementia which show no identifiable pathological lesions. He suggests that interaction between the amount of senile morphological changes, the proportion of neurons lost, and the site of the altered brain structure (rather than the interplay of morphological and personality factors) determines the extent of intellectual impairment.

Wang (63) sums up his own view of the current evidence on brain–behavior relationships in dementia by admitting that "it is still unresolved whether the difference among normal aging, senile dementia, and presenile dementia is an intensity, extensity, locational, or subtle qualitative ultrastructural difference." The localization of the lesions or their distribution between the cortex and subcortex could affect the brain–behavior relationship, although the majority of the dementias are characterized by diffuse degeneration. However, Wang goes on to say that, although the severity of cognitive deficit is usually correlated with the severity of brain changes, there are many discrepancies between these variables. He does not accept that the cognitive variable can be accounted for solely by the brain variable.

Validity of the MSQ Across Sociocultural Groups

Zarit et al. (67) studied the extent to which the MSQ is socioculturally fair as an indicator of a dementing process. The MSQ scores were compared with decrements in performance on a battery of psychological tests which are sensitive to cognitive impairment. The tests were applied to 113 consecutive admissions to a gerontology clinic and to 40 of their collaterals, all over 50 years of age. Level of education was strongly associated with cognitive deficit, but the MSQ "yielded an evaluation of cognitive functions that was relatively independent of education. Thus, although education was shown to affect the level of intellectual performance, positive ratings on [the MSQ] were usually associated with similar declines in cognitive function for all educational levels." In other words, a given level of MSQ score indicates an equivalent erosion of psychological performance in all educational groups. Of course the actual level of performance depends on the level of the subject's performance prior to the onset of the eroding process (i.e., dementia).

The practical and human consequences of the eroding process (presumably dementia) indicated by the MSQ measure are not, however, directly represented by psychological test performance but rather by such features as mortality rates or the incapacity to maintain an independent level of self-care or instrumental function. The US–UK Cross-National data (24) allow an examination of the

TABLE 3. *US–UK Cross-National Geriatric Community Study, New York: proportion of persons dependent at increasing dementia scores controlling for education*

Dementia[b]	Low education[c]		High education[c]		Total	
0, 1	22%	(29/129)	18%	(28/155)	20%	(57/284)
2, 3	36%	(23/64)	43%	(10/23)	38%	(33/87)
4+	77%	(31/40)	77%	(10/13)	77%	(41/53)
Total	36%	(83/233)	25%	(48/191)	31%	(131/424)

[a] Dependent = 4+ on Homogeneous Scale of Dependence.
[b] Homogeneous scale of dementia.
[c] Low education = $\leq$ 8 years. High education = $>$ 8 years.

relationship between MSQ (dementia scale) scores and incapacity for self-care (dependency scale) for high and low educational groups (Table 3). For the purposes of this analysis, subjects are called dependent if they score 4 or more on the dependency scale. By this token, the proportion of the New York community elderly who are dependent rises as the MSQ (dementia scale) scores increase and to about the same degree in the high as in the low educational groups. In both educational groups, dependency rates in those with dementia scale scores of 4+ are roughly four times higher than in those with dementia scale scores of 1 or less. It appears that a rise in dementia scale scores carries with it the same attendant risk of incapacity in both educational groups.

Nonverbal Psychological Tests

The relationship between sociocultural characteristics and psychological tests of dementia has been reported mainly with reference to the MSQ, which is obviously dependent on verbal communication. Confirmation of this relationship by relatively language-free tests, e.g., the face-hand test of Fink et al. (14), was reported by Kahn and his colleagues (34). Thus it seems less likely that the sociocultural correlates of dementia are merely an artifact of poor verbal performance on the part of socioculturally disadvantaged members.

Discrepancies Between the MSQ and the Clinical Diagnosis of Dementia

The MSQ, like other psychological tests of cognitive function, is subject to such factors as motivation, attention, communication problems, emotional disorder, physical health, and reaction to the test situation itself or the revealed deficits (63). Such factors may introduce noise into the assessment of cognitive status and thus undermine the construct validity of the test as an indicator of a dementing process. Moreover, the MSQ is primarily an indicator of an organic brain syndrome; only some organic brain syndromes are of the chronic, as opposed to the acute, variety, whereas Alzheimer's and related dementias are only a subset of chronic organic brain syndromes.

Similarly, the construct validity of the clinical diagnosis of Alzheimer's or related forms of senile dementia may be undermined by such factors as biased diagnosis, inadequate investigation and history-taking, poor reporting of symptoms on the part of the patient or an informant, and atypical presentations of the disorder. A study by the US–UK Cross-National Project (27) showed that the psychiatrists in a New York hospital frequently made a diagnosis of one or the other type of dementia in elderly patients even where the symptom patterns, psychological tests, and outcome were not characteristic of a dementing process. Furthermore, the clinical distinction between functional psychiatric disorder and chronic organic brain syndrome is more readily made than those between primary and secondary dementia and between Alzheimer's and the related dementias, including the arteriosclerotic type.

Since the MSQ and the clinical diagnosis of dementia are subject to reduction of their construct validity under various circumstances, and since they identify the Alzheimer and related dementias with differing degrees of precision, it is not surprising that the correlation between these two indicators of a dementing process is less than perfect. They are in fact sufficiently independent to permit the possibility that the documented relationship between sociocultural characteristics and the MSQ as an indicator of dementia would not be found when clinical diagnosis is used as the indicator of a dementing process.

With many reservations about the inferences that can be drawn from data based on hospitalized populations and routine hospital diagnoses, it is nonetheless of interest that the rate of organic brain syndromes as a primary diagnosis among admissions to the inpatient services of state and county mental hospitals in the United States during 1975 was 8.2/100,000 of the white population and 19.2/100,000 for all other races (43). These are not age-specific figures, but the majority of these organic brain syndromes occur in persons over the age of 55.

The small number of cases of dementia diagnosed in geriatric general population surveys makes sociocultural associations difficult to establish with confidence. It appears that the association between dementia and social class is weaker where diagnosis is the indicator than where the MSQ acts in this capacity. This is to say, among those persons who score high (make many errors) on the MSQ, a smaller proportion of the low than the high sociocultural groups receive a clinical diagnosis of dementia (i.e., cross-validation of MSQ by diagnosis is better for the high than the low sociocultural group). This is true in the US–UK Cross-National Geriatric Survey in New York (24). It also appears to be true of the Newcastle-upon-Tyne studies: Kay (37) reports that in the latter studies some elderly subjects who were initially classified as being demented were found 2 or 3 years later not to be deteriorated and were retrospectively reclassified as not demented; these initial misdiagnoses were concentrated in groups of subjects with low intelligence.

Pfeiffer (49) is also of the opinion that a high MSQ score at any given level warrants a clinical diagnosis of dementia less often among poorly educated than well educated elderly persons. However, Pfeiffer bases his opinion, and his recommendations for a corresponding calibration of the MSQ (i.e., for poorly educated persons the criterion score for dementia should be higher), on the assumption that similar proportions of each sociocultural group are demented.

Where there is conflict about the sociocultural associations of dementia, as indicated on the one hand by psychological tests such as the MSQ and on the other hand by clinical diagnosis, then a question arises as to whether credence should be given to the results obtained from one type of indicator while the results from the other type of indicator are dismissed. The answer may pivot on which of the two types of indicator is more reliable and valid with respect to identifying the presence of a dementing process (i.e., an accelerated progressive deterioration of intellectual-cognitive functions). When the persons under study are hospitalized or are clinic patients, then the relative merits of the indicators depend on how well the diagnoses are made in that particular location; the psychological tests are certainly more consistently administered across locations than are clinical diagnoses but are generally not as valid as a highly skilled clinical diagnosis can be. However, when the persons under study are randomly drawn from the general elderly population, then as many reservations must pertain to diagnosis as to psychological tests because the criteria for the diagnosis of dementia in community subjects have not yet been well worked out. Kay (37) points to the gross discrepancies in prevalence rates of dementia reported in various community surveys (from 1 to 7.2% for severe dementia in those over 65 years of age, and 2.6 to 15% for mild dementia). He suggests that differences in reported rates are mainly due to differences in method and criteria for diagnosis.

We already discussed the degree to which the MSQ is biased by sociocultural factors. Similar considerations apply to sociocultural biasing of diagnosis. The influence of demographic characteristics on bias in diagnosis has been shown for other diagnoses and other age groups (16); similar biases may be assumed to occur also for the diagnosis of dementia in the elderly. It is possible that when the diagnosis of dementia is loosely made there is a bias toward relative overdiagnosis of this condition in disadvantaged groups who may fail to arouse the clinician's therapeutic zeal or who may describe their symptoms poorly or give the impression that their intellectual level has deteriorated; but when the diagnosis is conservatively made, there is a tendency to diagnose as demented only patients with an obvious drop from their previous intellectual performance, leading to a relative underdiagnosis of dementia in the disadvantaged group.

In short, neither psychological tests nor clinical diagnosis can be accepted as culture-free indicators of a dementing process, but the extent of their sociocultural biases is not known.

Direct In Vivo Measures of Brain Function

So far, in the discussion of the relationship between psychological test performance and structural brain change, we have confined the measurement of brain change to quantification of morphological abnormalities at autopsy. At least two major methodological problems for an epidemiological study arise with the use of autopsy material as an indicator of a dementing process: (a) an uncertain sociocultural bias in the selection of persons whose brains are made available for autopsy; and (b) the heavy loading with patients who have reached an advanced stage of dementia. Sociocultural differences in the prevalence of dementias which might be apparent in a cross section of the elderly population, particularly if all degrees of severity of the dementing process are counted, could well be missed in a study based only on autopsied cases. Thus it would be desirable to examine also the sociocultural relationships of dementia as indicated in *in vivo* direct tests of brain functions.

Wang et al. (64) tested the relationship between cerebral blood flow (as measured by inhalation of ^{133}Xe) and WAIS verbal and performance scores of 20 elderly community volunteers grouped into equal numbers of low and high education–socioeconomic status. The only statistically significant correlation with blood flow was for performance IQ in the low status group ($r = 0.78$), although the corresponding correlation for the high status group was not low ($r = 0.54$) and there was less variance (to allow a high correlation) in blood flow in the latter group. These results tend in the direction of there being an equal fall-off in performance with decreasing blood flow in both socioeducational groups, but that, since the high-status group starts at a better performance level than the low status group, equal decrements in the two status groups may push the low group below the threshold for effective psychological functioning before the high group has fallen below this level. That is to suggest that sociocultural vulnerability is not an exaggeration of the degree to which noxious influences on the brain reduce psychological test performance; rather it is the lack of a margin of reserve for effective psychological functioning (or in the performance of the tasks of daily living). This says nothing about whether socioculture also increases the frequency of noxious influences on the brain; in the study cited above, the low-status group tended to have more subjects with low blood flow than did the high-status group, but the small sample size and the unrepresentative nature of the sample detracts from the significance of this finding.

Poitrenaud and his colleagues (51), employed radiotelemetric devices (EEG, EMG, ECG, and EOG) to study fluctuations in levels of arousal in 18 elderly subjects ranging across five educational levels. Educational levels were directly correlated with arousal levels ($r = 0.506$); and "the correlation between telemetric and behavioral data [on cognitive functioning] appears to support the hypothesis according to which disturbance of mental abilities might be due to arousal variations." The authors believe that memory impairment in the elderly is usually due to deficits of initial registration, and that the latter requires normal levels of attention and concentration, and a given degree of arousal.

POSSIBLE MECHANISMS OF ASSOCIATION BETWEEN SOCIOCULTURE AND RATES OF DEMENTIA

Selection, Survivorship, and Chronicity

It is necessary to question whether the reported relationship between sociocultural characteristics and the various indicators of dementia in the senium could be due to a biased selection of subjects. For example, it is inevitable that data gathered on community samples will omit cases of dementia in institutions. In that case, whichever sociocultural group maintained more of their dementing members at home [e.g., by dint of strong family support of the dependent elderly (25)] would appear to have higher rates of dementia. The converse argument would apply to samples from institutions. However, the studies cited here report the same sociocultural correlates of dementia whether the samples are drawn from the general population or from long-term care institutions.

Somewhat more complex is the effect on prevalence rates of dementia of differences in survivorship of sociocultural groups. Higher rates of dementia are found, if anywhere, in disadvantaged groups; these groups have a shorter life expectancy at birth than more advantaged sociocultural groups, although this differential is eliminated for life expectancy once old age is reached. A shorter life expectancy at birth would of course reduce the proportion of elderly and demented persons in the total population but not necessarily the proportion of elderly who are demented. It is conceivable that specifically those persons who are vulnerable to developing dementia, given their survival to the age of risk, die before reaching that age at such a high rate in a certain sociocultural group that the group is left with a low prevalence rate of dementia. There is no reason to believe that this occurs or that it would occur more often in the advantaged than in the disadvantaged group. It thus does not seem likely that differential attainment of the age of risk could account for the associations noted between socioculture and dementia.

Less easily disposed of is the possibility that differential survivorship *after* the onset of dementia may account for sociocultural differences in prevalence rates of dementia. Prevalence is a function of incidence multiplied by the duration of an episode of illness; clearly, increasing the duration of an illness increases the prevalence rate. Dementia occurring in the senium is usually an unremitting illness, so that increasing the duration can only be achieved by increasing survival after onset of dementia. Differences in such survival have been reported in relation to improved health care (22), but there is no evidence that this would operate in favor of disadvantaged groups and thus suffice to explain higher rates of dementia in those groups.

Brain Insults at Various Life Stages

Pasamanick (48) suggested that the higher rate of schizophrenia in disadvantaged sociocultural groups reflected a vulnerability to this disorder arising from fetal and neonatal trauma or disease and malnutrition during infancy and childhood. A comparable rationale could be advanced for alleged higher rates of dementia in disadvantaged groups. The rationale rests on the assumption that minimal, subclinical states of brain impairment, possibly eroding only the reserve capacity of the brain, predisposes the individual to show effects recognizable as dementia when an additional process of brain damage occurs later in life, either through the "normal" processes of aging or through a supervening pathological process. In support of this rationale, Netchine (44) showed that EEG maturation during infancy varies between sociocultural groups.

Less remote causes of dementia than those arising in early life might also occur more frequently in disadvantaged groups. Hypertension and stroke show higher prevalence rates in disadvantaged than in advantaged groups, as do chronic illnesses, e.g., anemia and kidney disease (41). These are examples of illnesses directly threatening the integrity of the brain or its adequate supply of oxygen and other nutrients.

Exposure to occupational hazards as yet unrecognized to be related to dementia could also be associated with sociocultural group membership, e.g., aluminum accumulation (7), chronic carbon monoxide inhalation, and other speculative precursors of dementia. Recently certain types of dementia have been attributed to a transmissable virus (62), raising the possibility that certain sociocultural groups may be more exposed than others to specific viruses causing dementia. As a final example, a genetic determinant of dementia has been postulated and some supportive evidence forthcoming (39), making it possible that certain cultural groups share a gene pool predisposing them to dementia.

The point of this speculation is to indicate that there do exist plausible potential mechanisms for an association between brain insults, sociocultural characteristics, and prevalence rates of a dementing process. It is important to attempt to identify these mechanisms so as to make the measures (operational definitions) of socioculture as relevant as possible to the mechanism we wish to study. In this way we hope to avoid spurious and misleading associations between socioculture and dementia and to increase the power of potential associations that reflect specific mechanisms relating the two areas.

Stress During Late Life

A proximate set of precursors of dementia was suggested by Amster and Kraus (1), i.e., life crises. The relationship between life crises (i.e., life events or stress) was previously demonstrated for various mental disorders and is regarded as relevant to understanding the sociocultural distribution of mental disorder (8). Amster and Kraus applied this model to mental deterioration in elderly persons: They examined 25 women with a deteriorated mental condition (i.e., 9 or more errors on the MSQ) and an equal number of women without mental deterioration (i.e., 0 or 1 error on the MSQ). The number of life events (as measured by the Holmes and Masuda Life Event Scale, modified for use with the elderly) during the preceding 5 years, or the 5 years preceding deterioration, was determined. There was a significant increase ($p < 0.01$) in number and magnitude of preceding life events in those women who were mentally deteriorated compared with those who were not deteriorated. Thus although the study is flawed in a number of ways (e.g., the possibility of retrospective falsification, confounding of early symptoms with life events), there appears to be a plausible (but by no means proven) possibility that life event stress may precipitate some cases of dementia. The subjective weights attached to the stress effects of life events is relatively constant across sociocultural groups, but the frequency of events is not necessarily constant, leaving it possible that life event stress may be one of the mechanisms for linking socioculture and the onset of dementia.

Bennett and Nahemow (2), in their studies of relocation stress among elderly persons being admitted to a long-term care facility, noted the occurrence of relocation reactions, which appear particularly in those persons who show a lack of skill in learning the rules required for adaptive functioning in the institution. This appears to suggest another potential mechanism for sociocultural associations of stress and its consequences. Bennett also described a type of isolated elderly person with a cognitive impairment that appeared to be partly a result of the isolation insofar as relieving the isolation by relocation in an institution improved the cognitive performance.

Sensory Deprivation

A relative decrease of sensory stimulation may occur during old age through age-related bodily impairments of such perceptual mechanisms as hearing, vision, taste, smell, touch, proprioception, and visceral sensation; through environmental changes involving loss of social contacts and enforced disengagement from activities; as well as through shifts in attitude, motivation, and capacities leading to withdrawal from previous interests. Some of these deprivations may be linked to social class and education through differences in morbidity rates or in the stability of social and activity patterns across age groups. It is thus of interest to examine the possible relationship between sensory deprivation and dementia.

Ernst et al. (13) stated that "There is . . . ample evidence to show that the general impact of the quality of perception is not merely a cognitive process, but has definite somatic implications . . . that interference with sensory function affects the morphology of the individual cell structure involved in the particular sensory process, as well as producing functional and biochemical changes in the organism." In support of this conclusion, the authors reviewed experimental sensory deprivation in the rat and rabbit, reporting that early deprivation of visual stimulation can cause altered electrical activity of the cortex and subcortex, polyribosome aggregation in the visual cortex, reduced density of synapses in the visual cortex, myopia, etc. Similar findings are reported for interruption of stimulation of other perceptual modalities. In humans, Tees (60) is said to have shown that visual deprivation produces a disturbance in depth perception; Downs (9) is cited as demonstrating that bed rest and sensory deprivation may produce changes in perception and behavior; and Oster (45) is quoted as noting that "cells require continuous stimulation in order to grow and function, and that sensory deprivation means a lack of stimulation which will hasten cell degeneration such as that associated with aging."

Coping and Adaptation

The socioculturally related precursors and precipitants of dementia have so far been considered mostly with the assumption that if sociocultural characteristics correlate with rates of dementia they do so because they promote the brain changes that underlie dementia or erode the reserve capacity of the brain and thus reveal a dementing process. Now we consider further the possibility that membership of a sociocultural group might be associated with a predisposition to impairment of adaptive behavior and thus to an increased rate of decompensated dementia without there necessarily being an increase in the frequency of the brain changes of dementia in that group relative to other sociocultural groups.

Education

Kahn, Fink, and Weinstein (15,32,65,66), among others, regard the effect of education on performance on the MSQ as a special case of a more general principle that premorbid personal, intellectual, and adaptive characteristics have a profound influence on the behavioral effects of altered brain function. They produced evidence in favor of this hypothesis from studies of acute brain damage, the recovery phase of electroconvulsive therapy, and chronic brain syndrome in the institutionalized elderly. They went so far as to predict that "the general [historical] increase in educational level . . . would also seem to forecast a decrease in the proportionate degree of mental impairment to be found in our aged populations in the future." Piercy (50) ascribed some of the presumed protection afforded by higher education to the stability of overlearned tasks.

Personality

Several other studies suggest that premorbid personality may influence the ability to adapt to a change in the functional capacity of the individual. Gianotti (19) tested this hypothesis in a study of adaptation to the memory loss of senile dementia. He described a personality type which predicted the tendency to confabulate (i.e., invent information) when the information was not available because of a failure of the memory retrieval system. Confabulation was regarded as a more adaptive alternative to admitting illness or incapacity; the confabulation is considered an adaptive reaction because the awareness of intellectual inadequacy by dementing subjects may lead to their becoming very anxious or angry, the so-called "catastrophic reaction." The premorbid personality of the confabulators was characterized as hard-driving, ambitious, and independent; and such persons tended to be found more often in the higher social classes and to be upwardly mobile. It is of special interest that the premorbid personality alleged to influence adaptive confabulation is thus hypothesized by Gianotti also to have sociocultural associations. Extrapolation from Gianotti's hypothesis might suggest that higher sociocultural groups would be also more adept at concealing the early effects of a dementing process than the lower sociocultural groups.

Sinnott (59) also argues that the capacity to adapt to the biological changes of old age is an enduring personality characteristic. He suggests that the crucial adaptive quality is flexibility in the assumption of roles, using evidence relating to sex roles as an illustrative example. Flexibility allows a satisfactory adjustment to role changes imposed by aging. The presence of this quality of flexibility is associated with longevity and arises possibly from social learning throughout life or as an expression of biological superiority. Thus the adaptive capacity described by Sinnott is regarded as possibly a socially learned attribute and related to sociocultural membership.

Intelligence

The hypothesis that low educational achievement and its correlates, low socioeconomic status and low intelligence, are associated with increased vulnerability to cognitive decline (i.e., dementia) draws some strength from evidence regarding an analogous vulnerability to physical decline and death.

Eisdorfer (10), in a review of predictors of longevity, pointed out that educational level and high intelligence are associated with a longer life span (21,28, 30,47,53). The brightest students outlive their classmates, and Supreme Court justices live longer than high-ranking politicians. He concludes that "this attests to the general significance of heightened intellectual-socio-economic class as a protector." As possible intervening mechanisms for this protection, he mentions higher financial status, more social activity, and more work and general life satisfaction but also the possibility that intellectual level itself is protective.

Savage et al. (56,57), working with data from the Newcastle-upon-Tyne epidemiological studies of the elderly, support the notion that higher intelligence enables an individual to retain the capacity for self-help and satisfying active interests.

Throughout this discussion on the protective effects of intelligence, it should be remembered that this refers to lifetime intelligence and not to the last year of life at which time a terminal drop in intelligence frequently occurs (58).

Arousal

Ostfeld (46) suggested that the link between educational level and mental impairment is the level of alertness. He states that "there is much evidence that mental alertness lessens the severity of loss of mental function. For instance, the higher the original educational level, and the more recent the extensive use of mental functions, the less the decline in mental function with disease." We have already discussed support for this hypothesis coming from the work of Poitrenaud et al. (51).

Labeling

A major factor leading to the overdiagnosis of dementia in the elderly is that many depressed elderly patients complain about their memory. Kahn et al. (35) showed that subjective "complaints about memory are not associated with impairment in performance in a series of tests but were significantly correlated with depression. Although family members usually concurred that the patient had a memory problem, in half the cases the 'patient' actually performed better than relatives on objective tests." Gurland et al. (26) supported this contention by finding that subjective (as opposed to objective) complaints of memory disturbance formed part of the factor of depression, not of cognitive impairment. Over and above these subjective complaints of memory disturbance, some cases of depression in the elderly show impairment of memory on objective testing (18).

It is tempting to presume that if depressed persons are misdiagnosed as being demented a self-fulfilling prophecy leads to an outcome characteristic of the progressive course of dementia rather than the recovery expected with depression. If such an effect occurred, it would offer another mechanism to explain possible sociocultural associations of dementia: Mislabeling persons as demented could occur relatively more often among the socioculturally disadvantaged group leading to a relative excess of dementia-like cases in that group.

Kramer (38), after examining the relatively high frequency with which diagnoses of dementia were made by the hospital psychiatrists in the United States as compared with the United Kingdom, asked whether this was an instance in which cases of remediable functional disorder among the elderly were being labeled as dementia with a consequent neglect of appropriate treatment for the patient and an unnecessary decline in their health. The US–UK Cross-National Geriatric Hospital Study (27) gave some support to Kramer's suggestion that mislabeling was occurring but failed to show that mislabeling of these elderly psychiatric inpatients as demented led to a decline in their health. The elderly patients in the particular psychiatric admitting service which was studied followed a course predicted by a careful "research diagnosis" regardless of the diagnosis given by the busy hospital psychiatrists, often a misdiagnosis of dementia. The push toward early discharge of patients in the service studied may have helped to counteract any deleterious effects of mislabeling.

IMPLICATIONS FOR THE PREVENTION AND ALLEVIATION OF DEMENTIA

Without prejudice to the issue of the presence and nature of the sociocultural associations of dementia, we may consider some of the implications for the prevention and alleviation of this condition that would flow from acceptance that such an association did in fact exist. Indeed it appears that there are already established a number of forms of treatment that, implicitly at least, draw on a sociocultural influence on dementia as a theoretical basis for therapeutic mechanisms.

We already discussed the possibility that disadvantaged sociocultural membership and low educational status may predispose to sensory deprivation. Ernst and his colleagues (13) concluded at the end of a lengthy review that "many of the effects of sensory deprivation in laboratory experiments [are] reversible [and, analogously, that] work with the elderly to counteract the effects of isolation and lack of sensory stimulation has proved successful in . . . alleviating . . . chronic brain syndrome." The basis for this conclusion was the work done by the authors themselves (11,12) in which they report that group therapy over a period of 3 months was associated with improved scores on cognitive tests, as well as the work of Folsom (17) with reorientation therapy, of Bowers (4) and Brook (5) with remotivation–resocialization, of Burnside (6) and McCorkle (42) with tactile stimulation of regressed patients, and of Powell (52) with exercise in demented subjects. Thus Ernst believes that "dementia" (organic brain syndrome) is sometimes due to sensory deprivation and "the therapist must not focus only on the organic factors of the aging brain but must stress the effects of the environment." Goldfarb (20) and Kahn (31) also indicated support for the view that an unstimulating social environment can cause excess disability in disorders of brain function and that this can be prevented or reversed if intervention is early enough.

The long-term effects of childhood education in promoting resistance to the declines of aging has also been receiving more consideration than it had previously been given. Birren and Woodruff (3) suggest that "consideration of life span development might lead educators to reflect upon the late-life consequences of early educational experience." He refers to educational intervention, during midlife and later, designed to reverse or prevent age decrements in cognitive performance (29).

Like the educational strategies, other potential interventions to prevent possible sociocultural deleterious influences on dementia may also be viewed in terms of the stage of the life cycle at which they can be initiated. The improvement of central nervous system (CNS) function through better health care and nutrition for disadvantaged groups during pregnancy and childhood is one possibility, as is protection during adult life from head injury, the noxious influence of alcohol and other CNS toxins, and hypertension. During mid-life and the retirement phases, the possibly harmful but preventable effects of disengagement, enforced idleness, poverty, poor health, uncontrolled stress, and institutionalization may have sociocultural associations.

None of this is meant to imply that these interventions have been proved effective, but rather that recognition that sociocultural variables may be associated with rates of dementia and its consequences opens up and encourages new avenues for treatment and prevention.

SUMMARY AND CONCLUSION: THE NEED FOR A SPECIFIC STUDY

The arguments presented in this chapter are intended to show that it is still an open matter whether there is an important sociocultural contribution to the prevalence of Alzheimer's and related forms of dementia occurring in the senium, but that the evidence now available is sufficiently intriguing to warrant further study of this issue. However, the uncertainties which remain after reviewing the current data suggest that a carefully designed study is required to allow further understanding of this issue.

A diagram of the interaction of sociocultural factors and other etiological factors in dementia is shown in Fig. 2 to emphasize that studies in this area should take into account: line A: correlates and mechanisms of sociocultural membership as well as conventional demographic factors; line B: several concepts of the way sociocultural factors could influence rates of dementia; and line C: four main indicators of dementia: impairment of adaptation, psychological test performance, brain changes, and diagnosis. In addition, prevalence and incidence should be considered and the various types of dementia specified.

Operational definitions can be found for each of the components in this model for the sociocultural etiology of dementia: For example (a) brain changes can be quantified by noninvasive techniques (e.g., computer assisted tomography and xenon inhalation brain scan) and perhaps by newer, more accurate methods which are emerging (e.g., proton emission tomography), thus avoiding reliance on autopsy material with the methodological limitations previously described; (b) impairment in adaptation can be measured by such instruments as the Katz Index of ADL (36) or the IADL scale of Lawton and Brody (40); (c) the MSQ with or without other psychological indicators of organic brain syndrome is a versatile tool for use in a wide variety of study situations; and (d) specific criteria for diagnosis of types of dementia are becoming available. Measures such as these applied to a representative sample of elderly persons stratified according to sociocultural membership and severity levels of dementia would, by their interrelationships, greatly advance our understanding of the sociocultural associations of dementia.

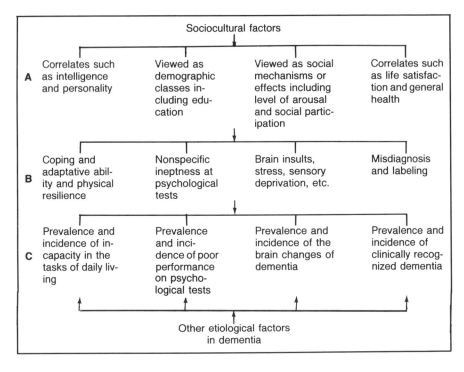

FIG. 2. Model for the interaction of sociocultural factors and other etiological factors in dementia.

ACKNOWLEDGMENTS

Roni Gurland, D.B.O., assisted in the literature review for this chapter.

REFERENCES

1. Amster, L. E., and Kraus, H. H. (1974): *Int. J. Aging Hum. Devel.,* 5(1).
2. Bennett, R., and Nahemow, L. (1965): In: *Proceedings of Institute on Mentally Impaired Aged,* edited by M. P. Lawton, pp. 88–105. Maurice Jacob Press, Philadelphia.
3. Birren, J. E., and Woodruff, D. S. (1973): In: *Life-Span Developmental Psychology: Personality and Socialization,* edited by P. B. Baltes and K. W. Schaie, pp. 305–337. Academic Press, New York.
4. Bowers, M. B. (1967): *J. Gerontol.,* 22:348–352.
5. Brook, P. (1975): *Br. J. Psychol.,* 127:42–45.
6. Burnside, I. M. (1974): *Am. J. Nurs.,* 73:2060–2063.
7. Crapper, D. R. (1974): In: *Frontiers in Neurology and Neurological Scientific Research,* edited by P. Seeman and G. H. Brown. University of Toronto Press, Toronto.
8. Dohrenwend, B. S. (1973): *J. Person. Soc. Psychol.,* 28:225–235.
9. Downs, F. (1974): *Am. J. Nurs.,* 7:434–438.
10. Eisdorfer, C. (1977): In: *Epidemiology of Aging,* edited by A. Ostfeld and D. C. Gibson, pp. 97–107. DHEW Publication No. NIH 75–711. U.S. Government Printing Office, Washington, D.C.
11. Ernst, P., Badash, D., Beran, B., Kosovsky, R., and Kleinhauz, M. (1977): *J. Am. Geriatr. Soc.,* 25:371–375.

12. Ernst, P., Beran, B., Badash, D., Kosovsky, R., and Kleinhauz, M. (1977): *J. Am. Geriatr. Soc.* 25:466–469.
13. Ernst, P., Beran, B., Safford, F., and Kleinhauz, M. (1978): *Gerontologist,* 18:468–474.
14. Fink, M., Green, M. A., and Bender, M. B. (1952): *Neurology,* 2:48–56.
15. Fink, M., Kahn, R. L., and Pollack, M. (1959): *J. Nerv. Ment. Dis.,* 128:243–248.
16. Fleiss, J. L., Gurland, B. J., Simon, R., and Sharpe, L. (1973): *Int. J. Soc. Psychiatr.,* 19:180–186.
17. Folsom, J. C. (1968): *J. Geriatr. Psychiatry,* 1:291–307.
18. Folstein, M. F., and McHugh, P. R. (1978): In: *Alzheimer's Disease: Senile Dementia and Related Disorders,* edited by R. Katzman, R. D. Terry, and K. L. Bick. Raven Press, New York.
19. Gianotti, G. (1975): *Psychiatr. Clin.,* 8:99–108.
20. Goldfarb, A. I. (1964): In: *The Evaluation of Psychiatric Treatment,* edited by P. Hoch and J. Zubin. Grune & Stratton, New York.
21. Granick, S., and Birren, J. E. (1969): Cognitive functioning of survivors versus nonsurvivors: 12 year follow-up of healthy aged. Presented at Eighth International Congress of Gerontology, Washington, D.C.
22. Gruenberg, E. (1978): In: *Alzheimer's Disease: Senile Dementia and Related Disorders,* edited by R. Katzman, R. D. Terry, and K. L. Bick, pp. 323–326. Raven Press, New York.
23. Gurland, B. J. (1980): In: *Handbook of Mental Health and Aging,* edited by J. E. Birren and R. B. Sloane. Prentice-Hall, Englewood Cliffs, N.J.
24. Gurland, B. J., Copeland, J. R. M., Kelleher, M. J., Sharpe, L., and Kuriansky, J. B. (1978): *A Preliminary Report on the U.S.–U.K. Geriatric Community Study.* Department of Geriatrics Research, New York State Psychiatric Institute, New York (mimeograph).
25. Gurland, B. J., Dean, L., Gurland, R. V., and Cook, D. (1978): In: *Dependency in the Elderly of New York City: Report of a Research Utilization Workshop, March 23, 1978,* pp. 9–45. Community Council of Greater New York, New York.
26. Gurland, B. J., Fleiss, J. L., Goldberg, K., and Sharpe, L., Copeland, J. R. M., Kelleher, M. J., and Kellett, J. M. (1976): *Psychol. Med.,* 6:451–459.
27. Gurland, B. J., Kuriansky, J., Sharpe, L., Simon, R., Stiller, P., Fleiss, J. L., Copeland, J., Kelleher, M., and Kellett, J. (1976): *Can. Psychiatr. Assoc. J.,* 21:421–431.
28. Hinkle, L., Whitney, L., Lehman, E., Dunn, J., Benjamin, B., King, R., Plakun, A., and Flehinger, B. (1968): *Science,* 161–238.
29. Hoyer, W. J., Labouvie, G. V., and Baltes, P. B. (1971): Operant modification of age decrements in intellectual performance. Presented at the 79th Annual Meeting of the American Psychological Association, Washington, D.C.
30. Jarvik, L. F., and Falek, A. (1963): *J. Gerontol.,* 18:173.
31. Kahn, R. L. (1977): In: *Readings in Aging and Death,* edited by S. H. Zarit. Harper & Row, New York.
32. Kahn, R. L., and Fink, M. (1959): *J. Neuropsychiatry,* 1:45–49.
33. Kahn, R. L., Goldfarb, A. I., Pollack, M., and Peck, A. (1960): *Am. J. Psychiatry,* 117:326–328.
34. Kahn, R. L., Pollack, M., and Goldfarb, A. I. (1961): In: *Psychopathology of Aging,* edited by P. Hoch and J. Zubin, pp. 104–113. Grune & Stratton, New York.
35. Kahn, R. L., Zarit, S., Hilbert, N. M., and Niederehe, G. (1975): *Arch. Gen. Psychiatry,* 32:1569–1573.
36. Katz, S., Ford, A. B., Moscowitz, R. W., Jackson, B. A., and Jaffe, M. W. (1963): *JAMA,* 185:914–919.
37. Kay, D. W. K. (1977): In: *Cognitive and Emotional Disturbance in the Elderly: Clinical Issues,* edited by C. Eisdorfer and R. O. Friedel, pp. 11–26. Year Book Medical Publishers, Chicago.
38. Kramer, M. (1961): In: *Proceedings of the Third World Congress of Psychiatry,* Vol. 3. University of Toronto Press/McGill University Press, Montreal.
39. Larsson, T., Sjogren, T., and Jacobson, G. (1963): *Acta Psychiatr. Scand. (Suppl. 167),* 39.
40. Lawton, M. P., and Brody, E. (1969): *Gerontologist,* 9:179–186.
41. Marquis Academic Media (1977): *Sourcebook on Aging,* 1st ed. Marquis Academic Media, Chicago.
42. McCorkle, M. (1974): *Effects of Touch in Seriously Ill Patients.* University of Iowa, Iowa City.

43. Meyer, N. (1977): *Mental Health Statistical Note No. 138.* DHEW Publication No. ADM 77–158. U.S. Government Printing Office, Washington, D.C.
44. Netchine, S. (1969): In: *Croissance de l'Enfant: Genese de l'Homme,* edited by Zasso. Presses Universitaires de France, Paris.
45. Oster, C. (1976): *J. Am. Geriatr. Soc.,* 24:461–464.
46. Ostfeld, A. (1977): In: *Epidemiology of Aging,* edited by A. Ostfeld and D. C. Gibson, pp. 129–135. DHEW Publication No. NIH 75–711. U.S. Government Printing Office, Washington, D.C.
47. Palmore, E., and Jeffers, F. (1971): *Prediction of Life Span.* Health Lexington Books, Lexington, Mass.
48. Pasamanick, B., and Knobloch, H. (1961): In: *Prevention of Mental Disorders in Children,* edited by G. Caplan. Basic Books, New York.
49. Pfeiffer, E. (1975): *J. Am. Geriatr. Soc.,* 23:433–439.
50. Piercy, M. (1964): *Br. J. Psychiatry,* 110:310–352.
51. Poitrenard, J., Hazemann, J., and Lille, F. (1978): *Gerontology,* 24:241–249.
52. Powell, R. R. (1974): *J. Gerontol.,* 29:157–161.
53. Quint, J., and Cody, B. (1970): *Am. J. Public Health,* 60:1118–1124.
54. Roth, M. (1971): In: *Recent Developments in Psychogeriatrics. Brit. J. Psychiat. Special Publication No. 6.* Headley Bros., Ashford, Kent, England.
55. Rothschild, D. (1937): *Am. J. Psychiatry,* 93:757.
56. Savage, R. D., Britton, P. G., Bolton, N., and Hall, E. H. (1973): *Intellectual Functioning in the Aged.* Methuen, London.
57. Savage, R. D., Gaber, L. B., Britton, P. G., Bolton, N., and Cooper, A. (1977): *Personality and Adjustment in the Aged.* Academic Press, New York.
58. Siegler, I. C. (1975): *Exp. Aging Res.,* 1:169–185.
59. Sinnott, J. D. (1977): *Gerontologist,* 17:459–463.
60. Tees, R. C. (1974): *J. Comp. Physiol. Psychol.,* 86:300–308.
61. Tomlinson, B. E. (1977): In: *Aging and Dementia,* edited by W. L. Smith and M. Kinsbourne, pp. 25–56. Spectrum Publications, New York.
62. Traub, R., Gajdusek, D. C., and Gibbs, C. J. (1977): In: *Aging and Dementia,* edited by W. L. Smith and M. Kinsbourne, pp. 91–172. Spectrum Publications, New York.
63. Wang, H. S. (1977): In: *Aging and Dementia,* edited by W. L. Smith and M. Kinsbourne, pp. 1–24. Spectrum Publications, New York.
64. Wang, H. S., Obrist, W. D., and Busse, E. (1970): *Am. J. Psychiatry,* 126:1205–1212.
65. Weinstein, E. A., and Kahn, R. L. (1955): *Denial of Illness: Symbolic and Physiological Aspects.* Thomas, Springfield, Ill.
66. Zarit, S., and Kahn, R. L. (1975): *J. Gerontol.,* 30:67–72.
67. Zarit, S. H., Miller, N. E., and Kahn, R. L. (1978): *J. Am. Geriatr. Soc.,* 26:58–67.

DISCUSSION

Sir Martin Roth: The first point that puzzles me, and perhaps I have not picked up the argument very clearly, is that on the one hand, the suggestion is made that sociocultural and educational factors may influence the diagnosis of dementia, and to this extent we may be labeling individuals of lower social class as demented on the basis of factors that have nothing to do with the phenomenon of dementia in a strict sense. However, conflicting with this particular claim was the observation that when psychiatrists were confronted with individuals of low social class status, they compensated for patients' failure in the MSQ and other tests, and were disinclined to diagnose them as suffering from dementia. In consequence, this contradicts the earlier point by suggesting that it is the members of the upper classes who are liable to be penalized for failure. I am bound to agree with George Bernard Shaw, "When it comes to the sufferings of the rich, I cannot bear to remain silent."

In relation to the findings about dementia and pathological change, I am uncertain about the study to which reference was made, and of course one is always very, very glad to be refuted by some other study, because if you have five or six refutations per year in psychiatry we will be making progress very fast. Let me say, before I proceed to the other point, that I believe that there may be some contribution by educational and social class factors. But I am not satisfied that Dr. Gurland has shown us anything concrete here.

To come to the other groups of findings in relation to dementia, I am unfamiliar with the studies being quoted. Of course it would be absurd to claim that all the correlates of dementia have been defined in pathological terms. But let me briefly recapitulate what the New Castle study did show. They showed in relation to one measure alone, a correlation not of 0.72, but of 0.77 between the recorded dementia score during life and plaque counts postmortem. This explains, in terms of one cerebral measure, over 60% of the variance in respect to psychological performance. This is a surprising figure, and it relates to measurement of psychological performance that was taken up to the preterminal stage of each individual's death by repeated testing. Now, if one claims that there is a significant association between pathological change on the one hand and personality measures on the other, one would wish for a study at least as complete as that undertaken in New Castle.

Can I just add a point that comes from clinico-pathological observations of pre-senile and senile demented subjects? To receive a brain in which the dementia remains a mystery when one has examined microscopic sections and the dementia has been properly documented and measured during life is exceedingly rare. One must be prepared to modify conclusions in the light of new data that are comprehensive both in relation to the psychometric measures and to the pathological findings. It is not good enough to be given impressions based on populations that are unspecified and measures that are incompletely described.

Finally, may I say that I don't know where Dr. Gurland obtained the idea that we had a homogeneous social class group in our sample. There is no basis for that view. And, if he wants to learn about the particular findings in relation to social class and dementia in our community studies (Dr. Bergmann may also be able to comment on this), there was no difference whatsoever in the prevalence of dementia as diagnosed by us in the community in the different classes. However, you are more likely to be admitted to the hospital if you are of lower social class, or if you are single and have relatives far away rather than near at hand.

I am sure there is something positive in social class and education because they appear to be associated with the maintenance of a good social facade and the preservation of personal habits that enable the old person with dementia to survive in the community for a longer period.

Socioeconomic factors may conceivably protect the individual with dementia in other ways. But such a view is unsupported by epidemiological and clinical data at the present time.

Dr. Bergmann: I agree with what Professor Sir Martin Roth has said. Perhaps one additional fact that might be worth considering is that the memory and information tests nearest to the MSQ test employed by Dr. Gurland did not correlate as highly with pathological findings as did the behavioral ratings, which does suggest that memory and information tests have a cultural component affecting variance of test scores.

Also, in our longitudinal studies, we found a group with low intelligence, low performance on memory and educational tests, and with an apparently low level of social function: They were diagnosed as having early dementia, but on follow-up, they did no worse than the normals. In fact, some had improved considerably. These were people who were simply misjudged because of their low social and cultural level, and I am sure that many of the so-called cures for dementia have been demonstrated on this group.

I would like to emphasize that the Folsom studies do not demonstrate a cure for dementia, but rather an improvement of function that Kahn from Holland and others very clearly indicated ceases with the discontinuation of the therapeutic procedure.

It is not valid to argue from these studies that dementia is amenable to treatment by behavioral and social methods—however valuable they may be in promoting better management.

Dr. Arie: I would just like to make two very brief points. First, of course, as Klaus Bergmann has said, everything turns on the difference between cross-sectional studies and follow-up studies, longitudinal studies.

And, the material that Dr. Gurland has presented is not, I think, homogeneous in that respect. People who function at borderline levels on a lifelong basis may well show a quite different progression between re-tests.

Secondly, the point that is being made about differential institutionalization levels is an interesting and probably a bi-model one, in that people of high social class are not necessarily less likely to be admitted to institutions. They may equally be more likely to be admitted to institutions through the capacity, financially, to cope with the costs, and through diminished tolerance of the burdens they pose in families with high standards.

The point is that they are admitted to different institutions, and they are informally institutionalized in various ways. Therefore the source of the cases is important. But at the same time it seems inconceivable, as Sir Martin and Klaus have said, that there is not something in this relationship between education and dementia. For if education means anything, it is the training in life skills and coping capacities, and this must in some way protect against the ravages of brain failure.

So, I think we have to be very grateful indeed to Barry Gurland for opening up this topic for us.

Dr. Clayton: I would like to make a similar comment. Even though a test score on the MSQ correlates with dementia, you are still not using specific diagnostic categories so that you might possibly have in your group some subjects with idiopathic dementias, and some with multi-infarct dementias, etc. If you are going to plan treatments or measure outcome, it is important to take these dimensions into consideration.

Sir Martin Roth: I am glad Klaus Bergmann mentioned this special group of women, the minority who were mistakenly diagnosed as suffering from dementia, but were subsequently identified as an underprivileged social group. To the extent that individuals who had been misdiagnosed in this manner might have been included in our clinical groups, the correlations between measures of dementia and pathological change would have been decreased. The real correlations would therefore be substantially greater than those estimated.

Dr. Lawton: It seems to me that the raw materials must be available from the substantial number of cases that Sir Martin (3), Corsellis (1), and Simon and Malamud (2) have studied in postmortem histological examinations, to tell us whether in fact these histological findings do correlate with some of the social background factors that we are studying.

Sir Martin Roth: Well, the answer is that the social background factors do not correlate strongly. There will have been an excess of lower socioeconomic classes in our own material because of bias in admission, so that we did not have a representative sample for study. But prevalence did not vary with social class in the community sample and histological appearances were unrelated to social factors in hospital cases.

Dr. Brody: I believe that epidemiologically this is almost a non-question. You really have to be someone special, such as someone wealthy or someone with a rare illness, to get your brain in the hands of a neuropathologist. And, so to determine socioeconomic class without having your study designed in advance to include all classes, and to get antemortem consent and cooperation at all levels to have the brain arrive at a neuropathologist are noble goals that may not be achieved.

Dr. Arie: Except in Britain, where neuropathology, like other things, is free when it is available.

Dr. Brody: I want to refer again to Dr. Gurland's association of sociocultural factors with senile dementia. First, we must accept that dementia associated with Alzheimer's-like neuropathology changes is a disease for which specific causes exist and hopefully will be found.

Sociocultural factors are very broad and because of the nature of the testing it is easy to think that the test itself is discriminating socioculturally. Certainly responses could be socially and educationally conditioned.

However, in search of causation, the apparent sociocultural association may be a clue. I am reminded of the history of pellagra, a mental disease with skin lesions that occurred primarily among children and women during a certain season, in a proscribed geographic area, and was assumed to be infectious. It turned out that sociocultural associations were the precipitating causes of the disease and, hence, of great epidemiologic importance.

The cause of pellagra, as we now know, is a niacin deficiency. The reason it occurred in women and children was that the economics, the sociocultural factors, were such that the best food had to be given to the strongest man who could earn money. If there was a little milk or meat, he got it and the rest of the family ate molasses and cornmeal, developed niacin deficiencies, and got pellagra.

The sociocultural suggestion is one of the very fragile clues we have as to causation of senile dementia, and I think it is worth following. I would think that at present, special effort should be made to identify and study populations at high risk of becoming demented. These might include native Guamanians, normal people over age 75, members of Huntington's disease families, prize fighters, perhaps people starting to have small strokes, and those exposed to potentially noxious chemicals and toxins such as lead or alcohol.

Dr. Weinberg: As a clinician who has come here to learn about clinical work, I felt rather encouraged as there was greater and greater disagreement among you as to how to arrive at a diagnostic classification. I believe we must not forget that, whether or not the individual is organically affected, it is the behavior of the individual that is of primary concern to us. I am impressed with the inventiveness of the human in being able to modalize pain, and to present us with confusion—which we add to sometimes by our own "systematic" methods of approach. Our patients are individuals with individual human experiences, and manifest two basically different types of personality structure—the core personality, which one incorporates from early infancy and early childhood, and the manifest personality, which one acquires through enculturation and adaptation to the environment. Many older individuals return to the core personality when dementing illness comes to the surface.

I would like to bring to your attention that earlier, when socioeconomic factors were being considered, there was quite a difference in approach between the British presentation and the American. In the United States, it's not just a question of socioeconomic factors, but also of different ethnic cultural groups. In Britain, you can talk in terms of socioeconomic levels, but here we must also take into consideration the fact that various generations have come from all parts of the world with differing ethnic derivatives, languages, and value systems. They differ far more widely in our country, in New York, say, than they do in a homogeneous society such as New Castle. We must attend to these variables, and to the fact that so many of our elderly have come from foreign lands and have had to integrate themselves into our society in a different fashion. These individuals may again return to previous modalities of adaptation once illness supervenes.

I should like to address a question to Dr. Brody at this point: Just how many studies have actually been made on the normal population? We here have been talking of people who have become ill, but what is it that we know of the normal process of aging?

Dr. Brody: There have been pitifully few studies on normality. Of course, Sir Martin's study in New Castle is one; Gruenburg's study in Syracuse is another. There is one that was alluded to this morning that will perhaps be the first endeavor in the United States in 20 years. A series of studies are being developed by the National Institute of Mental Health that are referred to as Epidemiology Catchment Area (ECA) Studies. They will be population studies in areas that include 200,000 to 400,000 people who are served by identifiable mental health facilities.

Yale University is conducting the first ECA with NIMH, and in collaboration with NIA and NINCDS, we are conducting an oversampling of the aged. The survey includes a sample of the general population and will also include those institutionalized persons who live within that catchment area. Field instruments are developed and will be upgraded as experience accumulates. Within the limits of survey techniques, we should know a lot more about mental illness and particularly dementia as it manifests itself in the elderly.

Dr. Gurland: In response to these remarks, I would like to state that there is no question that there is a relationship between MSQ scores and sociocultural characteristics. That has been shown by a number of epidemiological studies, including our own. These samples of elderly persons studied were randomly drawn and representative of both community and institutional populations. The relationship exists. I think the argument is about what it means.

I pointed out in my talk that diagnosis did not show as strong a sociocultural association as did MSQ scores. I tried to examime some reasons why this may be so. At this stage, there is nothing to indicate that the criterion validity of diagnosis is superior to that of MSQ scores in terms of independent indicators of dementia such as laboratory findings or outcome over time. These issues remain to be resolved. That being the case, I think it is an open matter whether a sociocultural association with dementia does or does not exist. I have chosen to come down in favor of it possibly existing. I don't think the argument has been definitively resolved at this stage. I have attempted to show that at least there is a body of research and treatment information that does draw implicitly on the possibility of a sociocultural relationship, and that there are some data that may support that possibility.

A question was raised suggesting that selective bias might be causing a spurious relationship between sociocultural indices and rates of dementia. I think the most straightforward answer is that such a relationship has been found in both institutional and community populations, and that, therefore, we have a universe if one puts those populations together. Thus the findings could not be a product of simple selective bias. The more complex aspects of this issue are discussed in my paper.

At present we have a longitudinal study built into our community survey, and I think that the outcome data will speak to whether we should have more confidence in the validity of the MSQ scores, or of the diagnoses. In the meantime, I would like to feel that the debate on the relationship between sociocultural indices and dementia is still open.

REFERENCES

1. Corsellis, J. A. N. (1962): *Mental illness and the Ageing Brain.* Oxford University Press, London.
2. Simon, A., and Malamud, N. (1968): Comparison of clinical and neuropathological findings in geriatric mental illness. In: *Psychiatric Disorders in the Aged.* Geigy Pharmaceutical Co., Manchester, England.
3. Tomlinson, B. E., Blessed, G., and Roth, M. (1970): Observations on the brains of demented old people. *J. Neurol. Sci.,* 11:205.

Clinical Aspects of Alzheimer's Disease and Senile Dementia, (Aging, Vol. 15), edited by Nancy E. Miller and Gene D. Cohen. Raven Press, New York 1981.

Neuropsychiatric Procedures for the Assessment of Alzheimer's Disease, Senile Dementia, and Related Disorders

H. S. Wang

Department of Psychiatry, Duke University Medical Center, Durham, North Carolina 27710

It is universally acknowledged that dementia is prevalent among the aged. Using the median figures derived from 17 reports in the literature (34), it is estimated that out of every 100 elderly (persons 65 years old or over) about 5 suffer from severe dementia and another 10 from mild dementia. The prevalence of dementia is expected to increase continuously as the result of further prolongation of the life span in the general population, which will eventually lead to a significant increase in the elderly group, especially those in the "very old" category (over 75 years old). It is projected that from 1970 to 2000 the increase in the over-74-year-old group will be 62%—twice as much as the increase in the 65-to-74-year-old group (31%).

Atrophy of the brain with unknown etiology—most likely due to Alzheimer's disease and senile dementia—accounts for the majority of dementias in late life. Based on three studies, Wells (38) calculated that about 51% of the cases with dementia could be attributed to Alzheimer's disease and senile dementia. This figure is consistent with findings of Tomlinson's pathological study of the brains of 50 demented patients (28). His study revealed that the morphological changes can be classified as senile dementia (Alzheimer's disease in old age) in 50%, arteriosclerotic (ischemic) dementia in 20%, and mixed senile and arteriosclerotic dementia in 18%. In other words, 68% of the brains in his 50 demented patients showed significant morphological changes of the Alzheimer's type.

Alzheimer's disease and senile dementia were considered to be different disorders largely because of the difference in their onset and natural course. Alzheimer's disease, as a rule, has an earlier onset and more rapidly deteriorating course than does senile dementia. From a morphological point of view, however, there are no significant quantitative or qualitative differences in these diseases. In both cases, the brain changes are characterized by cortical atrophy, widened cortical sulci, enlarged ventricles, and the presence of three characteristic histopathological changes: senile plaques, neurofibrillary tangles, and granulovacuolar degeneration of neurons (1). A recent workshop conference (12) recommended that "although the clinical and pathological manifestations of these disorders (Alzheimer's disease and senile dementia) are almost identical in the presenium and senium, different but as yet unknown etiological factors might be operative in, for example, a 50-year-old as compared to an 80-year-old. In order not to prejudge the etiological identity of the disease at different ages, the commission recommends that this disorder be termed Alzheimer's disease in the presenium and senile dementia of the Alzheimer's type in the senium." This recommendation, together with suggestions concerning diagnostic criteria, were forwarded to the American Psychiatric Association, which was working on the revised edition of the *Diagnostic Manual* (DSM-III).

In the recently published third edition of the *Diagnostic and Statistical Manual of Mental Disorders,* or DSM-III (1), the terms Alzheimer's disease and senile dementia are abandoned. These two disorders are classified under one category called "primary degenerative dementia," which is further subclassified as "primary degenerative dementia, senile onset" and "primary degenerative dementia, presenile onset" (including Alzheimer's and Pick's disease). The age of 65 is used as the criterion to separate these two subtypes.

The DSM-III clearly defines the diagnostic criteria for dementia, which include:

A. A loss of intellectual abilities of sufficient severity to interfere with social or occupational functioning
B. Memory impairment
C. At least one of the following:
   1. Impairment of abstract thinking, as manifested by concrete interpretation of proverbs, inability to find similarities and differences between related words, difficulty in defining words and concepts, and other similar tasks
   2. Impaired judgment
   3. Other disturbances of higher cortical function, e.g., aphasia (disorder of language due to brain dysfunction), apraxia (inability to carry out motor activities despite intact comprehension and motor function), agnosia (failure to recognize or identify object despite intact sensory function), "constructional difficulty" (e.g., inability to copy three-dimensional figures, assemble blocks, or arrange sticks in specific designs)
   4. Personality changes, i.e., alteration or accentuation of premorbid traits
D. State of consciousness not clouded (i.e., does not meet the criteria for delirium or intoxication, although these may be superimposed)
E. Either 1 or 2:
   1. Evidence from the history, physical examination, or laboratory tests of a specific organic factor that is judged to be etiologically related to the disturbance
   2. In the absence of such evidence, an organic factor necessary for the development of the syndrome can be presumed if conditions other

than organic mental disorders have been reasonably excluded and if the behavioral change represents cognitive impairment in a variety of areas

According to the DSM-III, the diagnosis of primary degenerative dementia, either presenile or senile, is made if the disorder demonstrates the core clinical feature of a dementia based on criteria described above and if it has an insidious onset with uniformly progressive deteriorating course—and all other specific causes of dementia have been excluded by history, physical examination, and laboratory tests.

The revision of the *Diagnostic Manual* (DSM-III) by the American Psychiatric Association clearly has considerably improved the defining of various mental disorders with more specific criteria, although there are still many controversies. This will definitely help enhance the consistency and reliability of the diagnosis of Alzheimer's disease and senile dementia (hereafter, both will be referred to as Alzheimer dementia). An accurate and reliable diagnosis, however, is not sufficient in the comprehensive planning of the treatment and management of patients with Alzheimer dementia, which from the clinical point of view is a complicated disorder influenced by various physical, psychological, and social factors (32,33).

Alzheimer dementia is caused by a degenerative process primarily involving the brain and is characterized by various microscopic as well as gross structural changes. Since these changes are not reversible, the prognosis of Alzheimer dementia is usually regarded as very poor. Consequently, patients with such a disorder are frequently neglected and given essentially custodial care in institutions.

A careful review of the literature and the findings from several recent studies indicate that dementias or related disorders are clearly associated with an excess mortality and a significantly shortened life span compared with the general population (35). The prognosis of dementia is better than it is commonly conceived to be if the patient's age as well as other factors that can be prevented or treated (e.g., pneumonia) are taken into consideration. In a longitudinal study of the relationship between brain disorder and longevity (35), slowed electroencephalographic (EEG) rhythm, diminished psychometric scores, and abnormal neurological findings correlated statistically with diminished longevity in a group of community elderly, but these three brain disorder indicators together account for less than 25% of the total variance affecting the longevity in the study. This finding is consistent with that of the NIH study (6), which found no correlation between longevity and several specific measurements of central nervous system (CNS) function, including cerebral blood flow, cerebral metabolic rate, and EEG. Libow (15) suggested that the excess mortality associated with dementia may be due to the following factors: pneumonia; benign neglect by physicians and nurses; nontreatment because of family wishes; incorrect and tardy diagnoses related to inability to obtain clear histories, physical examinations, and appropriate laboratory studies; organic brain dysfunction and death via yet undiscovered mechanisms; medication-related death; inanition; a systemic disease yet to be discovered that affects the brain and other vital organs; patient self-realization of serious illness and decline leading to death via this self-realization (i.e., "voodoo death").

According to the DSM-III, Alzheimer dementia can be viewed, for practical purposes, as consisting of three components: (a) memory and cognitive impairment—the core feature of dementia; (b) functional and structural impairment of the brain; and (c) behavioral manifestations that affect the patient's ability for self-care, interpersonal relationships, and adjustment in the community. These three components are grossly related but do not closely parallel each other. In some cases memory and cognitive impairment is rather severe although there is minimal or no evidence of brain impairment. In other cases the reverse may happen—there is little memory and cognitive impairment in the presence of significant brain impairment. Using clinical or psychometric measures as the only procedures in evaluating these demented patients frequently leads to false-positive diagnoses (the former cases) or false-negative diagnoses (the latter cases). As pointed out by Kahn and Miller (11), the false-positive diagnoses, which may be contributed by the common stereotype of the inevitability of senility in the elderly combined with poor physical health, poor cultural background, and depressed affect, can easily lead to acceptance of a spurious organic diagnosis and to overlooking possibilities for effective treatment. False-negative diagnoses, on the other hand, would be a clinical problem most often in patients with acute brain disorders where recognition of the physiological dysfunction may be critical to appropriate medical management.

It is well known that many physical diseases common in the aged can affect the brain (7). Superimposed brain disorders are not uncommon in Alzheimer dementia. The memory and cognitive functions are dependent on the status of the brain as well as many other psychological or emotional factors. The clinical manifestations, although determined to some extent by the degree of memory and cognitive dificits, are attributable to the pre-existing personality of the patient, socioeconomic factors, and the supporting system in the patient's environment.

From a clinical point of view, Alzheimer dementia, like other dementias, can be viewed as a bio-psycho-social disorder (32,33). To provide appropriate and effective treatment and care for patients suffering from such a dementia, a careful and thorough assessment of each of the three aspects of dementia—biological, psychological and social—is indispensible.

The measures and procedures currently available for the evaluation of various aspects of Alzheimer dementia, although numerous, can be grouped into four categories: history taking, psychiatric examination, neurological examination, and laboratory examination. There is considerable overlap among these four categories.

The present chapter does not intend to review all available evaluative measures and procedures; these are already described and discussed in detail in many standard textbooks on psychiatry and neurology and in several publications specifically concerning dementia (4,5,10,14,16–18,20–22,25–29,38). This chapter discusses several important areas, issues, and procedures related to a reliable and accurate assessment of the various aspects of Alzheimer dementia.

ASSESSMENT OF MEMORY AND COGNITIVE FUNCTION

Alzheimer dementia is primarily a disorder of the higher cortex. For this reason, innumerable clinical tests, procedures, and scales have been developed to assess the complex function of the higher cortex. Well organized clinical evaluative approaches were presented by Strub and Black (27) and Pearce and Miller (21), for example.

Regardless of the test, procedure, or scale used, the emphasis in the evaluation of the higher cortical function, either by psychiatrists or neurologists, is on the function of memory (immediate and delayed recall), abstract thinking (e.g., similarity, proverb), orientation (place, time, person, and situation), and judgment (decision-making). These are considered the core clinical features of dementia. In addition, calculation, comprehension, attention, language ability, and general information are also tested because they tend to become defective in Alzheimer dementia. One questionnaire designed originally by Weinstein and Kahn (37) has become a simple and practical clinical tool widely used by clinicians as a screening test for dementia. This questionnaire consists of 10 simple questions:

1. Where are you now?
2. What is the address of this place?
3. What is the date today (day of the month)?
4. What is the date (month)?
5. What is the date (year)?
6. How old are you?
7. When were you born (month)?
8. When were you born (year)?
9. Who is the president of the United States?
10. Who was the president before him?

The first five questions concern orientation; the latter five concern general information. This questionnaire is easy to administer clinically and provides a rough estimation of the patient's orientation and memory. It is more applicable to patients with relatively severe dementia and has the shortcoming of being poorly standarized. A similar version of this questionnaire with some modification was developed by Pfeiffer (23) for use with less demented elderly.

One should recognize that the many clinical tests used by psychiatrists and neurologists are not much different from the many psychological tests designed for the evaluation of higher cortical functions. Both evaluate the *behavioral* manifestations of brain function and are subject to influence by many socioeconomic, cultural, educational, and emotional factors. As a rule, the clinical approaches are simpler, less standardized, less structured, and therefore less reliable than the psychological testing. Accurate and reliable assessments of memory and cognitive impairments, especially those done over a period of time and those requiring repeated measurements, clearly require the several better standardized and more structured psychological tests.

In addition, two conditions require special attention in the assessment of memory and cognitive impairments whether the clinical or the psychometric approach is employed. These are depression and aphasia.

Depression

Depression is an affective disorder of varying severity that is quite common among the aged with or without Alzheimer dementia. In a portion of affectively impaired patients (approximately 10 to 15%), depression is associated with considerable deficits in memory, attention, and other cognitive functions indistinguishable from those observed in Alzheimer dementia alone. This "dementia" resulting from noncerebral disorder is often referred to as pseudodementia because it tends to show improvement when the depression is relieved. The differentiation between pseudodementia and true (organic) dementia has been discussed (39,40). As a rule, the memory and cognitive impairments in pseudodementia are most likely inconsistent, scattered, and limited to a few faculties with a rather fluctuating course. A therapeutic trial with antidepressants may be necessary in some cases to evaluate quantitatively and qualitatively the significance of the memory and cognitive impairment observed.

Aphasia

Speech ability is impaired when the speech center of the brain is affected by lesions of various types. The posterior language area, commonly referred to as Wernicke's area, primarily concerns the comprehension of spoken language. The anterior speech area (Broca's area) primarily concerns the function of language production. When either of these two speech areas is adversely affected, the patient has difficulty comprehending or speaking and therefore appears more confused, disoriented, and demented than what is expected from the severity of brain impairment. The confusion, disorientation, and inappropriate response to questions are usually worse under stress and questioning. Frequently, when all stress is removed and the patient is allowed to speak spontaneously, the speech may become more coherent, relevant, and logical; the patient may present him/herself as being in rather good contact with reality and as having a relatively good memory for remote and recent events.

ASSESSMENT OF BRAIN IMPAIRMENTS

The magnitude of memory and cognitive deficits as demonstrated by various neuropsychiatric examinations and psychological testing is only grossly correlated with that of brain impairment (30). In order to obtain a holistic picture of patients with Alzheimer dementia—an important element needed in the planning of appropriate and effective treatment and management of these patients—objective and accurate information regarding the functional and structural status of the brain in these patients is clearly essential.

The purpose of assessment of the brain status is to determine: (a) the presence or absence of brain impairment; and if brain impairment is present: (b) the extent of brain impairment, i.e., diffuse or focal; (c) the severity of impairment: the degree of histopathological changes and cortical atrophy; (d) the characteristics of impairment—degenerative or infarction; and (e) the causative and contributory factors to the brain impairment.

In routine psychiatric and neurological practice, the clinical neurological examination is the procedure most commonly employed in the evaluation of the CNS. Such an examination is, however, of only limited usefulness in Alzheimer dementia. This is due to the fact that Alzheimer dementia is a degenerative disorder of unknown etiology affecting the entire cortical tissue diffusely and presenting no pathognomonic neurological signs. The neurological examination nevertheless can elicit certain signs which are commonly associated with any brain impairment, whether due to degeneration, infarction, trauma, or mass lesion. These neurological signs include the presence of pathological, or the reappearance of certain primitive, reflex responses, and the presence of deficits in sensory or motor functions depending on where the brain tissue is most affected. The method of eliciting and interpreting the various abnormal reflex responses in dementia is described and discussed in detail by Paulson (20). The abnormal reflex responses include grasp reflex, tonic foot response, oral response (snout reflex), nuchocephalic reflex, palmomental reflex, corneomandibular reflex, and glabella tap reflex. Several of these reflexes (e.g., grasp reflex, tonic foot response, oral response) are considered characteristic of frontal lobe dysfunction, often referred to as frontal lobe syndrome, whereas others are more likely related to the diffuse brain dysfunction or subcortical lesion (e.g., glabella tap reflex).

Another group of neurological signs frequently seen in Alzheimer dementia as well as in other dementing disorders consists of apraxia, agnosia, and aphasia, to name a few important ones (21,27). Apraxia is a disorder characterized by an inability to correctly carry out single or successive purposeful movements in the absence of peripheral defects, e.g., weakness, sensory loss, and ataxia. There are two types of apraxia: motor and ideational. With motor apraxia the patient uses the wrong muscles and carries out inappropriate movements, although he may perform the requisite action in a reflex involuntary fashion.

Ideational apraxia is characterized by an impaired ability to carry out composite actions required for completing a complex sequence of movements (21).

Agnosia is a disorder of perception which may affect the tactile sensation, visual perception, and left-right orientation. With this disorder, the patient may neglect details when he is asked to draw simple pictures or describe what he sees in his immediate environment; fail to recognize, name, and point to individual fingers on one's self and on others; or fail to distinguish right from left on self and in the environment. A common test used by many neurologists and psychiatrists is the face–hand test developed by Bender (3). This test includes two series of 10 trials each, one with eyes closed and one with eyes open. Each series includes eight asymmetrical combinations of face and hand, four contralateral and four ipsilateral, and two trials of symmetrical stimuli, face–face and hand–hand. The detail of the testing procedure was described by Kahn and Miller (11).

Aphasia is a disorder of speech involving either its comprehension or its production. This disorder, as well as apraxia and agnosia, is most likely present with dysfunction of the parieto-occipital cortex of the dominant hemisphere. It can also be present in association with any diffuse cortical impairment of significant severity. For this reason, the presence of these neurological signs, like the presence of various abnormal reflex responses described above, provides little objective and useful information when assessing the severity of brain impairment in Alzheimer dementia.

The objective and accurate information regarding the functional and structural status of the brain in Alzheimer dementia is obtained primarily from the many laboratory procedures currently available and a few that are still under development (16,21,22,31,36). On the other hand, the importance of a thorough neurological examination and medical history cannot be minimized, as they can help rule out the presence of other disorders of the brain. The history is particularly helpful in the differentiation between Alzheimer dementia and multi-infarct dementia (8).

The following are some of the important laboratory procedures commonly used or being developed because of their great promise of providing an objective and accurate assessment of brain impairments (31,36).

Plain Skull X-Rays

The plain skull x-ray is readily available and is completely noninvasive and well tolerated by all elderly patients. It is of no significant usefulness for assessing the brain impairments in Alzheimer dementia, however, because it is usually normal or negative in this disorder. Nonetheless, this procedure is useful for ruling out skull fractures and detecting evidence of increased intracranial pressure and intracranial space-occupying mass.

Pneumoencephalography

Until recently, pneumoencephalography (PEG) was the procedure of choice to establish the diagnosis of Alzheimer dementia and to assess the severity of brain impairment. In this procedure, air, which has a much lower radiation absorption coefficient than brain tissue, is introduced into the space within and surrounding the brain through lumbar puncture. With the presence of air, the contour of the cortex and ventricle becomes much more clearly identifiable. A marked generalized ventricular dilatation and diffuse cortical atrophy which can be inferred from the atrophy of cerebral gyri and the widening of cerebral sulci are the characteristic findings of Alzheimer dementia. The magnitude of cortical atrophy and ventricular dilatation, in general, corresponds well with the severity of dementia. The interpretation of PEG is not always easy owing to the fact that there are considerable variations in normal ventricular size. This procedure also involves considerable discomfort and the risk in some patients that marked mental deterioration may develop after such a procedure. Since the recent development of computerized tomography (CT) scans, PEG is usually reserved for special cases when a more precise view of the cortex and ventricle is necessary.

Cerebral Angiography

In cerebral angiography a series of radiographic pictures are taken after a radiopaque contrast medium is injected by various routes into the cerebral vascular system. The position and arrangement of the deep veins may provide an estimation of the ventricular size but little help in the assessment of brain impairments. The main purpose of cerebral angiography is to evaluate the cerebrovascular system and to detect mass lesions, e.g., subdural hematoma and other intracranial tumors.

Radioisotope Brain Scan

The radioisotope scan is used to determine the distribution of radioisotope (technetium-99m pertechnetate or chlormerodrin labeled with ^{203}Hg or ^{197}Hg) in the brain after its is injected intravenously. The increased amount of radioisotope in a given area of the brain is believed to result from a change in the blood-brain barrier or from an increase in vascularity in the brain (e.g., brain tumor, infarction, arteriovenous malformation, brain abscess, subdural hematoma).

Radioisotope Cisternography

A radioisotope (e.g., ^{131}I-labeled human serum albumin), after being injected into the lumbar subarachnoid space, usually follows the circulatory pattern of the cerebral spinal fluid (CSF). This procedure, using sequential x-rays, is useful for evaluating the CSF dynamics and therefore the diagnosis of normal pressure hydrocephalus, which is characterized by the presence of ventricular stasis (i.e., an accumulation of the radioisotope in the ventricular system and its persistence there for 24 to 48 hr or more). The cisternography is usually normal in Alzheimer dementia.

Electroencephalography

EEG is the second most widely used procedure for evaluating the brain status of patients with Alzheimer dementia because of its noninvasiveness and ready availability. In Alzheimer dementia the characteristic change in EEG is neither specific nor pathognomonic. The EEG abnormalities, when present, usually consist of a slowing of the alpha rhythm and the presence of slow waves in the theta (4 to 7 Hz) and delta (1 to 4 Hz) ranges. These abnormalities, as a rule, are more severe in Alzheimer dementia of early onset than in that of late onset. Not infrequently the EEG changes are so minute they cannot be differentiated from those frequently observed in many elderly persons without Alzheimer dementia. Abnormalities in EEG correspond only grossly to memory and cognitive deficits. The presence of abnormalities is more reliable an indicator of the brain status than the absence of abnormalities, which is not uncommon among patients with Alzheimer dementia especially that of late onset. EEG abnormalities, however, can be caused by many drugs and metabolic disorders. Serial EEG examinations over a period of time often are more informative and reliable because they may detect the subtle but consistent gradual increase in rhythm-slowing commonly associated with Alzheimer dementia or the false-positive diagnoses due to drug or other factors not related to Alzheimer dementia which tend to fluctuate from time to time.

Echoencephalography

Echoencephalography is a relatively new diagnostic procedure utilizing ultrasonic waves for evaluating the internal structures of the brain. The procedure is completely atraumatic and noninvasive and was one of the promising procedures under development until the availability of CT scan. One of its greatest shortcomings is the difficulty of obtaining the correct echoes from different structures in the brain.

Cerebral Blood Flow Measurement

The human brain derives its energy almost entirely from the aerobic oxidation of glucose. Since the brain has little store of oxygen, it depends on an uninterrupted and sufficient blood flow to supply the oxygen needed. Under normal conditions, the cerebral blood flow (CBF) is directly under the control of the metabolic need of the brain, a phenomenon often referred to as autoregulation.

The amount of blood flowing through the brain therefore reflects the metabolic activity of the brain, which is known to decline significantly in Alzheimer dementia and other disorders of the brain.

Among the many methods that are currently available for measurement of CBF, the three most widely used are the nitrous oxide inhalation method, the carotid injection, and the inhalation method, the latter two using an isotope. The advantages of the inhalation method using ^{133}Xe are its complete noninvasiveness, its ability to provide a simultaneous evaluation of both cerebral hemispheres, and safety for repeat uses as compared to the nitrous oxide and carotid injection methods. The xenon inhalation method does have problems, however. The clearance curve obtained from a given region of the brain, after inhaling the radioactive xenon for a short period, contains a slow component attributable to the extracerebral tissue and considerable distortion resulting from the recirculation of the radioisotope that is unloaded from the entire body during the washout period. The sensitivity and reliability of this inhalation method, especially for detecting minor regional changes or differences, therefore need further evaluation.

A reduction of CBF may result from a depression of the cerebral metabolic activity as described above, cerebral vascular insufficiency most likely due to arteriosclerosis, or a combination of these two. The differentiation between these two conditions may not be easy. Cerebral vascular disease is suggested when (a) the blood flow is significantly reduced in one or few regions of the brain; (b) there is a marked reduction in CBF without clear evidence of cognitive impairment or marked EEG abnormality; or (c) there is an impairment of vascular reactivity to change of the carbon dioxide concentration in the arterial blood. In these cases the CBF is found to be reduced significantly, and the reduction generally parallels the severity of the brain change or cognitive impairments.

Brain Biopsy

To study the histopathological changes directly under a light or an electron microscope in the brain tissue is obviously the most accurate and reliable means available for establishing the diagnosis of Alzheimer dementia. However, in addition to the obvious practical difficulties and risk, such an approach is not always as informative as expected. False-negative diagnosis is not uncommon owing to the fact that only a small piece of brain tissue, most likely taken from the so-called silent area of the brain, is removed and used for such study. Furthermore, the usefulness of such a procedure is limited, as the histopathological changes characteristic of Alzheimer dementia observed at biopsy do not always reflect the severity of the brain impairment.

Computerized Tomography of the Brain

The CT scan, a new diagnostic procedure, has undergone much modification and improvement since its development by Hounsfield and initial application by Ambrose. It makes use of the most advanced progress in radiography and computer technology. The scanning system consists of an x-ray tube and two collimated sodium iodide scintillation detectors fixed on a common frame and in linear alignment with the x-ray tube across the patient's head. The common frame moves first linearly, thus making a linear scan of a "slice" of brain tissue. At the end of the linear scanning, the common frame is then rotated one degree and repeated as described above. During each linear scanning, x-ray transmissions through the head are recorded by the detectors and stored in a computer. The numerous readings from the input and both output detectors are then used to solve a great number of formulas simultaneously to yield the values of absorption coefficients for each small area (a cube) in every slice of brain tissue. Numerical values of absorption coefficient can either be printed out directly or displayed by a cathode ray oscilloscope as a gray-scale picture, which is in turn recorded permanently by a Polaroid camera.

CT scanning is harmless and can demonstrate the internal structures (normal and abnormal) of each slice of brain tissue. It is particularly useful for assessing the shape and size of ventricles and the contour of the cortex. For this reason it has become the most widely used and probably the most useful procedure for assessing brain status in patients with Alzheimer dementia and has consequently markedly reduced the need for cerebral angiography and PEG. Drawbacks of this useful procedure are the high cost of the equipment and sophisticated technology involved and the requirement of keeping the head still for 20 min or more to complete a routine CT scan, which may not be tolerable to some demented patients. The time to complete a CT scan has been greatly reduced as the result of the newly developed equipment.

Positron Emission Tomography

The potential of positron emitters for radionuclide imaging has long been recognized, but it has become possible, like CT scanning, only as the result of the many advances made in recent years in radiation detection and computer technology. The procedure, positron emission tomography (PET), still under development and often also referred to as emission computed tomography (ECT), is able to image the brain structures three-dimensionally (2,9).

The positron undergoes annihilation, resulting in the production of two photons of equal energy traversing in exactly opposite directions. The coincidence detection of short-lived positron-emitting radionuclides has the advantage of good attenuation correction so that true quantitative determination of radioactivity concentration is possible. The measurement, like CT scanning, consists of a series of rectilinear scans at multiple angles about a cross section of the brain. The data collected are a series of count-rate profiles, each point of which is proportional to the total activity along a line at that point perpendicular to the scan direction. The data are processed with a reconstruction algorithm, and the final result is the isotope distribution displayed as an image of the cross section. The greatest promising advantage is that isotopes and pharmaceuticals labeled with a positron-emitting radionuclide (e.g., ^{18}F-labeled 2-fluoro-2-deoxy-D-glucose) can be used and may provide a useful means of studying the normal cerebral physiology and metabolism of the brain *in vivo* as well as changes in a variety of disorders (e.g., stroke, epilepsy, schizophrenia, and dementia) which affect brain glucose utilization. In other words, PET has the power of displaying regional uptake of radioisotope or radiopharmaceuticals, whereas CT scanning is primarily a method of visualizing anatomy free of the shadows of overlying structures.

In summary, because of their noninvasiveness and safety and their relatively established reliability and validity, EEG, CBF measurement, and CT scan are probably the three most useful and practical procedures for the assessment of brain impairments in Alzheimer dementia. EEG and CBF provide information concerning primarily the functional status of the brain, and CT scans outline the structural status of the brain. One important factor when selecting an appropriate examination is the cost–benefit factor. The cost of CT scan is definitely much higher than either EEG or CBF measurement. It may be justified initially when an accurate assessment of the brain is needed for planning proper and effective treatment and for management of the patient with Alzheimer dementia. It may be too costly as a means of following the course of patients with this disorder. In contrast, EEG and CBF measurement may not provide as useful or precise information concerning the brain initially; they are more economical and practical as tools for following patients with Alzheimer dementia over a long period of time. For a more accurate assessment of the brain status, PEG may be indispensable. Several procedures (e.g., plain x-rays, angiography, cisternography, and isotope brain scans) are useful only in ruling out brain disorders other than Alzheimer dementia. Echoencephalography and PET need further development and evaluation before they can become a more useful and reliable procedure for the assessment of brain impairment.

ASSESSMENT OF BEHAVIORAL OR CLINICAL MANIFESTATIONS

A great number of elderly who have histopathological changes of the Alzheimer type and whose memory and cognitive impairments may or may not be detectable demonstrate little or no evidence of behavioral aberrations or evidence of dysfunctioning in their routine activities related to self-care or productive employment. These elderly do not meet the criteria of having a dementia, which is defined as a loss of intellectual abilities of sufficient severity to interfere with *social or occupational functioning*. In contrast, many other elderly with minimal histopathological changes of the Alzheimer type, or cortical atrophy, as well as little memory or cognitive impairments, may present a great variety of psychopathology and may be severely disabled in regard to self-care and social and occupational functioning. Multiple factors may contribute to the differences between these two groups. The important ones include the following.

Pre-existing Personality

How the elderly person copes with his life situation when he becomes aware of his mental decline is influenced by his pre-existing personality. Two important factors here are the ego defense mechanisms that are most familiar to him and his basic emotional needs. The role of pre-existing personality was first postulated by Rothschild (24). Later Kiev and his co-workers (13) found that patients who demonstrated a high order of adaptive versatility before their illness had less intellectual impairment in relation to loss of brain tissue than those who had for some time exhibited difficulties in overall adaptation with much anxiety. This is consistent with the observation of a positive association between compulsive traits and dementia (19).

Concurrent Brain Dysfunction

Various dysfunctions of the brain resulting from drugs, metabolic or hormonal disorders, nutritional deficiency, and cardiopulmonary and many other systemic diseases may be present in addition to the Alzheimer dementia. These dysfunctions, usually referred to as acute brain syndromes, tend to present a picture of confusion and delirium, often associated with visual or auditory hallucination and delusional ideation. These dysfunctions of brain are usually reversible and can be improved when the contributory or causative factors are removed.

Concurrent Emotional Disorders

Anxiety and depression are probably the most common concurrent emotional problems seen in patients with Alzheimer dementia. They may result from the awareness of the memory or cognitive deficits and the awkwardness and embarrassment experienced in the social setting. Anxiety is particularly acute and prominent when the patient is confronted with an unfamiliar or stressful situation (e.g., the catastrophic reaction under psychological testing). Depression may result from a lowering of self-esteem or social deprivation. Some patients with depression may demonstrate pseudodementia, as described above. The latter may further impair the memory and other cognitive functions of the patient.

Social and Environmental Factors

Patients with Alzheimer dementia of varying severity are less capable of coping with many life situations and solving conflicting issues than the normal individual. The amount of stresses and the support systems available to them in their environment play an important role in determining how well they can adjust and be managed in their immediate setting. Excessive stress and lack of support are usually the causes for many patients with Alzheimer dementia to be institutionalized.

CONCLUSION

A better treatment and management approach as well as better care facilities are urgently needed for taking care of the many elderly persons suffering from Alzheimer's disease or senile dementia (now called "primary degenerative dementia, presenile onset" or "senile onset," respectively, by the newly published DMS-III). To treat these patients appropriately and effectively, and to use the various care facilities properly, an accurate assessment of the three components of this disorder is essential. These three components include: (a) memory and cognitive impairment; (b) brain impairment; and (c) behavioral aberrations. The present chapter discusses only a few key issues and problems. It describes several basic principles and important practical measures and procedures for the formulation of an accurate assessment.

REFERENCES

1. American Psychiatric Association (1980): *Diagnostic and Statistical Manual of Mental Disorder,* 3rd ed. APA, Washington, D.C.
2. Atkins, H. L. (1976): *NY State J. Med.,* 79:1355–1359.
3. Benton, M. B. (1952): *Disorders in Perception,* Thomas, Springfield, Ill.
4. Botwinick, J. (1967): *Cognitive Processes in Maturity and Old Age.* Springer, New York.
5. Busse, E. W., and Blazer, D. (eds.) (1980): *Handbook of Geriatric Psychiatry.* Van Nostrand Reinhold, New York.
6. Gtanick, S., and Patterson, R. D. (eds.) (1971): *Human Aging II—An Eleven-Year Followup Biomedical and Behavioral Study.* DHEW Publ. No. (HSM) 71–9037. U.S. Government Printing Office, Washington, D.C.
7. Haase, G. R. (1977): In: *Dementia,* 2nd ed. edited by C. E. Wells, pp. 27–67. Davis, Philadelphia.
8. Hackinski, V. C., Iliff, L. D., Zilhka, E., DuBoulay, G. H., McAllister, V. L., Marshall, J., Russel, R. W. R., and Symon, L. (1975): *Arch. Neurol.,* 32:632–637.
9. Hoffman, E. J., and Phelps, M. E. (1979): *Med. Instrum.,* 13:147–151.
10. Jarvik, L., Eisdorfer, C., and Blum, J. E. (eds.) (1973): *Intellectual Functioning in Adults: Psychological and Biological Influences.* Springer, New York.
11. Kahn, R. L., and Miller, N. E. (1978): In: *The Clinical Psychology of Aging,* edited by M. Storandt, I. C. Siegler, and M. F. Elias. Plenum, New York.
12. Katzman, R., Terry, R. D., and Bick, K. L. (eds.) (1978): *Alzheimer's Disease: Senile Dementia and Related Disorders.* Raven Press, New York.
13. Kiev, A., Chapman, K. F., Guthrie, T. C., and Wolff, H. G. (1962): *Neurology,* 12:385–392.
14. Lezak, M. D. (1976): *Neuropsychological Assessment.* Oxford University Press, New York.
15. Libow, L. S. (1978): In: *Alzheimer's Disease; Senile Dementia and Related Disorders,* edited by R. Katzman, R. D. Terry, and K. L. Bick, pp. 315–319. Raven Press, New York.
16. Lowry, J., Bahr, A. L., Allen, J. H., Meachan, W. F., and James, A. E. (1977): In: *Dementia,* 2nd ed., edited by C. E. Wells, pp. 223–245. Davis, Philadelphia.
17. McFie, J. (1975): *Assessment of Organic Intellectual Impairment.* Academic Press, London.
18. Muller, Ch., and Ciompi, L. (eds.) (1968): *Senile Dementia—Clinical and Therapeutic Aspects.* Williams & Wilkins, Baltimore.
19. Oakley, D. P. (1965): *Br. J. Psychiatry,* 111:414–419.
20. Paulson, G. W. (1977): In: *Dementia,* 2nd ed. edited by C. E. Wells, pp. 169–188. Davis, Philadelphia.
21. Pearce, J., and Miller, E. (1973): *Clinical Aspects of Dementia.* Williams & Wilkins, Baltimore.
22. Peterson, H. O., and Kieffer, S. A. (1972): *Introduction to Neuroradiology.* Harper & Row, Hagerstown, Md.
23. Pfeiffer, E. (1975): *J. Am. Geriatr. Soc.,* 23:433–441.
24. Rothschild, D. (1941); *Am. J. Psychiatry,* 98:324–333.

25. Russell, E. W., Neuringer, C., and Goldstein, G. (1970): *Assessment of Brain Damage—A Neuropsychological Key Approach.* Wiley-Interscience, New York.
26. Smith, W. L., and Philippus, M. J. (eds.) (1969): *Neuropsychological Training in Organic Brain Dysfunction.* Thomas, Springfield, Ill.
27. Strub, R. L., and Black, F. W. (1977): *The Mental Status Examination in Neurology.* Davis, Philadelphia.
28. Tomlinson, B. E. (1977): In: *Aging and Dementia,* edited by W. L. Smith and M. Kinsbourne, pp. 25–56. Spectrum, New York.
29. Verwoerdt, A. (1976): *Clinical Geropsychiatry.* Williams & Wilkins, Baltimore.
30. Wang, H. S. (1973): In: *Intellectual Functioning in Adults: Psychological and Biological Influences,* edited by L. F. Jarvik, C. Eisdorfer, and J. E. Blum, pp. 95–106. Springer, New York.
31. Wang, H. S. (1973): In: *Mental Illness in Later Life,* edited by E. W. Busse and E. Pfeiffer, pp. 75–88, Amer. Psychiatric Assoc., Washington, D.C.
32. Wang, H. S. (1977): In: *Behavior and Adaptation in Late Life,* 2nd ed., edited by E. W. Busse and E. Pfeiffer, pp. 240–263. Little Brown, Boston.
33. Wang, H. S. (1977): In: *Dementia,* 2nd ed., edited by C. E. Wells, pp. 15–26. Davis, Philadelphia.
34. Wang, H. S. (1977): In: *Aging and Dementia,* edited by W. L. Smith and Kinsbourne, pp. 1–24. Spectrum, New York.
35. Wang, H. S. (1978): In: *Alzheimer's Disease: Senile Dementia and Related Disorders,* edited by R. Katzman, R. D. Terry, and K. L. Bick, pp. 309–313. Raven Press, New York.
36. Wang, H. S. (1980): In: *Handbook of Psychiatry,* edited by E. W. Busse and D. G. Blazer, pp. 285–304. Van Nostrand Reinhold, New York.
37. Weinstein, E. A., Kahn, R. L., Sugarman, L. A., and Linn, L. (1955): *Am. J. Psychiatry,* 109:889–894.
38. Wells, C. E. (1977): In: *Dementia,* 2nd ed., edited by C. E. Wells, pp. 247–276. Davis, Philadelphia.
39. Wells, C. E. (1979): *Am. J. Psychiatry,* 136:895–900.
40. Zung, W. W. K. (1980): In: *Handbook of Geriatric Psychiatry,* edited by E. W. Busse and D. G. Blazer. Van Nostrand Reinhold, New York.

DISCUSSION

Dr. Solomon: I recently had the experience of conducting some training workshops in rural southwestern Virginia, and I discovered all sorts of problems out there, such as how can you do a thorough history and physical when you are the only primary physician for 14,000 people?

How can you do any of the other aspects of the basic workup if your community hospital is not equipped with an EEG machine, if the nearest neurologist is 150 or 200 miles away, and the nearest psychiatrist is 150 or 200 miles away, et cetera?

What kind of recommendations would the respondents have in terms of that kind of health care delivery setting?

Dr. Arie: I would like to add a point that is perhaps of even wider significance. That is, even in countries that are very well provided with medical services, the numbers of the very old are so huge that it is inconceivable that every patient with a suspicion of dementia will be thoroughly investigated. I wonder if some of the speakers, could address themselves to this question. How far, and when, in the presence of what characteristic history and clinical picture is it necessary to investigate all patients further? I think that has great importance.

Dr. McLong: I am from Denver, Colorado, an internist who has gotten into geriatrics as my patients have grown older.

I would like to note that in our area we can seldom find a psychiatrist interested enough to see a patient over 65 years of age. I would say 90% of our senile patients are diagnosed and put in institutions by primary care physicians, either internists or family practice physicians. Most of these patients are not very carefully worked up. I think it would be extremely useful if we could emerge from this meeting with some minimal criteria that could be replicated in the physician's office simply because we do not have the numbers of geriatricians, of neuropsychiatrists, and of neurologists who are interested and skilled, at least in our part of the country, dealing with this problem.

Dr. Wisen: I am from Bloomington, Indiana, and am a practicing neurologist. I am not the neurologist 150 miles away: My practice has been always in a relatively small town. My comments pertain to both the medical and economic aspects of dementia. I'd like to make several points: First, Dreyfus published a paper in the *California Medical Journal* in 1974–1975 in which he reviewed 200 patients with a diagnosis of "arteriosclerotic cerebral vascular disease with organic brain syndrome." He could justify the diagnosis in only 4% of the sample. In 1975, in *JAMA* there was a paper describing four patients whose dementia was resolved with vascular surgery. I can second the comments made, that there has been an unfortunate blunting by entering in the differential diagnosis multiple infarctions as cause for dementia. It surely exists, but it is far less than we are accustomed to thinking. The problem is that it has created the image in the minds of many physicians that dementia is generally the result of small strokes. This state of affairs is also far more acceptable to the patient, and more palatable to the insurance companies, which often do not cover the diagnosis of organic brain syndrome or Alzheimer's dementia.

In addition, the focus on arteriosclerotic cerebral vascular disease is also associated with the prescription of millions of dollars of agents that "dilate blood vessels in the brain." This places an enormous economic burden on the patient with dementia, but to what effect? What I want to ask is in regard to the justification of using vasodilating agents in these conditions. It seems to me that the mere mention of arteriosclerotic cerebral vascular disease causes a reflex reaction in many physicians to use, and perhaps misuse, these agents. The last point that I wish to make is that CT scanning should not be considered the sole or primary instrument in diagnosing dementia. The lack of clarity regarding atrophy norms has brought grief to many people who are 65 or 70 and happen to have large ventricles. The radiologist's report of "large ventricles" is often interpreted as pathognomonic of early dementia. Such evidence should not be used in isolation in formulating a diagnosis.

Clinical Aspects of Alzheimer's Disease and Senile Dementia, (Aging, Vol. 15), edited by Nancy E. Miller and Gene D. Cohen. Raven Press, New York 1981.

The Nature of the Cognitive Deficit in Senile Dementia

Edgar Miller

Addenbrooke's Hospital, Cambridge CB2 2QQ, England

The term "dementia" implies a disturbance in cognitive functioning. The understanding of this cognitive impairment is therefore central to any consideration of dementia. This review attempts to set out the current position with regard to what is known about the cognitive changes that occur in dementia. In particular it concentrates on the experimental studies of cognitive functioning in dementia and ignores reports that are purely clinical in nature. As a general rule, investigations that involve only the application of standardized psychometric tests are also excluded except where they are central to the development of the main theme of this chapter.

It is useful to begin by defining terms. Here "cognitive" is being used to refer to most types of functioning that could be considered part of intellectual activity. This usage is somewhat overinclusive and extends beyond the boundaries of what is usually considered to be "cognitive psychology." However, the greatest emphasis is given to work that falls within the narrower definition. "Dementia" is also a term that has a varied usage. In this context it is taken to be those conditions that are characterized by cerebral atrophy, e.g., Alzheimer's disease and senile dementia.

This review begins by looking at the evidence first, after which the general problems of research in this field are considered together with the implications for future work and clinical practice. After a brief consideration of studies of general intellectual functioning, there is more detailed discussion of specific cognitive functions, especially memory.

INTELLECTUAL CHANGES

Despite the fact that this review is not primarily designed to cover psychometric work, it is difficult to give a comprehensive view of cognitive changes in dementia without at least briefly mentioning studies of general intellectual functioning. I recently dealt with these in greater detail elsewhere (50). Since that time nothing has occurred to change the general picture, so a summary of the previous and more detailed review is not unrepresentative.

As would be expected, groups of demented subjects show lowered mean IQ levels (50). The real interest lies not in showing that a decline in IQ occurs but in trying to analyze the nature of this change. In view of the central place that general intellectual decline holds in the concept of dementia, it is disappointing that this problem has received so little attention.

Among those reports involving the Wechsler scales (the Wechsler-Bellevue or Wechsler Adult Intelligence Scale), the typical finding is that verbal IQ is depressed and that performance IQ is even lower (8,15). Similarly, the use of the Mill Hill Vocabulary Scale and Progressive Matrices has shown that the biggest changes occur in the latter (38,39,59). There are a number of possible explanations of this differential change on the various types of IQ measure. On the Wechsler scales the performance items tend to be timed whereas the verbal ones are not. If it is assumed that the Mill Hill–Matrices difference reflects the same type of effect, then slowing becomes much less attractive as an explanation as these latter tests are untimed.

Two other possible explanations remain. The Wechsler performance subtests and the Matrices involve the manipulation of visuospatial relationships. It could be that this type of ability is especially vulnerable to decline in dementia. The other possibility rests with the fact that the Wechsler verbal subtests and the Mill Hill Vocabulary Scale relate to well-practiced verbal activities. The performance subtests and the Matrices involve items that are much less familiar and require the subject to adjust to new situations. The explanation of these discrepancies in terms of an inability to deal with new tasks is possibly the most plausible in the light of the very definite disturbances in acquisition that occur in dementia.

Some investigators have raised the question as to whether the intellectual changes that occur in dementia are the same as those produced at a slower rate in normal individuals as a result of the aging process. A number have examined the pattern of change in the Wechsler subtests in dements and normals. Some found that the pattern is the same (63,73), and others found that it is not (9,20). This issue remains open, but in passing it ought to be mentioned that attempts to answer this type of question raise important methodological problems which have yet to be satisfactorily resolved (48).

It is also of interest to know if the intellectual change in dementia can be considered to occur along a single dimension and so might be considered to be the result of the loss of one particular aspect of intellectual functioning. Again the evidence is not clear. Dixon (19) found that only one factor was required to account for a high proportion of the variance when a range of brief intellectual tests were given to subjects with varying degrees of dementia. Another factor analytic study used a large battery of intellectual and other types of test (28). No fewer than 14 factors were identified, of which three yielded a definite intellectual bias.

When all is considered, we can be reasonably sure that IQ is depressed in dementia and that the performance type of test is more vulnerable than verbal tests. Having shown this, the psychometric approach has gone very little farther in understanding the intellectual changes that occur in dementia. Statements that dements appear to have lost "fluid" rather than "crystallized" intelligence (in Cattell's sense) or that they have become more "concrete" in their intellectual functioning seem only to describe the findings in other terms and add little to the need for explanation of what is happening (23,31,61).

MEMORY

Memory is the best researched of the psychological changes that occur in dementia. It is also the only aspect in which individual investigators seem to have carried out a series of systematic and interlocking studies. Inevitably, research on memory processes in dementia carries over models and concepts from work on normal memory, which itself is a rapidly expanding and changing field (3,17). Applied research on memory disorders inevitably tends to lag behind the pure work in terms of the models of memory that are used. Because most of the work to be described has been carried out within the context of what Murdock (56) described as the "modal model," implying a multistage system with distinctions between such things as short- and long-term memory, it can most readily be presented within that framework. It should be remembered that the present position of work on normal memory makes this model rather less attractive than it was a few years ago. The present emphasis has moved toward the notion of considering memory in terms of "levels of processing" (17).

Beginning with the input end of the familiar multistage model, there appear to have been no studies of iconic memory in dementia within the tradition started by Sperling (68). The present writer's limited attempts suggest that such experiments are very difficult to carry out with demented subjects. I (51) made a preliminary attempt to look at the early stages of information processing in a tachistoscopic study. When presented with an array of six letters for a brief exposure (50 to 250 msec) followed by a "visual noise" masking stimulus, dements were less able to report letters than controls. This implies that dements are much less efficient at extracting information from brief displays, but why this is so is not clear from this particular experiment. It could be a defect in attention or iconic memory, an enhanced susceptibility to interference, or a combination of these things.

A large number of reports have implicated short-term memory. Inglis (33,34) started by looking at paired associate learning in elderly psychiatric patients. Demented subjects were slow to learn and were equally impaired regardless of whether the learning procedure required them to recall the correct response or to recognize it from a number of alternatives. They also showed very little retention of previously learned associates, as indicated by savings in later relearning. These results suggested to Inglis that the problem lay in acquisition rather than retention.

Inglis and his associates then went on to look at the acquisition process in greater detail using Broadbent's (10) dichotic listening technique. In this procedure different strings of digits are presented simultaneously to each ear. With an immediate recall the subject typically reports the digits presented to one ear before those presented to the other. At one time Broadbent postulated that the digits presented to the ear recalled first were processed by a "p-system," which is only able to pass information successively straight through the system. Digits presented to the ear that is reported second must be held temporarily in some form of short-term store until the first ear's stimuli have been reported. This short-term store is the "s-system" (11). Inglis (35) hypothesized that there might be a breakdown in short-term memory, as reflected by Broadbent's "s-system."

A series of experiments involving the dichotic listening technique were then reported (13,14,36), and all gave substantially the same results. When it came to their ability to recall digits from the ear that was reported first, dements generally did as well as controls. Digits from the ear to be reported second were recalled with very much reduced efficiency. This is precisely the result that Inglis had predicted (35). Unfortunately, the interpretation of these experiments no longer appears to be as clear as it was when they were first reported. What is being measured by dichotic listening is now open to dispute, and the situation is known to be more complex than was originally thought (12,16). Space does not permit this problem to be taken further save to comment that whatever it is that mediates the processing of the digits presented to the ear that is reported second is obviously closer to the short-term than the long-term end of the overall memory system.

I (44) also commenced with the hypothesis that short-term memory might be impaired. Using cases of presenile dementia (presumed to be Alzheimer's disease), the free recall of lists of words was studied. It was found that the demented group was impaired in the recall of words from the beginning and from the end of the list. Following Glanzer and Cunitz (26), the words recalled from the end of the list were considered to be the output from the short-term memory store. The experiment thus gave further evidence for a short-term memory impairment in dementia. According to the same model, recall of words from the beginning of the list was assumed to reflect those words that had successfully passed through the long-term store. Output from the long-term store was also reduced in dementia. This could be due to an additional impairment in long-term memory or to the fact that the short-term memory impairment could interrupt the flow of the first few words in each list through to the long-term store.

To test the latter possibility, it was then decided to examine recall as a function of rate of presentation of words in the list (44). If the reduced output from the long-term store was due solely to the short-term memory impairment reducing the flow of items from the beginning of the list through to long-term memory, then reducing the rate of presentation should give short-term memory a better chance to cope with the flow of words. More words would then be processed through to long-term memory, thereby increasing the amount recalled from the beginning of the list. The normal controls showed this effect very clearly, but the dements did not. This led Miller to suggest that the memory impairment in dementia had at least two components, involving short-term and long-term memory. The theoretical interpretation of free recall is no longer as certain as it seemed when these experiments were carried out (3,5), and the interpretation of the results is correspondingly less secure.

Fortunately, the same conclusions about the involvement of short-term and long-term memory can be derived from a further experiment based on a different technique (46). Dements were shown to be less able to give an immediate reproduction of a short list of words after a single presentation. This confirms the idea of an impaired short-term memory. Even with repeated presentations, dements were less able to learn lists of words that exceeded the word span (number that could be correctly recalled with a single presentation) by one, two, or three items. This supra-span learning would necessitate the use of the long-term store in order to cope with the excess items.

Before leaving short-term memory, it is appropriate to ask if the nature of the impairment in this aspect of memory can be defined in any greater detail. One possibility is that the short-term memory defect is really an artifact of a disturbance at the input end of the system that would reduce the efficiency with which information gets into short-term memory. Disturbed attentional processes or impaired iconic memory might have this effect, and the tachisto-scopic study using backward masking that has already been referred to gives data consistent with this possibility (51). Another possibility is that the efficiency with which material is coded in short-term memory might be reduced. Following Baddeley (2), an experiment was conducted looking at the effect of acoustic similarity on recall from short-term memory (45). It was found that acoustic similarity had a less drastic effect on the recall of the demented group, which is consistent with the notion that dements may be less able to utilize acoustic coding in short-term memory. This interpretation must be considered tentative as the demented and control groups were not equated for recall under the neutral condition and the effect of acoustic similarity might interact with overall recall efficiency.

Long-term memory in dementia has received rather less attention. We (49) presented a list of words to subjects three times. After an interval during which an attempt was made to distract the subjects and so prevent rehearsal of the words, retention was tested in one of three ways: a straightforward recall test, a recognition test in which the subject had to identify the correct word from a set of alternatives, and a partial information condition. The partial information condition consisted of giving the subjects the initial letters of the words to be recalled. As compared with the control group, dements performed very badly on the conventional tests of recall and recognition. On the partial information condition, the dements were indistinguishable from the controls. It was also evident that giving the controls the initial letters did not improve their recall over the level found for the conventional recall test, but a significant improvement was found in the case of the dements.

The results of this experiment on presenile dementia parallel findings obtained earlier using subjects with the amnesic syndrome (72). Because recall can be enhanced to normal levels, it suggests that (at least for the slow rates of presentation used in this experiment) the problem lies in retrieving information rather than in acquiring it. Even this assumption is open to dispute, as it has been suggested that the particular susceptibility of recall to enhancement by the provision of partial information is a feature associated with very weak and decayed traces, whether these exist in normal or abnormal groups (60,69,81). It could merely be that poor acquisition in dements leads to very weak traces in long-term memory, which are then susceptible to enhancement by partial information.

Regardless of the way in which the partial information effect ought to be interpreted, the possibility remains that there is a retrieval difficulty in dementia or some other problem associated with long-term memory. One possibility is that new information entering long-term memory might be coded in an inefficient or unusual way. Later recall might then be enhanced if cues given at the time of recall (e.g., the initial letters of the words to be recalled) give some indication as to how the information to be remembered was coded. This hypothesis is made slightly more plausible by the existence of evidence consistent with the notion that dements do not code efficiently in short-term memory.

A preliminary attempt to look at coding at long-term memory examined the types of error made by demented subjects in a recognition test in which the alternative stimuli differed from the correct one along different dimensions (47). The dements were certainly less able to select the correct response, but they showed no difference from the controls in the types of error they made when they did not select the correct response. This offers no support for the hypothesis of differences in coding. On the other hand, Whitehead (74) reported that the type of error in recall produced by demented subjects differed from those exhibited by elderly subjects with depression. It is not clear whether depressed patients can be regarded as "normal" as far as memory processes are concerned. Some further work in progress by the present writer is concerned with organization in free recall and has so far failed to yield any indication that dements organize or code information in long-term memory in an abnormal way.

The experiments showing the effect of partial information on recall (49,72) led to another interesting hypothesis. Warrington and Weiskrantz (72) suggested that disinhibition might account for the partial information effect. Especially where the to-be-remembered stimuli form a subset of a large range of familiar stimuli (common words in this case), successful performance may depend not only on the ability to recall the correct words but also on the ability to inhibit the recall of incorrect words. If this inhibitory function is lost, the subject may do badly because he recalls too much and he may then produce the wrong responses. Partial information would then enhance recall because it gives a cue for the correct word without providing an alternative which may be incorrectly recognized, as is the case with the conventional type of recognition test. We recently tested this hypothesis (53).

The first experiment examined intrusions in free recall based on the expectation that disinhibition of the type being considered would lead to a larger number of incorrect words (intrusions) appearing in the responses of the demented group. it was found that dements produced fewer responses than the controls, whether correct or incorrect, but there was a slight tendency for the demented group to have a higher proportion of intrusions. There is very little in this in the way of support for the disinhibition hypothesis. The second experiment was based on the fact that recognition tests typically show a decline in the efficiency of recognition as the number of response alternatives is increased. Because increasing the number of response alternatives would also increase the chance of one of these alternatives matching an erroneously recalled word resulting from disinhibition, it was predicted that the effect of manipulating this variable would be enhanced in dementia. This is just what was found: Dements became proportionately less able to recognize the correct word as the number of alternatives was increased. Because of the demonstrated possibility that the partial information effect could be merely a phenomenon associated with weak memory traces, whether these exist in normal or abnormal groups (60,69,80), it would be interesting to know if the effect of varying the number of response alternatives would change in normals as a function of the presumed strength of the trace.

It is sometimes felt that any discussion of possible deficits in long-term memory or retrieval runs counter to the common clinical impression that memory for remote events is reasonably well preserved. If this is the case, then remote memories also need to be retrieved and the retrieval process must be intact. This clinical impression of good preservation of remote memories also arises in the case of other conditions associated with memory impairment, e.g., the amnesic syndrome. In the latter case more objective investigations indicate that the recall of remote events probably is disturbed (67). It is quite possible that similar investigations carried out with demented subjects would give comparable results.

A final point in relation to memory concerns the possibility of other factors operating in dementia so as to produce an apparent memory defect. This is highlighted in an observation made by Whitehead (75). She used two types of recognition test in a memory experiment. Stimuli were shown one at a time, with a "yes" or "no" response being required. This was compared with a forced-choice format in which the correct item was always paired with an incorrect stimulus. There was a definite trend toward better performance with the forced-choice format. An analysis of errors implied that this was not because forced-choice testing reduced the number of false-positive identifications (as might be predicted from the disinhibition hypothesis dealt with above) but because it elicited responses of which the subject was unsure. It could be that in certain other experiments poor performance of demented groups was at least partially due to the adoption of different response criteria, e.g., an increased unwillingness to respond when unsure.

One study with elderly demented subjects used a signal detection analysis (55). Groups with depression and dementia were compared with normal elderly subjects on a recognition test. This study produced evidence that elderly depressives, who sometimes perform badly on memory tests, do exhibit a shift in their response criteria toward a situation in which they appear less ready to guess when not sure. As there was no evidence of a similar trend in the demented group, it does not seem that such factors are biasing the results in studies of memory processes in dementia.

There is good evidence that the ability to acquire new information is impaired in dementia. A tachistoscopic experiment implied that the problem starts at the earliest stages of the acquisition process (51). However, the dichotic listening experiments of Inglis and his associates, showing a particular vulnerability for material presented to the ear reported second, also suggest that there are deficits at a level approximating that of short-term memory in the familiar multistage model of memory. The evidence with regard to longer-term retention and retrieval is less certain, and more needs to be done in this area. At the very least, it would be premature to try to explain the whole of the memory disturbance in dementia as being due to difficulties in acquisition. So far there appears to have been no serious attempt to examine memory disorders in dementia in terms of the "levels of processing" model of memory (17).

LANGUAGE

Changes in language are often noted in clinical descriptions of dementia, and dysphasic phenomena are claimed to occur (18,70). Ernst et al. (21) carried out a detailed systematic examination of language functioning in a small group of demented patients. The only feature that all subjects seemed to have in common was a general poverty of vocabulary in narrative speech. Other than this there was no consistent pattern of dysphasic disturbance, although many subjects showed impairments in naming. Impaired naming is of course found in all types of aphasia (25).

Naming has been studied experimentally in demented patients (6,40). Subjects with senile dementia and age-matched normal controls were compared in their ability to name objects. In addition to being less able to provide appropriate names, the demented group revealed two other features. Although both groups were less able to name objects whose names were less frequently encountered in normal usage (as measured by either accuracy or latency), this effect was more marked in the demented group. In addition, demonstrating the use of the object improved naming in the demented group but had no effect on the controls.

Rochford (65) compared senile dementia patients with a younger group of subjects with aphasia due to focal lesions. When examining the types of error in naming that were made by the two groups, Rochford gained the impression that the aphasic group correctly identified the objects to be named but were unable to produce the correct word. In contrast the dements appeared more likely to give the incorrect name because they had misidentified the object to be named. Trying to test this further, Rochford argued that it was necessary to have a task which minimized any difficulty involved in recognizing the object that was to be named. This should benefit the dements but not the aphasics. The parts of the body are familiar and easily recognized, and subjects were therefore asked to name these. This made little difference to the aphasics, but it produced the expected improvement in the dements. This result fits in very nicely with the clinical observation that naming difficulties in dementia are unlike those occurring in the more usual forms of dysphasia, because in the latter, in contrast to the former, the patient gives the strong impression that he knows what the object is but just cannot find the right word to apply to it (70).

Other approaches have been used to study the production of words in dementia (54). Dements and controls were compared on a fluency test in which each subject produces as many words as he can beginning with the letter "S" within a 5-min period. The dements produced fewer words, although neither group seemed to have reached an asymptote in the cumulative total of words by the end of the 5-min period. Because of previous work on naming (6,40), the groups were also compared with regard to their tendency to produce words of different frequency of occurence in the language. The control group produced a significantly higher proportion of less common words. It is tempting to regard this as further confirmation of a particular vulnerability to the loss of rarer words in dementia. Unfortunately, further analysis revealed that the controls tended to start the task by producing common words and then passed on to the rarer ones later. It could be that the dements, being slower to produce words, had not worked through their repertoire of common words by the end of the 5-min period that was allowed.

In order to examine this possible frequency effect further, it was necessary to use a form of analysis that could not be contaminated in this way. Samples of conversational speech were recorded from each of a small number of demented and control subjects (54). Within each 2,000-word sample, separate counts were made of the number of words used only once in the sample, the number used twice, etc. There was no trend toward the demented group relying excessively on a small set of very commonly used words as might have been expected. In fact, the data from the two groups were indistinguishable. This experiment gives no encouragement to the notion that the pattern of word use might be different in dementia. In particular, it also failed to show the kind of changes that frequently occur when the speech of dysphasic subjects is subjected to this type of analysis (32).

There is little in the way of evidence relating to the receptive side of speech in dementia other than a single experiment based on the "verbal transformation effect" (57). The subject listens to a recorded word or phrase which is repeated over and over again. Subjects often report abrupt illusory changes in the stimulus and may "hear" other words or phrases. Elderly dements produced fewer transformations than controls and in this way behave as if they are older than they really are. On the other hand, those transformations that the dements did report involved a greater degree of phonemic change than was typical of the controls. In this respect the demented group behaved more like children in their responses.

Changes in language behavior do occur in dementia, but the experimental evidence, slight though it is, shows the change to be rather different from that which is typical of aphasia arising from focal lesions. Impairments of naming do occur, but these may be at least partly a consequence of misidentification of the object to be named (65). If subjects whose names are less commonly encountered in the language are also more difficult to recognize, this would explain Barker and Lawson's (6,40) ability to demonstrate a differential effect of word frequency whereas the analysis of conversational speech did not (54). This is because the question of recognition would not arise in conversation. It is unfortunate that the receptive aspects of speech have been neglected other than for the one experiment concerned with the unusual and somewhat bizarre phenomenon of the verbal transformation effect.

PERCEPTION

If the above analysis of naming disturbances is correct, it should be possible to find abnormalities in perception, especially in the visual modality. There was one direct study of visual perception that has claimed to find changes in visual perception, but the experimental design was very poor (78). Good evidence is hard to find, but two neuropsychological studies have some relevance (22,77). In one of these it was asserted that about 4% of a very large sample of patients with cerebral atrophy showed some perceptual distortion when asked to fixate on a particular object. The other involved a detailed examination of a small group of patients with presenile dementia for gnostic and praxic symptoms. A variety of minor abnormalities of a gnostic nature were elicited, but there was no consistent pattern of impairment (22). Other than the experiment on the verbal transformation effect described in the previous section, I know of no studies of auditory perception in dementia.

In view of the pointers that exist toward the possibility of perceptual abnormalities in dementia, this aspect of functioning needs further and detailed investigation. Any experiments in this field must also take into account the increased incidence of sensory impairments in patients with dementia (58).

OTHER COGNITIVE FUNCTIONS

Visuospatial deficits have been described by a number of investigators, but again there is a shortage of soundly designed experiments. Patients with senile dementia seem to have appreciable difficulty in solving paper and pencil mazes, and they also have an impaired appreciation of reflected space (1,79). For example, a demented subject who sees a reflection of an object situated over his left shoulder might try to reach through the mirror to grasp it. It has also been suggested that dements experience a disintegration of the body schema in that they show undue difficulty in fitting together pictures of different parts of the human body to make a whole (24).

Patients with many types of brain pathology have been claimed to be distractible. Lawson et al. (41) required their subjects to report back sets of digits presented either auditorily or visually. Distracting stimuli were also present on some trials (e.g., another voice reading a second set of digits). Subjects with presenile dementia proved to be distractible in the auditory modality but not in the visual. This does not necessarily mean that there is a true modality effect in the susceptibility of dements to distraction because the experimenters took no steps to equate the potency of the distractors used for each modality.

The concepts of information processing and information theory have been familiar to experimental subjects for some time but have been little exploited in this aspect of abnormal psychology. The only study I know of which directly applies these ideas to dementia is that of Hibbard et al. (30). The task used required the subject to make certain types of sensory discrimination. The demented group achieved lower scores on a measure of transmitted information than age-matched normal controls. Of peripheral interest in this context is the fact that an experiment on speed of movement indicated that dements were slow partly because they were slower to decide when and where to move (50). This is consistent with the notion of an information-processing impairment.

Many aspects of cognitive functioning in dementia either remain untouched or, at best, are only very tentatively explored. It is difficult to draw meaningful conclusions from the data that do exist for such parameters as visuospatial ability, information processing, and distractibility other than the obvious need for much further work.

COGNITIVE DEFICITS IN RELATION TO OTHER ASPECTS OF DEMENTIA

Cognitive impairments are not the only changes produced by dementia. It is important therefore to consider how well they correlate with other variables. In particular, it is of interest to examine the relationship between cognitive deficits and the physical changes that take place in the brain because it has been suggested that these two things are not directly related (66). It is the basis of Rothschild's thesis that the pathological changes in dementia are merely those of normal aging. The dement differs from the normal elderly person only in being less able to adapt to normal pathological changes (66).

A number of investigations have found a relationship between the degree of atrophy as revealed by air encephalography and various indices of intellectual functioning (27,43,76). More recently Roberts and Caird (64) found similar relationships where the measures of brain dimensions have been based on computerized tomography. In general these relationships do not appear to be very large when measured in terms of correlation coefficients, although they are definitely significant in the statistical sense. In addition, it should be noted that a small proportion of the subjects in a number of the relevant investigations were probably not cases of dementia as it is being considered here.

The most impressive correlations relate to neuropathological changes. Blessed et al. (7) report substantial correlations between scores on a series of simple tests and rating scales of mental functioning on the one hand and plaque counts on the other. This was initially done in a sample of elderly subjects that included normal elderly people as well as those with dementia. Even when those with low plaque counts and good scores on the tests were removed from the analysis (presumably leaving a group that was mainly demented), the correlations were still appreciable. Many other variables (e.g., cerebral blood flow and peripheral nerve conduction) have also been shown to be associated with psychological measures (29,42,50).

There can be no doubt that the cognitive deterioration in dementia occurs in step with the physical changes that take place in the brain and other parts of the nervous system. Apart from the pathological investigation of Blessed et al. (7), the measured association is often not large although it is typically statistically significant. I (50) have argued on methodological grounds that the problems inherent in this type of correlational study are such that the obtained correlations are likely to be small despite the fact that a strong underlying association may exist.

DISCUSSION

Almost paradoxically one of the problems involved in evaluating research into dementia is that groups of demented and age-matched normal controls can be shown to differ on almost any cognitive variable that the research worker cares to investigate. This can make the few instances in which differences fail to occur of even greater interest than some of the circumstances in which positive results can be readily obtained. This is a situation not often encountered in the study of pathological groups.

The wide range of functional deficits that can be so easily demonstrated raises a fundamental question. It is tempting to view the study of psychological disturbances in any clinical condition as the search for a single, defining deficit that can explain all the manifest phenomena. An example is the attempt to explain all the behavioral consequences of schizophrenia as being the result of an impairment in attentional mechanisms, or those of frontal lobe lesions as being due to a fault in the processes underlying the planning and control of behavior. It may be that ultimately all the varied manifestations in dementia will prove capable of being understood as the by-products of a single fundamental deficit, e.g., malfunctioning arousal system (37,62). However, this need not necessarily be the case, and it can be argued that such an outcome may not even be likely.

Dementia, as conceived here, is associated with diffuse and wide-ranging pathological changes in the brain, and these are certainly not confined to any one part of subsystem of the brain. It is therefore to be expected that there will be disruption of the brain systems underlying most, if not all, aspects of behavior. The resulting picture may be one of a general disintegration of functional capacities right across the board rather than a series of manifestations of one or more fundamental or underlying variables. If this argument is accepted, the search for a single behavioral theory of dementia would be misplaced. Psychological research into the consequences of dementia should be either descriptive or based on explanatory models that are confined to a single behavioral subsystem. Only if work on a number of different aspects of behavior should start to converge on similar underlying mechanisms would it be worthwhile to start considering the possibility of a single, grand psychological model of dementia.

Characteristics of the Work Reviewed

When the whole body of research into cognitive deficits in dementia is considered, a number of general characteristics can be discerned. Each of these has in its own way contributed to obscuring our understanding of cognitive deterioration in dementia. A number of those that seem of greatest significance are considered in this section.

Dementia is hardly a popular area of research. Possibly because of this there has been a tendency for researchers to carry out one or two investigations in the field and then move on to other things. This lack of commitment has meant that there are few examples of systematic attempts to explore a particular problem in depth. In consequence, there is a relatively high proportion of experiments that are inevitably superficial and which are difficult to fit into the context of anything else. It is to be hoped that the growing realization of the importance of dementia as a social problem in Western society with its ever-increasing proportion of elderly members, will mean that more individuals or groups will emerge who are willing to make a sustained commitment to research into dementia.

A major methodological problem when evaluating studies of dementia is that of the selection of subjects. All too often the subject populations are poorly described, and the criteria on which their selection is based varies considerably. Variables such as age and length of illness can show wide variation. Until quite recently some workers have labored under fallacious assumptions, e.g., the idea that nearly all organically produced deterioration in the elderly is the result of cerebral arteriosclerosis. Although the identification of dementia is not without its problems, there can be no doubt that future work can, and should, be based on better definition of the subject populations used than is the case at present.

A second methodological issue relates to experimental design. At least two kinds of question can be asked. The first is concerned with the ways in which dements may differ in their cognitive functioning from either normal subjects or other pathological groups. The appropriate experimental design involves applying the same experimental procedure to different groups of subjects so that the performance of different types of subjects can be compared. Usually age-matched groups of demented and normal subjects are involved, with the possible addition of other pathological groups. In passing, it might be noted that age-matched control groups may not always be appropriate when concern lies in testing certain theoretical ideas about dementia (48).

A second type of question that can be posed relates to the way in which the performance of demented subjects varies under different experimental conditions. This approach is of particular relevance when the problems involved in the management of dementia are being considered. Recently attention was drawn to the fact that elderly demented patients do seem to be responsive to environmental manipulations (50,52,80). When the problem of management is highlighted, the point of interest shifts from trying to define the deficits that exist to establishing under what circumstances performance is maximized or minimized. This requires a different type of research design. Instead of comparing a demented and a control group on a particular memory task, it becomes more appropriate to study how well groups of demented subjects retain the same information under different conditions of acquisition. Although research based on dement–normal comparisons will continue to be of significance in understanding cognitive deficits in dementia, it is now important that some consideration be given to answering questions relating to the variation in performance of demented groups under different conditions.

Even within the commonly used dement–normal comparison type of research, there is a further methodological problem that has yet to be satisfactorily resolved. This can probably best be described in the context of a specific example. When trying to explore short-term memory deficits in dementia, I (45) wished to test the hypothesis that effective short-term memory capacity might be reduced in dementia because of inefficient coding. Building on the work of Baddeley (2), efficiency of the immediate recall of very short lists of words was compared using lists of unrelated words and lists of acoustically similar words. If dements are less able to utilize acoustic coding in short-term memory, then it would be expected that the normal tendency for less efficient recall of the acoustically similar lists would be reduced in dementia. This was indeed found, and the results are undoubtedly consistent with the hypothesis. Unfortunately, the demented group were also less able to recall the unrelated lists than the controls. It could be that the effect of acoustic similarity is itself a function of how well the subject can recall unrelated lists. To control for this, it would be necessary to ensure that dements and controls were matched for the recall of the unrelated lists. Given the extremely poor memory performance of demented subjects, this is very difficult in practice, if not actually impossible under some circumstances. This kind of methodological difficulty can arise in many contexts, and there is no sure way of getting around it.

A final issue of research methodology concerns the point that dementia is a slowly progressive disease. Most investigations look at a group of dements at one point in time. There is a lack of work which systematically tries to follow the development of cognitive impairments to see how they change with different stages in the disease process.

Other than the methodological issues outlined above, there is another aspect of research into cognitive impairments in dementia that is a major cause for concern. Attempts to describe the cognitive impairment need to be built on a sound model of normal functioning. There are no well established models with clearly acceptable measures of their constituent functions. The discussion of memory given above illustrates this problem, although space did not permit the issues to be explored in any depth. Most work on memory processes in dementia has been based on the familiar multistage model of normal memory. Not only is this model now seriously in dispute, but there are significant objections that can be raised against any chosen measure of any one of its aspects, e.g., short-term or primary memory. It remains to be seen if the currently more fashionable levels of processing model of memory (17) will provide a sounder theoretical base in the long term despite the criticisms that have been leveled against it (4). However, the basic point remains that the extent to which memory or any other cognitive function is understood in terms of its normal functioning is likely to set a limit to our understanding of the same processes as they operate in abnormal groups.

Future Directions

It is difficult to speculate on what will be the most fruitful lines of development. The previous section outlined some of the less desirable features of the work that has been carried out so far. Future work should be able to improve on some of these things without much difficulty, but others will not be so easily dealth with. This section briefly considers a few more areas of research that I believe are particularly in need of development.

Memory is the cognitive function that has received the greatest attention so far. As already indicated, research into memory processes in dementia has not yet caught up with thinking about normal memory, and the levels of processing model needs to be applied to dementia. In addition, it is my belief that the earliest levels of processing (e.g., attentional mechanisms and iconic memory) might well be of considerable significance for understanding memory processes in dementia. A problem is that many of the experimental paradigms for this type of study would be extremely difficult to use with demented patients. Even with early cases of presenile dementia the simple backward masking technique (51) did not prove easy in practice. Fortunately, some examples of simpler techniques can be found, and one has already been used successfully in the investigation of normal age changes (71).

Looking beyond memory, and with the single other exception of langue, the overriding impression is that many important aspects of cognitive functioning have been virtually ignored. There have been few if any soundly conducted experiments relating to such things as perception, information processing, visuospatial abilities, and thinking. These gaps obviously need to be filled. It is impossible to latch on to any specific features as being in particular need of information when looking at what is almost a total vacuum.

Finally, and at the risk of repetition, the desirability of developing research which not only identified deficits but explores the conditions under which they are maximized or minimized must be stressed. The predominant practical problem presented by dementia is that of management. The study of cognitive processes can contribute to this by finding ways in which the impact of cognitive deterioration can be diminished, thereby ensuring that the afflicted individual retains his functional capacities for as long as possible.

CONCLUSIONS

To date, research into cognitive processes in dementia has been very uneven in its development. There has been a considerable emphasis on memory and some work on language but an almost total neglect of many other important aspects of cognitive functioning. There are a number of important methodological and other limitations in this work, not all of which will be easily rectified. It is possible to make some suggestions as to what might be the most appropriate ways to develop work in this field.

REFERENCES

1. Ajuriaguerra, J. de, Strejilevitch, M., and Tissot, R. (1963): *Neuropsychologia,* 1:59–73.
2. Baddeley, A. D. (1966): *Q. J. Exp. Psychol.,* 18:362–365.
3. Baddeley, A. D. (1976): *The Psychology of Memory.* Harper & Row, New York.
4. Baddeley, A. D. (1978): *Psychol. Rev.,* 85:139–152.
5. Baddeley, A. D., and Hitch, G. (1974): In: *The Psychology of Learning and Motivation,* Vol. 8, edited by G. H. Bower, pp. 47–90. Academic Press, New York.
6. Barker, M. G., and Lawson, J. S. (1968): *Br. J. Psychiatry.,* 114:1351–1356.
7. Blessed, G., Tomlinson, B. E., and Roth, M. (1968): *Br. J. Psychiatry,* 114:797–811.
8. Bolton, N., Britton, P. G., and Savage, R. D. (1966): *J. Clin. Psychol.,* 22:184–188.
9. Botwinnick, J., and Birren, J. E. (1951): *J. Gerontol.,* 6:365–368.
10. Broadbent, D. E. (1954): *J. Exp. Psychol.,* 47:191–196.
11. Broadbent, D. E. (1958): *Perception and Communication.* Pergamon Press, Oxford.
12. Broadbent, D. E. (1971): *Decision and Stress.* Academic Press, London.
13. Caird, W. K., and Hannah, F. (1964): *Dis. Nerv. Syst.,* 25:564–568.
14. Caird, W. K., and Inglis, J. (1961): *J. Ment. Sci.,* 107:1062–1069.
15. Cleveland, S., and Dysinger, D. (1944): *J. Abnorm. Soc. Psychol.,* 39:368–372.
16. Craik, F. I. M. (1977): In: *Handbook of the Psychology of Aging,* edited by J. E. Birren and K. W. Schaie. Van Nostrand, New York.

17. Craik, F. I. M., and Lockhart, R. S. (1972): *J. Verb. Learn. Verb. Behav.*, 11:671–684.
18. Critchley, M. (1964): *Br. J. Psychiatry*, 110:353–364.
19. Dixon, J. C. (1965): *J. Gerontol.*, 20:41–49.
20. Dorken, H., and Greenbloom, G. C. (1953): *Geriatrics*, 8:324–333.
21. Ernst, B., Dalby, A., and Dalby, M. A. (1970): *Acta Neurol. Scand. [Suppl.]*, 43:99–100.
22. Ernst, B., Dalby, M. A., and Dalby, A. (1970): *Acta Neurol. Scand. [Suppl.]*, 43:101–102.
23. Eysenck, M. D. (1945): *J. Neurol. Psychiatry*, 8:15–21.
24. Gailliard, J. M. (1970): *J. Psychol. Norm. Pathol.*, 67:443–472.
25. Geschwind, N. (1971): *N. Engl. J. Med.*, 284:654–656.
26. Glanzer, M., and Cunitz, A. R. (1966): *J. Verb. Learn. Verb. Behav.*, 5:351–360.
27. Gosling, R. H. (1955): *J. Neurol. Neurosurg. Psychiatry*, 18:129–133.
28. Gustafson, L., and Hagberg, B. (1975): *Acta Psychiatr. Scand. [Suppl.]*, 257:1–36.
29. Gustafson, L., and Risberg, J. (1974): *Acta Psychiatr. Scand.*, 50:516–538.
30. Hibbard, T. R., Migliaccio, J. N., Goldstone, S., and Lhamon, W. T. (1975): *J. Gerontol.*, 30:326–330.
31. Hopkins, B., and Post, F. (1955): *J. Ment. Sci.*, 101:841–850.
32. Howes, D. (1964): In: *Ciba Foundation Symposium on Disorders of Language*, edited by A. V. S. Reuck and M. O'Connor, pp. 142–176. Churchill, London.
33. Inglis, J. (1957); *J. Ment. Sci.*, 103:796–803.
34. Inglis, J. (1959): *J. Abnorm. Soc. Psychol.*, 59:210–215.
35. Inglis, J. (1960): *Nature*, 186:181–182.
36. Inglis, J., and Sanderson, R. F. (1961): *J. Abnorm. Soc. Psychol.*, 62:709–712.
37. Kendrick, D. C. (1972): *Br. J. Soc. Clin. Psychol.*, 4:63–71.
38. Kendrick, D. C., Parboosingh, R-C., and Post, F. (1965): *Br. J. Soc. Clin. Psychol.*, 4:63–71.
39. Kendrick, D. C., and Post, F. (1967): *Br. J. Psychiatry*, 113:75–81.
40. Lawson, J. S., and Barker, M. G. (1968): *Br. J. Med. Psychol.*, 41:411–414.
41. Lawson, J. S., McGhie, A., and Chapman, J. (1967): *Br. J. Psychiatry*, 113:527–535.
42. Levy, R., Isaacs, A., and Hawks, G. (1970): *Psychol. Med.*, 1:40–47.
43. Matthews, C. G., and Booker, H. E. (1972): *Cortex*, 8:69–72.
44. Miller, E. (1971): *Neuropsychologia*, 9:75–78.
45. Miller, E. (1972): *Neuropsychologia*, 10:133–136.
46. Miller, E. (1973): *Psychol. Med.*, 3:221–224.
47. Miller, E. (1974): *Bull. Br. Psychol. Soc.*, 27:173–174.
48. Miller, E. (1974): *Age Ageing*, 3:197–202.
49. Miller, E. (1975): *Br. J. Soc. Clin. Psychol.*, 14:73–79.
50. Miller, E. (1977): *Abnormal Ageing*. Wiley, Chichester.
51. Miller, E. (1977): *Br. J. Soc. Clin. Psychol.*, 16:99–100.
52. Miller, E. (1977): *Br. J. Soc. Clin. Psychol.*, 16:77–83.
53. Miller, E. (1978): *Br. J. Soc. Clin. Psychol.*, 17:143–148.
54. Miller, E., and Hague, F. (1975): *Psychol. Med.*, 5:255–259.
55. Miller, E., and Lewis, P. (1977): *J. Abnorm. Psychol.*, 86:84–86.
56. Murdock, B. B. (1971): In: *The Psychology of Learning and Motivation*, Vol. 5, edited by G. Bower, pp. 67–127. Academic Press, New York.
57. Obusek, C. J., and Warren, R. M. (1973): *J. Gerontol.*, 28:184–188.
58. O'Neil, P. M., and Calhoun, K. S. (1975): *J. Abnorm. Psychol.*, 84:579–582.
59. Orme, J. E. (1957): *J. Gerontol.*, 12:408–413.
60. Piercy, M. F. (1977): In: *Amnesia*, edited by C. W. M. Whitty and O. L. Zangwill, pp. 1–51. Butterworth, London.
61. Pinkerton, P., and Kelly, J. (1952): *J. Ment. Sci.*, 98:244–255.
62. Post, F. (1966): *J. Psychosom. Res.*, 10:13–19.
63. Rabin, A. I. (1945): *J. Gen. Psychol.*, 32:149–162.
64. Roberts, M. A., and Caird, F. I. (1976): *J. Neurol. Neurosurg. Psychiatry*, 39:986–989.
65. Rochford, G. (1971): *Neuropsychologia*, 9:437–443.
66. Rothschild, D. (1942): *Arch. Neurol. Psychiatry*, 48:417–436.
67. Sanders, H. I., and Warrington, E. K. (1971): *Brain*, 94:661–668.
68. Sperling, G. A. (1960): *Psychol. Monogr.*, 74:No. 498.
69. Squire, L. R., Wetzel, C. D., and Slater, P. C. (1978): *Neuropsychologia*, 16:339–348.

70. Stengel, E. (1964): *Proc. R. Soc. Med.,* 57:911–914.
71. Walsh, D. A., and Thompson, L. W. (1978): *J. Gerontol.* 33:383–387.
72. Warrington, E. K., and Weiskrantz, L. (1970): *Nature,* 228:628–630.
73. Whitehead, A. (1973): *Br. J. Psychiatry,* 123:203–208.
74. Whitehead, A. (1973): *Br. J. Soc. Clin. Psychol.,* 12:435–436.
75. Whitehead, A. (1975): *Br. J. Soc. Clin. Psychol.,* 14:191–194.
76. Willanger, R. (1970): *Intellectual Impairment in Diffuse Cerebral Lesions.* Munksgaard, Copenhagen.
77. Willanger, R., and Klee, A. (1966): *Acta Neurol. Scand. [Suppl.],* No. 42.
78. Williams, M. (1956): *Br. J. Med. Psychol.,* 19:270–279.
79. Williams, M. (1956): *J. Ment. Sci.,* 102:291–299.
80. Woods, R. T., and Britton, P. (1977): *Age Ageing,* 6:104–112.
81. Woods, R. T., and Piercy, M. (1974): *Neuropsychologia,* 12:437–445.

Clinical Aspects of Alzheimer's Disease and Senile Dementia, (Aging, Vol. 15), edited by Nancy E. Miller and Gene D. Cohen. Raven Press, New York 1981.

The Differential Psychological Evaluation

Edgar Miller

Addenbrooke's Hospital, Cambridge CB2 2QQ, England

Psychological assessment, once the major stock in trade of the clinical psychologist, has become increasingly unfashionable. The psychologist's drift away from assessment has been partly due to the increasing development of therapeutic techniques of a psychological nature that have demanded his attention (e.g., behavior therapy and the various forms of psychotherapy). Another reason for the decline in interest in assessment has been the feeling that the conventional techniques of psychological assessment, especially psychometrics, have severe limitations in solving clinical problems (24). The swing away from psychological assessment is exemplified by the need of recent writers on one aspect of assessment to start by justifying their continued concern (72).

Despite the general dissatisfaction with the conventional forms of psychometric assessment, this does not mean that psychometric techniques are of no value or that other forms of assessment cannot be devised to solve the same problems. What is evident is that some caution is needed in evaluating the effectiveness of assessment devices. It is also worth noting that these can never be considered effective or ineffective in a general sense. They can be evaluated only in relation to the specific assessment problems that they are used to resolve.

It seems sensible to commence the discussion of the psychological evaluation of dementia by considering the problems to which assessment might be directed. Traditionally there has been an appreciable interest in trying to measure change, particularly in intellectual functioning. This has largely been directed toward devising ways to measure the change in intelligence that has occurred from the premorbid level. Being able to determine that the patient's intelligence quotient (IQ) has declined by a certain number of IQ points may help in the diagnosis of dementia. Once the diagnosis has been made, this particular type of information probably contributes little further. The increasing interest in trying to halt or slow down the progression of dementia by drugs or other means (13,17,34, 51,85) means that these methods of intervention need to be evaluated. There is therefore a major need for means of assessment that can measure change in this context.

A second major concern of psychological assessment in relation to dementia has been with the problem of differential diagnosis. In elderly populations the differentiation between dementia and functional psychiatric disorder, especially depression, is of particular concern. The need to discriminate between dementia and depression not only arises frequently but has important implications for management and prognosis (50). In addition, dementia of the Alzheimer's/senile type can be difficult to distinguish from a number of other organic disorders that may have a deleterious effect on general mental functioning.

A final set of assessment problems arises out of the need to make decisions about management. The increasing use of psychological and social methods in order to try to maintain the afflicted individual's functioning at as high a level as possible also makes its demands for assessment (51,85). Decisions must be made about which patients might benefit from the various programs and in what way. Similarly, some form of assessment is also required to make decisions about the placement of an individual in the various types of care facility that are available.

It will be seen that work on the psychological assessment of dementia has contributed to the solution of these various problems with varying levels of success. Much effort has gone into developing ways of measuring the decline in IQ and in discriminating dementia from depression. Other assessment needs have been very much neglected.

METHODOLOGICAL ISSUES

Before passing to a more detailed examination of the various approaches to the psychological evaluation of dementia, it is sensible to begin by considering the methodological issues in this field. This is not a comprehensive exposition on methodology but concentrates on issues that tend to arise in the assessment of the individual patient who has, or who might be suspected of having, a dementing illness.

A simple point which is often overlooked is that reliable group differences on a given measure do not necessarily mean that the measure is useful when making decisions about individuals. For example, it can readily be demonstrated that the mean height of a randomly selected group of women is lower than that of a randomly selected group of men. However, knowing that a given person's height is, for example, 68 inches is not a very useful piece of information for determining that individual's sex. Not only is height a poor indicator of sex in the single case, but there are better and quicker ways of making this differentiation! This raises another point that Cronbach and Gleser (10) emphasized in a very different assessment context. The practical usefulness of any assessment device depends not only on its validity in the formal psychometric sense but also on how it relates to the other means that are available for reaching the same assessment goal.

In validity studies a number of complications surround the selection of subject groups. These are discussed using the validation of diagnostic tests as an example, but the same points may apply to a greater or lesser degree in the validation of assessment procedures designed to serve other purposes. It is tempting to select groups that consist of clear-cut examples of the relevant conditions. On the other hand, the nature of clinical practice means that the test is most useful in making diagnostic decisions about cases that are more problematical. The validity of the test with this latter type of case may well be lower than it is for the more obvious members of one category or the other. The diagnosis of dementia, at least in the early stages, is never completely accurate (57). As a result, some cases used in diagnostic validation studies may not really be members of the class to which they are assumed to belong. In cases where the need is to discriminate between dementia and depression, it would be possible to follow up the subjects used to confirm the diagnosis since the long-term outcome for the two conditions is very different.

The problem of contamination in diagnostic studies has also received attention. Direct contamination, whereby the test is partially used as the criterion against which it is validated, is, in principle if not in practice, easy to eliminate. It can happen where a test is used on a trial basis to help in diagnosis and the cases are later analyzed retrospectively to see if the test results relate to the diagnosis that was achieved. If the test contributed in any way to the decision-making process that was used to arrive at the diagnosis, then it is not surprising if later analysis reveals some validity. More subtle and much more difficult to eliminate is the kind of indirect contamination to which Shapiro et al. (75) drew attention. Poor memory is a common feature of dementia, and the use of tests of learning and memory to distinguish dementia from functional psychiatric disorders is an obvious development. It may happen in a validity study that there is no direct contamination between the test under examination and the diagnosis, yet some other form for evaluating memory may be used to reach the diagnosis. In this case the test under examination may correlate with the indices of memory used in reaching the diagnoses, and because of this a spuriously high impression of validity may be obtained.

Another factor that is rarely taken into account is that of antecedent probabilities or base rates (47). In any given situation the chances of an individual patient being depressed or demented may not be equal. For example, in two separate British psychogeriatric services, it was found that admissions contain approximately two depressives for every dement (23,39). The mathematical basis to the argument is set out quite clearly by Meehl and Rosen (47), but intuitively it can be seen that changes in the base rate can affect the usefulness of the test. A test that correctly identifies 90% of the cases with dementia and 90% of those with depression may be quite useful where the base rate is 50:50. If the base rate were to alter to 90:10, then the same level of overall diagnostic accuracy could be achieved just by assigning the most common diagnosis to all cases.

The problem of where to set the cut-off point is not as simple as it may seem. Typically test constructors set a cut-off point that achieves the maximum overall correct classification. However, this typically involves some incorrect classifications in both directions. For example, when trying to discriminate between dementia and depression, the two types of error may not be considered equally undesirable. It could be argued that since depression is a treatable condition it is much more serious an error to misdiagnose a depressed patient as demented than for the reverse to occur. If this argument is taken to its logical conclusion, it would be appropriate to set the cut-off score to minimize this type of error even at the expense of a greater risk of falsely classifying a demented patient as depressed. Altering the cut-off point in this way typically does not result in the same cut-off point that would achieve the minimum overall level of misclassification.

A final methodological point in relation to diagnostic assessment concerns the need for cross-validation in assessment research. In a recently reported investigation, several tests were given to groups of demented subjects with vascular and nonvascular etiology (62,64). The statistical analysis yielded a formula which enabled the two types of dementia to be discriminated with a 70% level of accuracy. This is an impressive level of diagnostic discrimination for psychological tests in these circumstances. On the other hand, it is likely that in a study of this nature the analysis has capitalized on some chance variations in the test scores between these two groups. Experience suggests that a repetition of this study would probably yield a much less encouraging result. For this and other reasons, validation data must be treated with some caution until cross-validation has been achieved, preferably by other workers in a different center.

When the literature on the psychological evaluation of dementia is examined with the above methodological issues in mind, it rapidly becomes clear that there is little evidence that can safely be assumed to be free from most of the possible pitfalls. The most sophisticated work from this point of view is probably that of Kendrick and his associates, which was originally published over a decade ago (39,40). Possibly the lack of further work of this quality reflects the low status that is now accorded to research into assessment.

A rather different kind of issue that arises in the use of psychometric tests with elderly populations is the adequacy of test norms. Not only do many potentially useful tests lack norms for the elderly, but where such norms are available they may be less well derived than those relating to younger age ranges. The latter situation appears to be the case with the commonly used Wechsler Adult Intelligence Scale (WAIS) (15). Even if the norms for cognitive tests are well established initially, there is good reason to believe that they can become out of date and unrepresentative of later generations of elderly subjects (52).

The evaluation of changes associated with aging presents considerable methodological problems (6), but there is now appreciable evidence that cross-sectional studies wherein groups of elderly subjects are directly compared with younger adults overestimate the decline in cognitive functioning that occurs as a result of normal aging (6,50,70). The reason for this is that the older group differs from the younger on other variables besides age. The older group was born at a time when ante- and postnatal care were less satisfactory, infant nutrition was less adequate, and educational opportunities were much more limited than was the case for the younger subjects. These things can have an impact on cognitive functioning, and successive generations would be better placed with regard to these factors. In consequence, later generations of old people should be able to perform better on cognitive tests, and there is evidence that the age at which intellectual decline starts to become manifest is increasing generation by generation (71). The likely result is that a test such as the WAIS, published in 1955, is likely to have norms for elderly subjects based on a mean level of performance which is below that of similarly aged subjects today. In other words, the danger is that the test will now overestimate IQs in the elderly.

MEASUREMENT OF CHANGE

A common early goal in the assessment of patients with organic disease of the brain was to measure the decline in intellectual functioning that had occurred from premorbid levels. Only rarely are patients encountered for whom psychometric data are available from some previous time which is recent enough to be considered reliable and not too close to the onset of the condition to be possibly contaminated by it. Direct measurement of decline by comparison of data obtained on two occasions is usually feasible only from the time at which the patient comes into contact with the service. The initial assessment of the patient can then be compared with assessments made on later occasions to see if there is any further decline in functioning. This is sometimes useful where a diagnosis of dementia remains in doubt.

Although apparently simple in conception, any comparison of psychometric data obtained on two occasions involves technical complications. The test used must be very reliable. If it is not, a very large change in score must occur between the two testings in order to be outside the range of possible chance variation. A subject's score also changes from one testing to another because of such things as practice effects regardless of any true change on the variable being measured. Ideally, appropriate test–retest data should be available for the test being used, and it is then possible to predict how the subject should perform on a second exposure to the test after a given interval. The subject's actual later performance can then be compared with this prediction (60). Suitable test–retest data are extremely sparse even for the most commonly used tests. An indication of likely changes on retesting and test–retest correlations can be obtained for the Wechsler-Bellevue Scales, the WAIS, Raven's Progressive Matrices, and the Primary Mental Abilities (14,19,26,27,46,73). Only in the case of the Primary Mental Abilities were the data actually obtained from elderly subjects, and the rest must be treated as only rough indications because of this.

Since the direct measurement of decline is difficult, there have been a number of attempts to devise indirect methods. These are inevitably based on the assumption that some aspects of intellectual functioning are more prone to decline as a result of disease than others. Those functions that are resistant to decline are then used to estimate the premorbid level, and those more susceptible to decline can give an indication of the present level of ability. A comparison between premorbid and present estimates can then be achieved.

The earliest scales designed to measure intellectual decline were based on the assumption that vocabulary is resistant to decline, and so scores on vocabulary tests were used to indicate premorbid levels. The well known instruments based on this principle are the Babcock Examination for the Efficiency of Mental Functioning, the Hunt Minnesota Test for Organic Brain Damage, and the Shipley Institute of Living Scale (2,32,76). The most detailed review of the validity of tests based on the use of vocabulary in this way was provided by Yates (86), but there are some more recent, if less detailed, discussions (45,50).

In brief, these instruments depend on certain assumptions which are only rough approximations to the truth. A number of studies have shown that vocabulary does not always remain unaffected by cerebral pathology, although it may be more resistant to decline than many other facets of cognitive functioning (1,50,55). The correlation between vocabulary scores and IQ is usually substantial but not so high as to avoid there being appreciable error in basing an estimate of IQ solely on vocabulary (86). Finally, the instruments under discussion must assume that were there no pathology the IQ estimated from vocabulary would be the same as that estimated from the tests used to indicate the present level of functioning. In fact, this is often not the case, and it is common experience that normal subjects can show definite differences in ability on different types of intellectual test. The effect of such deviations from the underlying assumptions is cumulative, and it is therefore not surprising that instruments using vocabulary in the measurement of intellectual decline are not accurate enough for clinical use with individual patients.

A very recent development in this type of approach is to use the score on a reading test as the index of premorbid intelligence. It is claimed that reading remains relatively intact in dementia (at least in the early stages) and is much less likely to show deterioration than vocabulary. Nelson and O'Connell (56) published regression equations having fairly small standard errors which enable the various WAIS IQs to be predicted from errors on a reading test. They also attempted to validate their work by comparing demented and normal groups on the amount of intellectual decline indicated by this technique. The level of discrimination was quite good, although there was still some overlap between the two groups. The use of a reading test as a basis for the estimation of premorbid IQ may have minimized some of the problems inherent in the use of vocabulary, but it almost certainly did not eliminate them. It remains to be seen if the same discriminatory power will remain when the technique is cross-validated.

Another popular indirect way of measuring intellectual deterioration is the use of "deterioration indices" based on various combinations of subtest scores from the Wechsler intelligence scales (11,29,82). Wechsler (82) noted that the various subtests of the WAIS tended to decline at different rates as a function of age. In effect, Wechsler's index uses four of the subtests showing least decline with age as indicators of premorbid levels and another four, more sensitive to the effects of age, as measures of the present level. In addition to the gratuitous assumption that the psychological consequences of dementia or brain damage are the same as those of normal aging, the Wechsler deterioration index (together with the many suggested alternatives) involve assumptions similar to those outlined above for the instruments based on vocabulary. Again the assumptions are at best only roughly correct, and the deterioration indices typically do not emerge very well from validation studies when they have been attempted (50). One of the few investigations of Wechsler's index that specifically used elderly demented patients was that of Savage (69). The group mean of the elderly demented subjects was significantly different from that of the controls in the expected direction. The problem is that the amount of overlap was such that one-fourth of the demented group emerged as having less deterioration than the mean level for the controls. Again this does not inspire great confidence when interpreting data obtained from the single case.

Another possible way of estimating the extent of intellectual decline is to use the patient's educational and occupational level as a basis for judging what his IQ must have been. The main difficulty with this method is the considerable variation in IQ found in subjects with given educational or occupational records (28). This variation is not only large, it is greatest among those of lower occupational levels, who inevitably tend to be encountered more often in clinical practice.

It must be concluded that the measurement of intellectual decline from premorbid levels is unsatisfactory. The most promising technique at this point is that based on the use of reading tests. This may be because it has only just been published and others have not yet had a chance to cross-validate it (56). It is possible to test for further intellectual change after the time of initial assessment, but even here there are difficulties caused by the absence of sound test–retest data relating to the various instruments that might be used. To date there appears to have been little or no attempt to measure deterioration in cognitive functioning in a way that is comparable to the means discussed above for estimating decline in general intelligence.

Ongoing Measurement of Change

The preceding section is largely concerned with measuring the amount of decline in cognitive functioning from premorbid levels. A further and relatively neglected aspect of the measurement of change is that relating to ongoing changes. This is particularly important in the evaluation of therapeutic or management techniques (e.g., drugs or behavioral treatments). Such interventions are of course applied after a dementing illness is known to have occurred or is at least strongly suspected, and the need is to monitor the effect of the intervention.

Instruments considered suitable for this role must meet certain characteristics. To avoid "floor effects," they must be pitched at such a level that even moderately demented individuals can achieve more than minimal scores. This may well mean that most conventional psychometric tests are unsuitable for this purpose. Appropriate instruments must also be sensitive to the kind of ongoing changes in functioning likely to be manifest in demented patients and particularly to those that are likely to be influenced by the treatment or intervention under consideration.

Rating scales are one type of measure that could prove useful. A large number of these have been devised for, or used with, the elderly, and many are listed by Salzman et al. (68). Very few seem suitable for the measurement of change (21). An exception is the Stockton Geriatric Rating Scale (48). The original developers of this scale did not envisage it as a measure of change, but an adapted version has been used successfully in this way (21).

Measures based on direct observation are ideally suited to detecting change and have been commonly used for this purpose in many clinical settings. There are very few examples of the use of direct observational techniques with demented patients, but they must have considerable potential because they can be readily adapted to the circumstances of the patient and to dealing with behavior that is of direct clinical relevance. The principles involved in using measures based on direct observation do not vary with the subject population being studied, and these have recently been set out in detail (42).

Another technique with some potential in the ongoing measurement of change is automated assessment (18,44,65). The work in this field is somewhat tentative as yet, but the general technique offers many opportunities to develop indices that are sensitive to alterations in cognitive state. There is also some evidence that automated testing can be used with subjects who are too deteriorated to perform adequately on the usual types of psychometric tests of cognitive functioning (18).

DIAGNOSTIC TESTING

Probably the most common differential diagnosis concerning dementia for which psychological assessment might be appropriate is that between dementia and the functional psychiatric disorders, especially depression. This differential diagnosis is not infrequently encountered in psychogeriatrics. It is also worth taking pains over because, unlike some differential diagnoses in psychiatry, it has marked implications for prognosis and management.

Unless the patient is so deteriorated clinically that specialist investigations to detect cognitive decline would be superfluous, it is unlikely that the single administration of an intelligence test such as the WAIS would be of diagnostic significance. IQ is depressed in dementia but probably not to a great extent in the early stages. The range of IQs found in groups of dements is also large, and hence an IQ is of little value in itself (50,52).

Memory is the function whose decline is mostly readily detected in the early stages of dementia, and therefore tests of verbal learning and/or memory have an obvious rationale as diagnostic tests. Depressed patients may also complain of memory impairments. It has proved difficult to decide whether memory is truly impaired in depression or is merely a by-product of such factors as a generally discrepant reporting of symptoms or alterations in response criteria. The evidence is unfortunately conflicting (30,37,53,54), but it can be stated with confidence that any memory impairment in the functional psychoses is certainly much less severe than that which occurs in dementia.

One of the first memory/learning tests to be devised specifically for use with the elderly was the Inglis Paired Associate Learning Test (33). This test has two parallel forms, and Inglis showed that it gave worthwhile discrimination for patients with and without dementia. Cross-validation studies have been carried out that substantially confirm Inglis' original findings (8,58). Although now somewhat dated, this test continues to have some popularity in studies of dementia, especially in Britain.

Shapiro and Nelson (74) suggested a learning test which involves choosing a set of words the subject is unable to define. These are usually determined by administering one of the standard vocabulary tests such as that in the WAIS. The subject is then taught the meanings of these words by a set procedure. The score on the test relates to how quickly the subject can learn the meanings to a given criterion. The first successful test based on this principle of new word learning was that of Walton and Black and was devised with a view to distinguishing all "organic" from "nonorganic" patients regardless of age (78). It has been used with the elderly and emerges as having a useful level of validity which was confirmed by cross-validation (5,79).

A rather more sophisticated version of the new word learning approach to tests of learning and/or memory was developed by Kendrick specifically for use with psychogeriatric patients (38). This is the Synonym Learning Test (SLT). It is based on the Mill Hill Vocabulary Scale together with an extended list of more difficult words should the subject emerge as being able to define too many of the words in the original Mill Hill scale. The SLT is not used on its own but is administered together with a simple test of motor speed, the Digit Copying Test (DCT).

This small test battery is more sophisticated than most in that its normative data are based on Bayesian statistics (41). The Bayesian model allows base rates to be taken into account. When developing the SLT it was considered that there was an antecedent probability that approximately one-third of those on whom the test battery was used would be demented. This base rate was estimated from psychogeriatric admissions to the Bethlem Royal Hospital, which is a prestigious teaching unit linked to the Institute of Psychiatry in London. A more recent study showed that this proportion is also about right for a much more typical British psychiatric hospital (23). Obviously any users of the SLT and DCT would be well advised to check on the base rates in their own institution and, if necessary, make the appropriate adjustments. The original standardization of the tests and a further cross-validation by Kendrick and his associates showed that very encouraging levels of diagnostic discrimination can be obtained when the SLT and DCT are administered on two occasions a few weeks apart (38,39). Other reports have not been quite so encouraging (83).

Learning tests, and in particular the SLT, have run into a number of problems. They tend to misclassify functional patients with low IQs as demented, and this starts to be a problem when the IQ drops to around 80. Another difficulty is that subjects can find learning tests stressful, which in turn can make them unpleasant to administer. An appreciable minority of elderly subjects refuse to persevere with the SLT until the criterion is reached. To surmount this problem, Kendrick and his associates devised an alternative to the SLT (20,40), the Object Learning Test (OLT), which requires the subject merely to recognize pictures of common objects that they were shown previously. The OLT is quicker to administer than the SLT, is not similarly stressful, and subject refusal is rare. However, a full and detailed report has yet to appear in the literature, and so no final judgment can be made. A diagnostic study in which the OLT and DCT were administered to over 100 psychogeriatric patients was claimed to yield an accuracy level for diagnostic discrimination in excess of 90% (40).

Tests of learning and/or memory are among the most useful diagnostic aids when trying to distinguish between dementia and functional disorders. It has been possible to give only a very brief account of some of the learning/memory tests commonly used in the diagnosis of dementia. A great variety of other memory tests have been devised for use in a variety of circumstances (16), and some of these might also be of value in the diagnosis of dementia. Experimental studies of memory disturbances in dementia might also supply ideas for tests. For example, the free recall procedure appears to give good discrimination between demented and nondemented subjects and also has a high level of subject acceptability (49).

Another group of tests that can be applied to the diagnosis of dementia are the various design-copying tests devised by Bender (3), Benton (4), and Graham and Kendall (25). These tests are usually considered when distinguishing between "organic" and "nonorganic" subjects of all types, but they do have some validity when used to detect dementia. Unfortunately, their discriminatory efficiency is much less impressive than that often obtained for the verbal learning tests (7,12). The main advantage of the design-copying tests seems to be their ease and speed of administration. This also leads to a higher level of subject compliance than is found with some learning tests.

Various forms of neuropsychological assessment can be of assistance in the diagnosis of dementia. Basically the forms of neuropsychological testing tend to remain rather similar regardless of the subject population being studied. A general account of neuropsychological assessment techniques is beyond the scope of this chapter, but suitable descriptions are available elsewhere (45,81). Although early cases of dementia may preserve reasonable levels of orientation, an inability to give satisfactory answers to straightforward questions relating to orientation in space and time must raise suspicions of an organic disorder of some kind (84). Patients with dementia often perform badly on tests of spatial perception and praxis (50,61). Language defects may also be worth looking for, as there is evidence of dysphasic types of disorder in dementia (50). Naming seems to be the most consistently impaired function (67).

One neuropsychological test that has proved to be of particular value in the diagnosis of dementia is the Face-Hand Test (35,36). In this test the subject is touched simultaneously on one hand and one cheek and has to report where he has been touched. This is done initially with the eyes closed and then later, if necessary, with the eyes open. The indications are that this gives worthwhile levels of discrimination between demented and functional patients. However, like many neuropsychological tests, the Face-Hand Test could benefit from better standardization.

Finally, a number of rating scales and questionnaires can be useful in diagnosis. Two instruments appear to be of particular note. The first is the Mental Status Questionnaire, which involves 10 questions relating to orientation and general information (35,36). Three or more errors on this scale are indicative of some degree of organic impairment. In Britain, Pattie and Gilleard have been developing scales which also have useful levels of diagnostic validity and appear to have better normative data than most (22,59). This work was in fact built on an earlier American scale, the Stockton Geriatric Rating Scale (48).

So far the discussion of diagnostic testing has concentrated only on the discrimination of dementia from functional psychiatric disorders. Dementia is not the only form of organic disease of the brain that may occur in older people. In particular, various forms of vascular disease may affect the brain in old age. Some claim to be able to distinguish between the intellectual deterioration produced by Alzheimer's disease and that resulting from vascular etiology (62,64). In a recent discussion of this problem the present writer argued that it is overly optimistic to expect to make this type of discrimination on psychological grounds (52). Psychological assessment may be able to give some hints as to the differential diagnosis between the various forms of organic impairment, but these are limited. For example, the Alzheimer's type of dementia is unlikely to give signs as focal in nature as those of a stroke or tumor, but the power of the discrimination is probably not sufficient to place a great deal of confidence in the findings.

DECISION-MAKING FOR MANAGEMENT

Accurate diagnosis and the measurement of change are important but do not exhaust the decision-making needs when dealing with demented patients. Decisions must still be made about management. The patient may need any of a range of provisions, varying from total residential care in an institution to living as before in the community but with occasional contact by domiciliary services. The patient may benefit from some kind of therapeutic regimen or management program. Decisions about these things are needed, and psychological assessment might have a contribution to make. Psychologists working with demented patients have given comparatively little attention to this aspect of assessment, which probably reflects the underlying attitude of therapeutic nihilism, which is still all too prevalent. Because of the paucity of established work, this section is necessarily somewhat speculative.

One interesting and possibly relevant development is occurring in the field of behavior therapy. After an initial period of development in which the question of assessment was ignored and concern was concentrated on therapeutic techniques, behavior therapists are now trying to develop methods of assessment that will allow them to identify the client's problems, select suitable means of intervention, and monitor effectiveness. The loosely defined selection of techniques that have been proposed for these purposes are subsumed under the title "behavioral assessment" and a recent overview was provided by Ciminero et al. (9). Many of these techniques could have some relevance to work with the demented patient, but the most immediately relevant is probably the form of assessment based on direct observation (42).

Again, behavior rating scales could be of considerable use when making decisions about management if properly designed with this end in view. In fact, many such scales have been developed for this purpose in work with the mentally retarded, and a number have proved extremely useful in clinical practice. Unfortunately, most of the scales that are applicable to older and demented patients (e.g., the Stockton Geriatric Rating Scale) were not designed for use in making this kind of decision (48,77). As a result, they do not cover all the possibly relevant aspects of functioning in a systematic way. In work with children, the use of criterion referenced scales has become quite popular (66,80). In conventional scales and tests, the emphasis is on how well the subject performs on an item in relation to a reference group. Criterion referenced scales ask a question of more immediate practical value—which is whether the subject can perform what is described by the item at an adequate level. For example, the usual norm referenced scale asks how well the subject can tie his shoes, feed himself, etc., in relation to other people his age. The criterion referenced test merely asks whether he can tie his shoes within an appropriate length of time. The particular criterion would presumably be chosen in relation to how competent the subject needs to be to manage independently for this item. If the subject cannot meet the criterion, the criterion referenced scale can then go on to examine whether the subject can adequately carry out certain other activities which might be needed in order to achieve the main task. Criterion referenced scales can therefore be readily directed to everyday skills that might be important in the functional adaptation of the demented patient and, if necessary, extend the analysis by breaking the task down into its constituent parts so that the crucial aspect can be identified for therapeutic intervention.

Despite the established value of this type of scale in work with other handicapped groups (e.g., the mentally retarded) and their obvious relevance for elderly handicapped people where difficulties in the skills required for everyday living also arise, there have been remarkably few attempts to develop the criterion referenced type of scale for use with demented patients. A notable exception are some of the scales developed at the Philadelphia Geriatric Center by Lawton (43). His "Activities of Daily Living Scale" is particularly apposite but probably does not analyze the relevant aspects of behavior in quite enough detail for the planning of any remedial programs aimed at the restitution of lost skills.

In general terms the decision-making processes for making decisions about management in dementia are not different in principle from those appropriate to other patient groups. The types of assessment technique that have proved useful in this role with other handicapped groups (e.g., the mentally retarded) are also likely to be of value with demented patients. What is now required is much more effort in putting these ideas to work with the problem of dementia.

GENERAL DISCUSSION

It can be seen that work on psychological assessment in relation to dementia has had its greatest success in the differential diagnosis of dementia and especially when distinguishing dementia from the functional psychiatric disorders. Much work has also gone into attempts to find ways of measuring the decline in IQ from premorbid levels. The latter exercise has proved difficult, and in my opinion it is doubtful if a clinically satisfactory indirect means for the measurement of decline will ever be found. The problem of devising measures sensitive to change that can be used as dependent variables in the evaluation of various forms of intervention has received little systematic attention. Investigators trying to evaluate any form of treatment or management program tend to use their own *ad hoc* measures, and the measurement of change for this purpose needs to be put on a sounder basis. Another area in need of much more extensive attention is that of methods of assessment which can be used as a basis for making decisions about the detailed management of individual patients and the design of intervention programs where appropriate.

A difficulty that can arise in the psychological assessment of demented patients is in dealing with the more advanced cases who are often regarded as "untestable" (52). By this is usually meant the patient who cannot be tested adequately on the usual kinds of psychometric test. In such cases the diagnosis has typically become so obvious that assessment with a view to differential diagnosis is irrelevant. On the other hand, it may still be useful to be able to measure change (e.g., the response to an altered environment), and decisions may still have to be made about management. It may be possible to extend downward to a limited degree the level at which conventional psychometric tests can be used satisfactorily. The way that elderly subjects respond to psychometric tests can be influenced by operant conditioning procedures, and it may then be possible to shape up subject behavior necessary for testing (31). Nevertheless, the assessment techniques most likely to be of value with the more deteriorated cases will be rating scales and methods based on the direct observation and recording of behavior.

Another development with potential in the assessment of patients for whom conventional psychometric testing is impossible is that of automated testing (18,63). The automated testing devices used so far have been based on the "matching-to-sample" technique developed in the animal laboratory. The subject faces a screen (or set of screens), and a stimulus (or "sample") is projected onto the upper part. Concurrently with this, or after a delay, two "match" stimuli are presented below the "samples." The subject then indicates by pressing a button, or even touching the appropriate part of the screen, which of the two alternatives matches the original sample. It can readily be seen that a very wide range of difficulty can be introduced by manipulating the nature of the stimuli, and a memory element can be introduced by having a delay between "sample" and "match" stimuli. Accurate automatic recording of response latencies on individual trials is also possible and the order of presentation of stimuli can be controlled by computer. Preliminary results have shown that elderly subjects too deteriorated for conventional psychometric testing can perform adequately on such a device (18), and there are reports which indicate that further work along these lines would be worthwhile (44,63).

In conclusion, it appears that many problems involved in the psychological evaluation of the demented patient still require resolution. When conventional forms of psychometric test directed at the traditional problem of differential diagnosis are used, much greater attention needs to be given to the methodological issues outlined earlier in this chapter. Many of the most useful developments in the assessment of dementia may well come from the application of other forms of assessment technique (e.g., rating scales, automated testing, and direct observational methods) to the problems of measuring change and making decisions about management. Rating scales and direct observational methods also have the important advantage that they can be directly related to the kinds of behavioral disturbance or incompetence which make the demented individual a social problem.

REFERENCES

1. Acklesberg, S. B. (1944): *J. Abnorm. Soc. Psychol.,* 39:393–406.
2. Babcock, H. (1930): *Arch. Psychol.,* No. 117.
3. Bender, L. (1946): *Instructions for the Use of the Visual Motor Gestalt Test.* American Orthopsychiatric Association, New York.
4. Benton, A. L. (1963): *The Revised Visual Retention Test.* State University of Iowa Press, Iowa City.

5. Bolton, N., Savage, R. D., and Roth, M. (1967): *Br. J. Psychiatry,* 113:1139–1140.
6. Botwinick, J. (1977): In: *Handbook of the Psychology of Aging,* edited by J. E. Birren and W. K. Schaie, pp. 580–605. Van Nostrand, New York.
7. Brilliant, P. J., and Gynther, M. D. (1963): *J. Consult. Psychol.,* 27:474–479.
8. Caird, W. K., Sanderson, R. E., and Inglis, J. (1962): *J. Ment. Sci.,* 108:368–370.
9. Ciminero, A. R., Calhoun, K. S., and Adams, H. E. (1977): *Handbook of Behavioral Assessment.* Wiley, New York.
10. Cronbach, L. J., and Gleser, G. C. (1965): *Psychological Tests and Personnel Decisions.* University of Illinois Press, Urbana.
11. Crookes, T. G. (1974): *Psychol. Rep.,* 34:374.
12. Crookes, T. G., and McDonald, K. G. (1972): *Br. J. Soc. Clin. Psychol.,* 11:66–69.
13. Davies, G., Hamilton, S., Hendrickson, E., Levy, R., and Post, F. (1977): *Age Ageing,* 6:156–162.
14. Desai, M. (1952): *Br. J. Med. Psychol.,* 25:48–53.
15. Eisdorfer, C., and Cohen, L. D. (1961): *J. Abnorm. Soc. Psychol.,* 62:520–527.
16. Erickson, R. C., and Scott, M. L. (1977): *Psychol. Bull.,* 84:1130–1149.
17. Fine, E. W., Lewis, D., Villa-Landa, I., and Blakemore, C. B. (1970): *Br. J. Psychiatry,* 117:157–161.
18. Gedye, J. L., and Miller, E. (1970): In: *The Psychological Assessment of Mental and Physical Handicap,* edited by P. J. Mittler, pp. 735–760. Methuen, London.
19. Gerboth, R. (1950): *J. Consult. Psychol.,* 15:365–370.
20. Gibson, A. J., and Kendrick, D. C. (1976): *Bull. Br. Psychol. Soc.,* 29:200–201.
21. Gilleard, C. J. (1978): An investigation into the nature of behavioral change in the dementias of old age. Ph.D. thesis, University of Leeds.
22. Gilleard, C. J., and Pattie, A. (1977): *Br. J. Psychiatry,* 131:90–94.
23. Glaister, B. R. (1971): *Br. J. Soc. Clin. Psychol.,* 10:367–374.
24. Goldfried, M. R., and Kent, R. N. (1972): *Psychol. Bull.,* 77:409–420.
25. Graham, F. K., and Kendall, B. S. (1960): *Percept. Motor Skills,* Monogr. Suppl. No. 11.
26. Guertin, W. H., Rabin, A. L., Frank, G. H., and Ladd, C. E. (1962): *Psychol. Bull.,* 59:1–26.
27. Hamister, R. C. (1949): *J. Consult. Psychol.,* 13:39–43.
28. Harrell, T. W., and Harrell, M. S. (1945): *Educ. Psychol. Meas.,* 5:229–239.
29. Hewson, L. R. (1949): *J. Nerv. Ment. Dis.,* 109:158–183.
30. Hilbert, N. M., Niederehe, G., and Kahn, R. L. (1976): *Educ. Gerontol.,* 1:131–146.
31. Hoyer, W. J., Labouvie, G. V., and Baltes, P. B. (1973): *Hum. Devel.,* 16:233–242.
32. Hunt, H. F. (1943): *J. Appl. Psychol.,* 27:375–386.
33. Inglis, J. (1959): *J. Ment. Sci.,* 105:440–448.
34. Jacobs, E. A., Winter, P. M., Alvis, H. J., and Small, S. M. (1969): *N. Engl. J. Med.,* 281:753–757.
35. Kahn, R. L., Goldfarb, A. I., Pollack, M., and Peck, A. (1960): *Am. J. Psychiatry,* 117:326–328.
36. Kahn, R. L., and Miller, N. E. (1978): In: *Clinical Psychology in Gerontology,* edited by E. Siegler, M. Storandt, and M. Elias, pp. 246–259. Plenum Press, New York.
37. Kahn, R. L., Zarit, S. H., Hilbert, N. M., and Niederehe, G. (1975): *Arch. Gen. Psychiatry,* 32:1569–1573.
38. Kendrick, D. C. (1965): *Br. J. Soc. Clin. Psychol.,* 4:141–148.
39. Kendrick, D. C. (1967): *Br. J. Med. Psychol.,* 40:173–178.
40. Kendrick, D. C., Gibson, A. J., and Moyes, I. C. A. (1978): *Bull. Br. Psychol. Soc.,* 31:177–178.
41. Kendrick, D. C., Parboosingh, R.-C., and Post, F. (1965): *Br. J. Soc. Clin. Psychol.,* 4:63–71.
42. Kent, R. N., and Foster, S. L. (1978): In: *Handbook of Behavioral Assessment,* edited by A. R. Ciminero, K. S. Calhoun, and H. E. Adams, pp. 279–328. Wiley, New York.
43. Lawton, M. P. (1971): *J. Am. Geriatr. Soc.,* 29:465–481.
44. Levy, R., and Post, F. (1975): *Age Ageing,* 4:110–115.
45. Lezak, M. D. (1976): *Neuropsychological Assessment.* Oxford University Press, London.
46. Matarazzo, R. G., Wiens, A. N., Matarazzo, J. D., and Monaugh, T. (1973): *J. Clin. Psychol.,* 29:124–197.
47. Meehl, P. E., and Rosen, A. (1955): *Psychol. Bull.,* 52:194–216.
48. Meer, B., and Baker, J. A. (1966): *J. Gerontol.,* 21:392–403.

49. Miller, E. (1971): *Neuropsychologia,* 9:75–78.
50. Miller, E. (1977): *Abnormal Ageing.* Wiley, London.
51. Miller, E. (1977): *Br. J. Soc. Clin. Psychol.,* 16:77–83.
52. Miller, E. (1980): In: *Handbook of Mental Health and Aging,* edited by J. E. Birren and R. B. Sloan. Prentice-Hall, Englewood Cliffs, N.J.
53. Miller, E., and Lewis, P. (1977): *J. Abnorm. Psychol.,* 86:84–86.
54. Miller, W. R. (1975): *Psychol. Bull.,* 82:238–260.
55. Nelson, H. E. (1953): An experimental investigation of intellectual speed and power in mental disorders. Ph.D. thesis, University of London.
56. Nelson, H. E., and O'Connell, A. (1978): *Cortex,* 14:234–244.
57. Nott, P. N., and Fleminger, J. J. (1975): *Acta Psychiatr. Scand.,* 51:210–217.
58. Parsons, P. L. (1965): *Br. J. Prev. Soc. Med.,* 19:43–58.
59. Pattie, A., and Gilleard, C. J. (1975): *Br. J. Psychiatry,* 127:489–493.
60. Payne, R. W., and Jones, H. G. (1957): *J. Clin. Psychol.,* 13:117–121.
61. Pearce, J., and Miller, E. (1973): *Clinical Aspects of Dementia.* Bailliere Tindall, London.
62. Perez, F. I., Gay, J. R. A., Taylor, R. L., and Rivera, V. M. (1975): *Can. J. Neurol. Sci.,* 2:347–355.
63. Perez, F. I., Hruska, N. A., Stell, R. I., and Rivera, V. M. (1978): *Can. J. Neurol. Sci.,* 5:307–312.
64. Perez, F. I., Rivera, V. M., Meyer, J. S., Gay, J. R. A., Taylor, R. L., and Matthew, N. T. (1975): *J. Neurol. Neurosurg. Psychiatry,* 38:533–540.
65. Perez, F. I., Stell, R. I., Hruska, N. A., and Rivera, V. M. (1978): *Can. J. Neurol. Sci.,* 5:307–312.
66. Popham, W. J., and Husek, T. R. (1969): *J. Educ. Meas.,* 6:1–9.
67. Rochford, G. (1971): *Neuropsychologia,* 9:437–443.
68. Salzman, C., Shader, R. I., Kochansky, G. E., and Cronin, D. M. (1972): *J. Am. Geriatr. Soc.,* 20:209–214.
69. Savage, R. D. (1971): In: *Recent Developments in Psychogeriatrics,* edited by D. W. Kay and A. Walk, pp. 51–61. Royal Medical Psychological Association, London.
70. Savage, R. D. (1973): In: *Handbook of Abnormal Psychology,* edited by H. J. Eysenck, pp. 645–688. Pitman, London.
71. Schaie, K. W., and Gribbin, K. (1975): *Annu. Rev. Psychol.,* 26:65–96.
72. Schaie, K. W., and Schaie, J. P. (1977): In: *Handbook of the Psychology of Aging,* edited by J. E. Birren and K. W. Schaie, pp. 692–723. Van Nostrand, New York.
73. Schaie, K. W., and Labouvie-Vief, G. V. (1974): *Devel. Psychol.,* 10:305–320.
74. Shapiro, M. B., and Nelson, H. E. (1955): *Br. J. Med. Psychol.,* 4:205–280.
75. Shapiro, M. B., Post, F., Löfving, B., and Inglis, J. (1956): *J. Ment. Sci.,* 102:233–246.
76. Shipley, W. C. (1940): *J. Psychol.,* 9:371–377.
77. Taylor, H. G., and Bloom, L. M. (1974): *J. Gerontol.,* 29:190–193.
78. Walton, D., and Black, D. A. (1957): *Br. J. Med. Psychol.,* 20:270–279.
79. Walton, D., White, J. G., Black, D. A., and Young, A. J. (1959): *Br. J. Med. Psychol.,* 22:213–220.
80. Ward, J. (1970): *Br. J. Educ. Psychol.,* 40:314–323.
81. Warrington, E. K. (1970): In: *The Psychological Assessment of Mental and Physical Handicap,* edited by P. J. Mittler, pp. 261–288. Methuen, London.
82. Wechsler, D. (1958): *The Measurement and Appraisal of Adult Intelligence.* Williams & Wilkins, Baltimore.
83. Whitehead, A. (1971): An investigation of learning in elderly psychiatric patients. Ph.D. thesis, University of London.
84. Williams, M. (1970): In: *The Psychological Assessment of Mental and Physical Handicaps,* edited by P. J. Mittler, pp. 319–339. Methuen, London.
85. Woods, R. T., and Britton, P. G. (1977): *Age Ageing,* 6:104–112.
86. Yates, A. J. (1956): *J. Ment. Sci.,* 102:409–440.

DISCUSSION

Dr. Goldman: I was struck, as I am sure many others were, by the relative competence of the dements in Dr. Miller's presentation. While there is a large body of literature on memory impairment with age, on the other hand, the dements whom I have had the opportunity of having to work with can hardly remember their names, let alone a series of words.

I wonder what the criteria were for dementia in his presentation, and whether the extreme form of dementia that I see is an extension of ordinary senile loss of memory or whether it is an entirely different process?

Dr. Miller: With regard to this, I really should have pointed out that in the experimental studies that I had been involved with, the patient population consisted of individuals from a neurological unit. They were presenile cases who had been referred early in order to exclude the possibility that they suffered from something treatable. Accordingly, they were not the sort of demented patients you get in a large institution; they were not chronically hospitalized demented patients. That is why they could do the sort of things that many other populations of demented patients couldn't.

Dr. Halpe: The analysis of the breakdown of the brain may lead to more powerful theories about a mechanism of cognitive function. Professor Roth, would you care to speculate on the possibility of using the studies of dementia that we listened to today to produce theories about human cognition and human behavior in general?

Sir Martin: I should like to select first one point that links up with something that Dr. Miller said.

There is an unexplained sequence that occurs in virtually every form of dementia. I don't see that it need necessarily be that we always find recent memory, or the ability to acquire and retain new knowledge, is impaired more severely than remote memory from the outset. The deficit then becomes more extensive, involving general intellectual functions, power of abstraction and reasoning, problem solving and numerical ability, perceptual accuracy, and so on.

The deterioration always proceeds in this direction, so that one may find relatively pure amnestic syndromes. But one never finds general intellectual deficit with memory intact in individuals undergoing deterioration. If an explanation for this sequential order could be discovered, it would probably shed important light on cognitive functions in general. For there is no reason why the change should always proceed in this direction. There must be something fundamental about the memory disturbance. Most psychiatrists are familiar with one or two individuals who have a vast memory store relating to restricted fields of knowledge but who are mentally subnormal. I am referring to the "idiot savant." On a quite different intellectual level, there are people capable of remarkable feats of calculation, with phenomenal memories who are not particularly gifted mathematicians. In contrast, the creative mathematician may not excel in arithmetic. The point I am making is that memory and general intelligence seem to vary independently to some extent. Yet the process of dementia appears to always afflict the former with selective severity before it affects problem solving and reasoning ability. All this is, of course, highly speculative.

Dr. Gustafson: To Dr. Miller, I would like to comment on aphasia in patients with dementia. I agree that the classic focal types of aphasia are rare in this patient group. However, I think it is very important to analyze speech disturbances in dementia. Our group in Lund has followed the development of aphasia and other dysfunctions in patients with presenile dementia. We found that the type of aphasia, like other subsymptoms, gave important information for differential diagnosis. Aphasia in patients with Alzheimer's disease is different from that in patients with diffuse cortical atrophy predominating fronto-temporally, what we usually call Pick's disease. I think that the designation "global aphasia" should be avoided when describing dementia.

Dr. Merskey: In regard to Dr. Miller's presentation, I would like to say that I do get substantial help from psychologist colleagues who use systems of qualified scaling that go beyond the point where the Wechsler leaves off.

It may be that the systems they have developed so far are limited to the patients we have in our own facility. But, for example, the extended scale for dementia described by Ed Hersch (3) and the London psychogeriatric rating scale (1,2) both yield reliable information about the degree of dementia of the patient.

They change appropriately with time as deterioration proceeds, and give us appropriate prediction as to the best ward placement of individual patients. I think there is valuable work going on, in terms of psychological quantification of change in dementia.

Dr. Miller: Dr. Mersky has suggested that some of the kinds of things that I denied were going on, are going on with regard to assessment.

I will half take his point. I agree that there are some interesting developments in measurement, but generally speaking, I stand by my point. Very little, I think, is being done in terms of solving important problems relating to assessment.

Dr. Gurland: I would like to single out one point for reply. That is the contrast between the usefulness of rating scales and of diagnosis for various purposes.

Earlier, I was discussing the use of these devices for studying an epidemiological phenomenon. I was not wishing to convey any primacy for rating scales as opposed to diagnosis for every situation. Several of the US-UK Cross National Project's studies have considered the relative strengths of rating scales and diagnosis.

We have found that rating scales are more valid than are some diagnostic concepts in the hands of some groups of psychiatrists. In the hands of other psychiatrists, diagnosis is a better predictor than is a rating scale. We have seen this with respect to predictive outcome or the selection of treatment, and even with respect to the relationship between physiological tests and the classification of psychopathology.

In our epidemiological studies, we have used a wide variety of techniques for classifying people, including rating scales, and face-to-face diagnosis. We look to find a plausible convergence in the results of these different methods of classification for whatever issue we are studying. Our series of studies has shown that we have no a priori way of being able to determine the correct or best method of classification. When these results do not converge, we are left with a research challenge: Which is right or which is the most useful research lead. Thus, the issue is not whether the MSQ is more or less valid than diagnosis, but what sense can be made out of the fact that one obtains certain sociocultural correlations with MSQ and somewhat different ones with diagnosis.

REFERENCES

1. Hersch, E. L. (1979): Development and application of the extended scale for dementia. *J. Am. Geriatr. Soc.,* Vol. 27.
2. Hersch, E. L., Csapo, K. G., and Palmer, R. B. (1977): Development and usefulness of the London Psychogeriatric Rating Scale. In: *Proceeding of the Fourth Annual Meeting of the Ontario Psychogeriatric Association,* pp. 141–144.
3. Hersch, E. L., Kral, V. A., and Palmer, R. B. (1978): Clinical value of the London Psychogeriatric Rating Scale *J. of Am. Geriatr. Soc.,* Vol. 26.

*Clinical Aspects of Alzheimer's Disease and
Senile Dementia*, (Aging, Vol. 15), edited by
Nancy E. Miller and Gene D. Cohen.
Raven Press, New York 1981.

Drug Treatment of Cognitive Impairment in Alzheimer's Disease and the Late Life Dementias

*H. Harris Funkenstein, **Robert Hicks, †Maurice W. Dysken,
and †John M. Davis

*Department of Medicine (Neurology), Peter Bent Brigham Hospital, Department of
Neurology, Boston Children's Hospital and Harvard Medical School, Boston, Massachusetts
02115; **Department of Clinical Psychopharmacology and Section on Geriatric Psychiatry,
Department of Psychiatry and Behavioral Sciences, The University of Texas Medical School
at Houston, Houston, Texas 77025;†Illinois State Psychiatric Institute and Department
of Psychiatry, University of Chicago School of Medicine, Chicago, Illinois 60612*

Normal aging produces a number of changes in the central nervous system with important consequences for the optimal functioning of the individual. In terms of gross structure, the brain may lose 20% of its weight with age (11) as sulci widen and ventricles enlarge (110). Early studies (69) noted a decline in cerebral blood flow and oxygen utilization with normal aging, but more recent investigations (123) observed no such decrements when the effects found in patients with vascular or degenerative disease are excluded. The degree to which these changes represent normal aging as opposed to senile cortical atrophy is difficult to specify, especially during the eighth and ninth decades, when the changes frequently accelerate and are found in a substantial proportion of the population (67). Studies of neurotransmitter changes in the aging and senile brain (25,68,88) hold special potential relevance for the pharmacologic treatment of cognitive decline: It may become possible, by restoring diminished precursors or the actual transmitter themselves, to facilitate synaptic function in a manner similar to that already employed in, for example, Parkinson's disease.

Psychologically, aging brings a number of important changes in behavior and intellectual function. As Critchley (20) reviewed, the basic neurological examination is changed in many important respects, resembling to lesser degree the alterations seen in frontal lobe atrophy and Parkinson's disease. Intellectually, some decline is inevitable, although the precise nature and extent remain controversial (70,112). Cross-sectional studies show a tendency for a gradual decline in scores on the Wechsler Adult Intelligence Scale (WAIS)—with declines in the performance subtests (especially digit symbol, picture arrangement, and block design) exceeding those on the verbal subtests, and with vocabulary and information remaining relatively intact (12). Recent studies show that aged individuals are frequently more cautious in their approach to problems, striving for a low

---

** Deceased.

error rate at the expense of markedly slowed performance (15,16). Eisdorfer et al. (34) suggested that alterations in autonomic arousal (as measured by pulse rate, galvanic skin reflex, and plasma free fatty acid mobilization) may play a role in the learning deficits of elderly males, although this observation is not confirmed by a similar study employing a slightly different methodology (116). This suggestion, although little explored in the literature, has nonetheless considerable potential importance for the treatment of cognitive decline in view of the large number of psychotherapeutic agents thought to alter the level of arousal.

In addition to the problems posed by normal aging, further problems are posed for the drug treatment of cognitive decline by the large and growing number of demented persons. Recent work appears to argue against the simple view of dementia as an inevitable outcome of aging. Studies of 800 patients in institutional settings over 10 years, beginning at ages 75 or 80 on the average, show only a small incidence of senile dementia in those free of the disease at the onset of the study (72). The Duke Longitudinal Study provides further support for the notion of functional integrity in aging (94,95). Females with senile dementia are overrepresented in the demented population, even after one corrects for their greater longevity. A number of psychometric studies indicate that the memory and performance deficits of individuals with senile dementia are qualitatively different from those of age-matched otherwise normal elderly (86,126). This is especially true of tasks requiring instrumental modalities, e.g., the manipulation of objects in space and complex visual and linguistic discriminations. Despite the obvious importance of a detailed analysis of the cognitive deficit in dementia, there are very few longitudinal studies of dementing persons.

A large number of pharmacologic attempts to improve cognitive performance were predicated on the assumption that most such patients suffer from a variant of cerebrovascular disease. This assumption is clearly untrue. Most cases of senile dementia [70 to 80% by the estimate of Tomlinson et al. (129)] reflect the histopathological changes in the cortex and hippocampus characteristic of Alzheimer's disease: neurofibrillary tangles, senile plaques, and granulovacuolar degeneration. The evidence that these changes bear no relation to the degree of atherosclerosis has been provided by a number of studies (113,129). Their relationship to the clinical deficits of dementia is clearly established (105,129). The mental changes of dementia embrace memory, intellect, mood, personality, and behavior (86). Disorientation, agitation, psychosis, and paranoia can also be observed (116), especially in the presence of sensory deficits or after the injudicious use of sedative medications which impair reality testing. Depression is a frequent accompaniment of dementing processes. Alleged successes for some drugs in improving cognitive performance may reflect concurrent improvement in either mood or motivation.

The following sections review the major classes of drugs employed to improve cognitive function and the studies that have attempted to assess their usefulness. In some cases, the selection of drug is based on certain physiological or psychological theories regarding the nature of impaired cognition in the elderly and/or demented (e.g., oxygen, vasodilators, stimulants, anticoagulants, and choline). In other cases, however, this selection is based on the clinical observations of individual investigators (e.g., procaine, isoprinosine, piracetam). As mentioned above, even the "logically" chosen drugs often involve a selection process based on erroneous conceptions regarding the nature of the aging process and the underlying pathology involved in dementing illness. Fortunately, as indicated below, the drugs under consideration rarely have a single action, and beneficial effects may issue from alterations in cerebral metabolism or neurotransmitter systems rather than from dilatation of the cerebral vasculature or protein anabolism.

SPECIFIC AGENTS

Cerebral "Vasodilators"

Drugs which increase blood flow by an action on blood vessels constitute an important line of therapeutic investigation in the treatment of the elderly. The mechanism of all of these agents involves a direct effect on vascular smooth muscle, resulting in decreased cerebral vascular resistance and increased cerebral blood flow (64). Rationale for their use relies on the observation that cerebral blood flow declines with age (123) and in the most common forms of dementia (91). Most authorities, however, consider cerebral blood flow reductions in dementia to reflect a diminished metabolic need of a shrunken cerebral tissue rather than a primary step in the pathogenesis of the disease. It is also doubtful if vasodilating drugs are really efficacious for either improving cerebral perfusion or stimulating increased oxygen consumption (111). Nonetheless, a number of studies seem to demonstrate that some of these agents may be efficacious in treating elderly patients with dementing illness. Drugs in this class include the following.

Papaverine (Pavabid®)

There are uncontrolled studies (e.g., refs. 32,74,85) suggesting a clinical effectiveness for papaverine in the treatment of mood disturbance, cognitive impairment, and social dysfunction in the elderly. However, of six controlled studies on this agent, only two reported positive results (102,125). Of the others, two (9,104) found papaverine to be less effective than the vasodilator Hydergine® (discussed in more detail below). One study (81) found it to be no more effective than either the central nervous system (CNS) stimulant pentylenetetrazol (Metrazol®) (see below) or niacin, and one (18) found it no greater than placebo in clinical effect. The two positive studies, moreover, raise several methodological questions. Stern's study (125) involved a double-blind crossover approach which found papaverine moderately superior to placebo in improving 13 of 15 symptoms associated with chronic brain syndrome. These conclusions, however, were based on combined ratings by six staff members. The charge nurse was the only one privy to the code. Her ratings were included in the consolidated weekly scores but were weighted only 25%. Ritter et al. (102) compared symptoms before, during, and after treatment with either placebo or papaverine 600 mg/day in a state hospital population. The placebo and drug groups improved, with significantly greater improvement in the drug-treated group for conceptual organization, mannerisms, and degree of cooperation but not for memory. These findings raise the question of how much improvement could be considered simply the result of increased attention. [Shader has unpublished data on seven treatment subjects and eight controls showing no apparent effect of papaverine when given at 600 mg/day (114). However, he raises the question of whether the negative results found in his study and in other negative studies employing a similar research design might reflect inadequate dosage (115)].

Pharmacological evidence suggests that papaverine is a dopamine antagonist. Duvoisin (27) reported a case in which papaverine interfered with the therapeutic response to L-DOPA in a patient with Parkinson's disease. In addition, Gardos et al. (42) observed that papaverine had a beneficial effect in tardive dyskinesia. Both reports are consistent with a proposed antidopaminergic action in man. There is also evidence that papaverine acts by phosphodiesterase inhibition (53).

Isoxsuprine hydrochloride (Vasodilan®)

Uncontrolled studies (10,137) appear to confirm the efficacy of isoxsuprine hydrochloride in senile patients, but the only controlled studies thus far have concentrated on cerebral arteriosclerosis (3) and episodic disorders (e.g., headache and dizziness) which can be attributed to cerebral ischemia (23). A recent study (18) showed no benefit with isoxsuprine in the treatment of senile dementia.

There is evidence that this drug acts primarily by beta-receptor stimulation (89).

Cyclandelate (Cyclospasmol®)

Clinical studies of cyclandelate, uncontrolled (122,132) and controlled (2,6, 38,39,51,63,138), appear to demonstrate benefits in some groups of geriatric patients. The drug has been shown to increase cerebral blood flow and cortical perfusion rates (41,42) by acting predominantly at the arteriolar and capillary levels (33). It should be noted, however, that no invariable improvement in ischemic brain damage results when cerebral blood flow is increased (33). The controlled studies, utilizing double-blind conditions and placebo use, employed doses ranging from 400 to 1,600 mg daily. Not every positive study indicated improvement from baseline in the drug-treated group. In their 12-month study of 21 patients suffering from cerebral arteriosclerosis, Young et al. (138) showed that patients on placebo deteriorated significantly on various psychometric, behavioral, and neurological parameters, whereas such a decline was absent in the cyclandelate-treated group.

A more recent double-blind, placebo-controlled, crossover study, however, casts doubt on the efficacy of cyclandelate: Westreich et al. (135) studied 24 demented patients with cerebral atherosclerosis who were subjected to an extensive medical screening battery and a number of psychometric tests designed to assess visual spatial perception, memory, intelligence, and logical thinking. During the 12-week study, there were no significant differences between drug and placebo in improving higher cortical function. Further work needs to be done to establish whether cyclandelate has any practical benefit.

Dehydroergotoxin (Hydergine®)

Dehydroergotoxin, a mixture of ergot alkaloids (dihydroergocristine mesylate, dihydroergokriptine mesylate, and dihydroergocornine mesylate), is usually administered sublingually. It is probably the most frequently prescribed drug for the treatment of cognitive impairment secondary to cerebrovascular insufficiency and senile dementia. Marketed initially as a vasodilator by virtue of its adrenolytic and direct vasomotor activity, recent evidence suggests that its actions include: stimulation of nerve cell metabolism (87), interference with norepinephrine uptake (93), and inhibition of phosphodiesterase activity (17). Increases in jugular pyruvate/lactate ratio suggest that increased cerebral blood flow may result from improved cerebral metabolism, rather than vice versa (57).

Table 1 presents a total of 18 Hydergine efficacy studies that meet criteria for a carefully controlled study. Fourteen of these studies found Hydergine superior to placebo in disturbances of memory, mood, and social function. Of the three negative studies, one employed a low daily dose of drug (40), and the other two did not hold up in attempts at replication, which in one case (106) involved a longer period of study and in the other (100) employed a parallel group instead of a crossover design.

The actual therapeutic effect of Hydergine, however, is unclear, particularly in terms of the symptoms that are suggested to improve. For example, the "target symptoms" followed in these studies are heterogenous, including poor memory, apathy and other mood disturbance, and dyssocial behavior. Some of these studies (e.g., refs. 30,44,106) specifically found no improvement in memory function despite apparent gains in mood, confidence, and sociability. Many of these studies, moreover, do not make it possible to assess whether Hydergine actually acts by improving mood and lessening anxiety, thus improving test performance that was depressed for emotional reasons. This possibility is suggested by the observations of Shader and Goldsmith (115), who compared Hydergine and imipramine to placebo. They found both of the drugs superior to placebo, but only after 9 weeks of therapy—a time course suggesting antidepressant action as a possible, at least partial, basis for Hydergine's efficacy. [We presented typical data showing that, with continuous treatment over a time

TABLE 1. *Summary of adequately controlled studies on Hydergine*

Study	Year	Ref.	No. of pts.	DB/placebo	Max. daily dose (mg) and route of admin.[a]	Duration (weeks)	Results
Hofstatter et al.	1955	56	35	Yes/Yes	3.0 (?)	6	+
Hollister	1955	57	26	Yes/Yes	4.0 (s.l.)	8	+
Forster et al.	1955	40	15	Yes/Yes	1.5 (s.l.)	?	−
Gerin	1969	44	39	Yes/Yes	3.0 (s.l.)	12	++
Triboletti & Ferri	1969	130	59	Yes/Yes	3.0 (s.l.)	12	++
Grill & Broicher	1969	49	31	Yes/Yes	3.0 (?)	6	++
Ditch et al.	1971	24	40	Yes/Yes	3.0 (s.l.)	12	+++
Rao & Norris	1971	97	57	Yes/Yes	3.0 (s.l.)	12	+++
Banen	1972	8	78	Yes/Yes	3.0 (s.l.)	12	++
Roubicek et al.	1972	106	4	No/No	0.6 (i.v. & s.c.)	15 days	−
Roubicek et al.	1972	106	44	Yes/Yes	4.5 (?)	12	+
Jennings	1972	62	50	Yes/Yes	3.0 (s.l.)	12	−
Arrigo et al.	1973	4	20	Yes/Yes	4.5 (?)	12	++
Rehman[b]	1973	100	46	Yes/Yes	4.5 (?)	12	+++
Rehman[c]	1973	100	30	Yes/Yes	4.5 (?)	12	++
McConnachie	1973	84	52	Yes/Yes	4.5 (?)	12	+++
Thibault	1974	128	48	Yes/Yes	6.0 (?)	12	++
Gaitz et al.	1977	43	54	Yes/Yes	3.0 (s.l.)	24	+

[a] s.l. = sublingual. i.v. = intravenous. s.c. = subcutaneous.
[b] Crossover design at 8 weeks.
[c] Parallel-group study (no crossover).

period of 12 to 24 weeks, Hydergine produces continued improvement (Figs. 1 and 2). The longer the study, the greater is the difference between improvement means. Figure 1 presents mean factor scores along four dimensions derived from the Sandox Chemical Assessment Geriatric Scale, or SCAG (43). The cognitive dysfunction axis is characterized by confusion, mental dullness, memory impairment, disorientation, and lack of self-care. It should be noted that this score is based on observer ratings and not on the results of psychological testing. Although the drug-placebo differences are small, they appear consistently in a large number of patients, giving a clear, statistically significant difference.]

As noted, studies by Bazo (9) and Rosen (104) compared the response to Hydergine to that produced by papaverine and found a superior effect for the former drug in most aspects of patient performance. It is tempting to hypothesize that in this population papaverine lacks significant antidepressant effects, which may account for the difference. This notion is consistent with the conclusions of Shader and Goldsmith (115), who extensively reviewed some of the studies on Hydergine and other "vasodilators."

In summary, it appears that Hydergine does benefit some elderly or mildly demented subjects, although it probably does not do so by virtue of any vasodilator action. Evidence in favor of this conclusion comes from the above studies, which were carried out in a number of centers, academic and nonacademic, and resulted in consistent findings along a variety of objective outcome measures. Further research should attempt to define the nature of the psychological function affected, particularly the degree to which improved attention and memory (both measurable) reflect improved mood.

Nicotinic acid

Nicotinic acid has for some time been known to possess vasodilating properties, which manifest chiefly as peripheral flushing after large doses of the drug. In an initial study, Lehmann and Ban (79) reported apparent improved performance on a number of perceptual and psychomotor tasks which correlated with a beneficial response to carbon dioxide inhalation. However, their subsequent follow-up report (30) was not as optimistic for a larger group of geriatric patients.

Miscellaneous Vasodilators

A recent review by Ban (7) included several other vasodilators. Many had theoretically possible but essentially undocumented therapeutic efficacy; these included carbon dioxide, either by inhalation or as a result of increased blood concentration secondary to carbonic anydrase inhibitor administration; tocopherol (vitamin E); and serotonin antagonists, e.g., methysergide.

CNS Stimulants

The CNS stimulants—which include pentylenetetrazol (Metrozol®), caffeine pipradrol, methylphenidate (Ritalin®), and the amphetamines—have been used

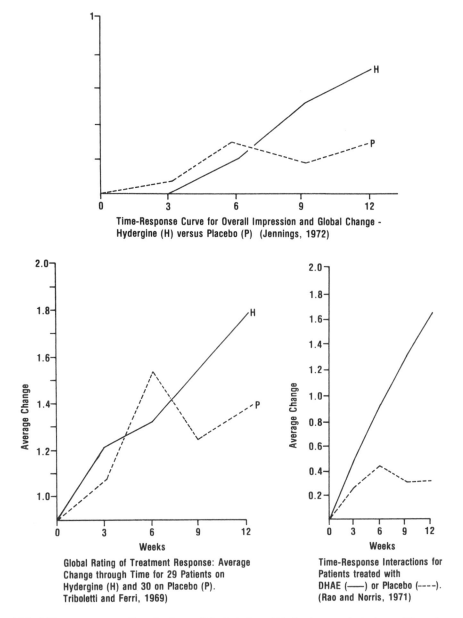

Time-Response Curve for Overall Impression and Global Change -
Hydergine (H) versus Placebo (P) (Jennings, 1972)

Global Rating of Treatment Response: Average
Change through Time for 29 Patients on
Hydergine (H) and 30 on Placebo (P).
Triboletti and Ferri, 1969)

Time-Response Interactions for
Patients treated with
DHAE (——) or Placebo (----).
(Rao and Norris, 1971)

FIG. 1. Time response ratings for three clinical studies of Hydergine conducted over 12 weeks. (From refs. 62,97,130.)

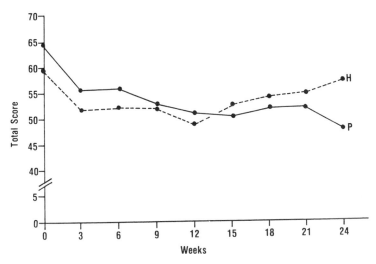

FIG. 2. Time response ratings of hydergine over 24 weeks. (From ref. 43.)

alone or in combination with vitamins as a means of improving mood and psychomotor performance (pipradrol combined with vitamins in an alcohol elixir goes by the name of Alertonic®).

The literature on the efficacy of the CNS stimulants is extensive, especially that on pentylenetetrazol, which Lehmann and Ban (79) comprehensively reviewed. There are numerous uncontrolled studies reporting benefits of this agent to institutionalized, and hence severely affected, subjects. However, the controlled studies are for the most part negative. For example, in 16 controlled studies reviewed by Lehmann and Ban, only 5 showed clear improvement over placebo. This improvement, moreover, was manifest only in ratings of ward behavior and/or global scales, with improvement on psychological testing being only minimal at best. Some of the better controlled studies cited were unequivocally negative (76,81). In a more recent study on pentylenetetrazol, Cole and Branconnier (18) administered 600 to 800 mg/day for 12 weeks to elderly community volunteers with mild memory difficulty. Although they found a modest advantage over placebo on the results of a neuropsychological battery of tests, many patients were unimproved.

Magnesium Pemaline (Cylert®)

The serious side effects accompanying stimulant medication in the elderly led some investigators to try magnesium pemaline (Cylert®), a compound sometimes used in the treatment of hyperactive children because of its mild stimulant effect (60). Early optimism (96), however, was not borne out by subsequent clinical trials (31,127). (See also *RNA-like Compounds,* below).

Procaine Hydrochloride (Gerovital-H3®)

Jarvik and Milne (61) provide a review of the history of the "elixir" procaine hydrochloride beginning with its introduction in Rumania during the late 1950s. Although "special qualities" for Gerovital-H3 have been claimed, it apparently differs little from procaine hydrochloride solutions commercially available in the United States; any differences that do exist are probably quantitative and not qualitative.

The drug, given by intramuscular injection, is rapidly absorbed from the injection site. It is hydrolyzed by pseudocholinesterase (plasma cholinesterase procaine esterase)—mainly in the plasma but also to some degree in the liver— to form para-aminobenzoic acid (PABA) and diethylaminoethanol (DEAE), which are eliminated by urinary excretion and/or further biotransformation(s) (61). It is therefore contraindicated in patients on anticholinesterases (e.g., neostigmine, Prostigmin®) or who are known to have a pseudocholinesterase deficiency. It also interferes with sulfonamides, which act by blocking bacterial synthesis of folic acid from PABA.

In terms of effect, this agent was reported in East European medical centers to improve mood and reduce confusion in senile patients. Sakalis et al. (108) found that Gerovital had a mild euphoriant effect in 10 senile patients with depression. However, Kral et al. (71) carried out a more extensive trial in senile and arteriosclerotic patients with largely negative results.

Renewed interest in this drug has resulted from the observation that it is a reversible monoamine oxidase (MAO) inhibitor (83). Since aging has been associated with decreasing MAO activity (103), this provided a rationale for Gerovital's use and an explanation for its purported activity (5).

Anabolic Substances

As noted earlier, brain weight and cell number decline with age; attempts to reverse this decline by prescribing agents capable of producing protein anabolism or by improving cellular metabolism have occasionally been reported. None of these agents, however, succeeds in actually restoring brain tissue.

Fluoxymesterone is anabolic and androgenic. Given to institutionalized patients, it produces an improved sense of well-being and greater appetite, with mild sedation (73). The drug was given over a 6- to 9-month period, during which recall of meaningful material improved while memory for visually presented arbitrary material declined. Other investigators have commented on the favorable results of increased motivation on the learning of material familiar or relevant to the subject in geriatric patients. There is also evidence that improvement on fluoxymesterone is seen primarily in individuals with mild impairment on other tests of cognitive function (78).

Pyritinol (or *Pyrithioxine*) is reported to improve glucose metabolism in subjects with depressed metabolism secondary to organic dementia and even in those with normal rates of metabolism (126). Scattered reports of its use have been encouraging (e.g., refs. 52,55) as have reports of the closely related compound *naftidrofuryl* (13,45). Obviously, further studies employing these compounds in a wider variety of geriatric patients are needed before their possible usefulness can be defined.

RNA-like Compounds

Interest in the possibility that memory may be encoded in the sequence of nucleic acids comprising RNA in a manner similar to the encoding of genetic information in DNA has led to efforts aimed at enhancing nucleic acid synthesis by giving *RNA, DNA,* or *magnesium pemaline* (Cylert®), a precursor of tricycloaminopropene. The last is easiest to administer. As pointed out earlier, magnesium pemaline may act as a CNS stimulant rather than a stimulator of RNA synthesis (60), and hence it is discussed in the previous section. It is difficult to see how nonspecific facilitation of RNA synthesis, even if this view of memory were correct, could lead to specific memories being encoded. If it could be shown that memory retrieval or storage depends on an RNA transcription and that this step limits the functioning of the memory system in the elderly or demented, then such efforts might rest on a sounder footing. Food, of course, contains these substances in abundance but has yet to be shown per se to have any therapeutic effect on memory.

Anticoagulants

Walsh (133) proposed that anticoagulants, especially *warfarin* (Coumadin®), may, by preventing blood sludging in narrow vessels, offer some benefit in treatment of senile and presenile dementias. Walsh and Walsh (134) claimed improved intellectual performance in an uncontrolled study. However, Lukas et al. (82) found no difference between papaverine and anticoagulant-treated groups over 4 months; indeed, further intellectual deterioration was documented during the period. Similarly, Ratner et al. (99) found no difference over 1 year in a placebo-controlled double-blind study assessing 25 variables apparently reflecting mental and cognitive function. Given these doubtful results and the admitted dangers of anticoagulants in the elderly, there is little justification for their use at present.

Vitamins

Lehmann and Ban (77) recommended large amounts of B-complex and C vitamins in the management of the elderly. It is not clear if this represents a response to the frequently marginal diets of the elderly or a specific treatment for cognitive dysfunction. At present, no link between cognitive failure and vitamin deficiency has been established for the majority of elderly individuals.

Chelating Agents

Reports by Crapper et al. (19) that aluminum is increased in brains with Alzheimer's disease and that aluminum administered to animals produces neuro-fibrillary degeneration has stimulated interest in chelating agents (e.g., *dimercaprol, British antilewisite, BAL*). No large-scale study has evaluated this possibility as yet, although preliminary work indicates that dimercaprol does not reverse the dementia following repeated hemodialysis, where the aluminum intoxication theory is on strong ground. Moreover, experimental aluminum intoxication produces an acute encephalopathic state, whereas senile and presenile dementias evolve much more slowly.

Piracetam (Nootropil®)

Stegink (124) reported positive clinical effects with piracetam in elderly human patients suffering from vertigo, physical fatigue, and mental asthenia. Lagergren and Levander (75) showed that piracetam counteracts the impairment of mental function caused by decreased pulse in patients with an artificial pacemaker. Mindus et al. (87) found that the drug was not superior to placebo in protecting against retrograde amnesia following electroconvulsive therapy (ECT) in depressed patients. The effects of piracetam on mental functions and regional cerebral blood flow were investigated by Gustafson et al. (50) in a controlled study of eight patients who displayed symptoms of moderate presenile dementia. They found that the drug had no significant effect on either mental function or regional blood flow. In another double-blind placebo-controlled study, Abudzzahab et al. (1) reported negative results with 56 hospitalized geriatric patients who showed mild deterioration in mental functioning.

Cholinomimetic Drugs

A number of normal volunteer studies associated impaired learning with anti-cholinergic drug administration and learning enhancement with cholinergic drug administration. Drachman and Leavitt (29) compared the pattern of memory impairment induced by scopolamine in normal volunteers with cognitive performance of aged subjects. The results is both groups were strikingly similar, showing impairment of memory storage and possibly retrieval despite normal immediate memory span. Drachman (28) also found that *physostigmine* counteracted the scopolamine-induced impairment, particularly in tests of memory storage. This is supported by the results of Davis et al. (22), who produced modest improvement in storage and retrieval of material from long-term memory following physostigmine administration in normal humans. Also supportive is work such as that by Sitaram et al. (118), who found that *arecholine* and *choline* enhanced serial learning in normal subjects.

Several clinical studies have been performed in which choline or its naturally occurring precursor *lecithin* has been given to patients with Alzheimer's disease or senile dementia or the Alzheimer type. Boyd et al. (14) gave choline chloride, 5 and 10 g/day, to seven patients in an uncontrolled pilot study and found no improvement in cognitive performance at the end of 2 and 4 weeks, respectively. Smith et al. (119) carried out a double-blind placebo-controlled study with 10 patients who were given choline bitartrate, 9 g/day. Although no significant difference between drug and placebo emerged on cognitive testing, three patients seemed to be less confused after 2 weeks of choline treatment. In an uncontrolled study, Signoret et al. (117) studied the effect of choline citrate administration in eight younger patients with early Alzheimer's disease and noted improvement in cognitive functioning at the end of 3 weeks on a regimen of 9 g/day.

Etienne et al. (35) administered choline (base), 8 g/day, to three patients with Alzheimer's disease and assessed cognitive improvement while measuring plasma levels of choline. Plasma choline levels increased five- to sixfold after 2 weeks of this dose; and on a block design test, the least demented patient showed improvement that coincided with the peak plasma level. Renvoise and Jerram (101), in a double-blind placebo-controlled study, found no significant improvement in cognitive performance after 8 weeks of choline chloride (15 g/day) in 18 demented patients. Etienne et al. (35) administered oral lecithin to seven outpatients with Alzheimer's disease of less than 3 years' duration. An initial dose of 25 g/day was increased by 25 g/week up to the maximum amount the patients could tolerate. Plasma choline levels increased from a mean level of 10.9 nM/ml to 38.2 nM/ml at the end of the 4-week trial. Three patients showed improvement in new learning ability, as evidenced by their scores on the paired associate learning test of the Wechsler Memory Scale. The best scores coincided with peak choline levels. In two of these patients there was some improvement in a measure of visual retention.

Several studies examined the effect of physostigmine, a centrally active anticholinesterase, on cognitive performance in dementia. Smith and Swash (121) administered single doses of 1 mg physostigmine subcutaneously to a 42-year-old man with biopsy-established Alzheimer's disease. Although there was no improvement on tests of memory, physostigmine reduced significantly inappropriate behavior on these tests. Muromoto et al. (90) found a remarkable improvement in a 57-year-old man's ability to accurately copy geometric figures. These observations are consistent with the idea that cognitive improvement may be the result of an increase in central cholinergic activity.

Consistent with these clinical findings is evidence that Alzheimer's disease is accompanied by a disproportionate reduction, in selected areas of the brain, of the enzymes associated with cholinergic transmission, i.e., acetylcholinesterase and choline acetyltransferase (21,120,136).

Hyperbaric Oxygenation

The observation of reduced cerebral blood flow and reduced cerebral oxygen utilization in aging brains has led to a direct effort to make more oxygen available.

Jacobs et al. (59) administered 100% oxygen at 2.5 atmospheres for 3 hr a day for 15 days and claimed improved memory in the subjects. Goldfarb et al. (46) failed to confirm these findings, as did Raskin et al. (98). The transient nature of the improvement, even if it could be documented, would seriously limit this approach.

Propranolol (Inderal®)

We discussed the pharmacokinetics of propranolol—including age-related changes—in detail elsewhere (53).

Although never followed up, Eisdorfer et al. (34) reported improved learning in aged volunteers as a result of administering propranolol. The possibility that learning deficits in the elderly or the demented might reflect inappropriate levels of arousal has not received the attention it deserves, especially in view of the ease with which attentional variables, psychologic and physiologic, can be measured.

The use of propranolol in the elderly is of course problematic because of its toxicity, particularly cardiac, which is largely not dose-related (48).

Electroconvulsive Therapy

Despite its long history, electroconvulsive therapy (ECT) continues to represent a viable and effective means of dealing with depressive symptoms of widely divergent causes. The use of transient anesthesia, neuromuscular blockade with succinylcholine and unilateral nondominant application, has greatly improved its safety and reduced the incidence of physiologic and psychologic sequelae. Greenblatt et al. (47) found a superior response to ECT in older patients as compared to drugs. This is especially notable in view of the side effects, especially cardiac, and drug interactions to which the elderly are especially sensitive. In the elderly group, ECT is an effective alternative (107,131). Our unit (33) reported the case of a 69-year-old man whose symptoms of Parkinson's disease improved in a fashion parallel to those of his depression following a course of ECT, suggesting that ECT acts by increasing catecholamine synthesis (dopamine and norepinephrine). For the elderly individual with primary mood disturbance or with a combination of early dementia and depressive symptoms, ECT may offer a means of improving cognitive performance by substantially improving the mood disorder.

DISCUSSION

Attempts to improve cognitive functioning in aging and dementia patients have met with modest success at best, as indicated by the numerous studies described above. Even those drugs which appear to improve function, either behavioral or intellectual, do not possess clear-cut indications or an optimal dose regimen. Yet these and other drugs will undoubtedly continue to be tried, and it is therefore appropriate to discuss some of the principles that should guide future studies if beneficial drugs are to be recognized and other drugs avoided.

A major drawback of the clinical literature to date is the diversity of patient populations addressed by the studies and the lack of precision in the characterization of the patients treated. References to "institutionalized" or "nursing home" patients without further information regarding cognitive and behavioral status foreclose the possibility of direct comparisons between studies. Many study populations are given incorrect diagnoses; this is especially common, as mentioned earlier, in the population alleged to suffer either transient vascular insufficiency or dementia on a vascular basis. Further studies on more homogenous but smaller populations may permit readier recognition of significant effects.

The choice of drugs has not always been guided by an understanding of the pathophysiology of the disease or the precise details of the psychological deficits tested. Some recent investigations with stimulants and with choline have proved exceptions to this general practice. Even at the present uncertain state of neuropsychology, one can identify different processes contributing to the overall cognitive function of the individual, e.g., attention, perception, recognition, detection, psychomotor reaction time, span of apprehension, short-term memory, storage and recall of learned material. Tests exist for the quantification of deficits in each of these areas. The choice of drug studies should be guided by likely effects, e.g., choline on memory consolidation or CNS stimulants on psychomotor reaction time.

Fortunately, the number of retrospective or uncontrolled drug trials appears to be diminishing. Good intentions do not always guarantee, however, that all double-blind, placebo-controlled studies will produce valid results. Many drugs have recognizable side effects which defeat the attempt to make the study double-blind. With rating scales it is particularly important that the individuals doing the rating remain blind to the actual drug employed. The use of different dosage levels and a crossover design may improve the chance of significant results. A crossover design where patients and family members can elect at several alternative points to switch or not may permit the inclusion of observations by relatives concerning the subject's improved mental status or further mental decline. This is one way to ensure that improved psychometric performance is in fact reflected in better daily functioning at home. Finally, efforts should be made to avoid a practice effect from the repeated administration of the same tests by a suitable randomized design.

Agreement on a standard set of psychometric tests would facilitate comparison of results in different studies and permit earlier recognition of significant effects on particular psychological functions. Selection of the test should depend on the sensitivity of the test to altered psychological function and on the postulated role of the drug in altering psychological processes. In some cases, where drugs appear to have a nonspecific facilitatory effect on cerebral metabolism (Hydergine, pyritinol) the latter factor may be less important. The design of tests should take into account the interests and motivation of the subjects tested: For example a version of the Wechsler Memory Scale logical memory subtest which relates the story of a South Boston washerwoman elicits much higher and more reliable scores in Boston than a description of shells falling on a French schoolhouse.

When selecting potential dependent variables, it is important to keep the number small. If a sufficient number of hypotheses are explored concurrently, a subset of hypotheses will be proved "true" at the 5% confidence level merely by chance. This effect probably accounts for many of the preliminary results that could not be confirmed on subsequent drug trials.

Few studies control for the effects of medication on mood and motivation. The frequency of depression among the aging and the dementing populations is recognized. The terms used to describe the beneficial effects of drugs in some studies clearly indicate a noncognitive locus of action: "brighter," "more sociable," "less irritable," "fewer mannerisms," reduced dizziness and headache. Although such beneficial effects are not to be ignored, the failure to separate secondary cognitive gains due to improved mood from primary effects on cognitive processes may ultimately cloud the usefulness of so-called "cognitive" drugs by multiplying the number of conflicting studies.

Finally, it is important to specify variables other than age or diagnosis when characterizing the clinical populations under study. Educational and ethnic variables may markedly affect the skills and motivations which subjects bring to the testing situation. The very interpretation of test directions may depend on subtle factors in the subject's background, on his perception of the person administering the test, and on his previous acquaintance with such testing situations. The project of undertaking an experimental study may alter environmental variables (e.g., increased attention, greater encouragement, more modern and spacious quarters) that may, by themselves, alter cognitive performance. A large number of studies agree on the undoubted effect of placebo on performance, possibly operating through such a chain of circumstances. [For example, see the study of Westreich et al. (135) on cyclandelate in dementia.]

CONCLUSIONS

The evidence thus far compiled appears to indicate that no drug has demonstrated any clear efficacy in reversing the cognitive decline of old age or the cognitive failure of dementia. Promising results are either refuted by equally carefully conducted studies or are too preliminary for a final assessment. Certain drugs (e.g., Hydergine, certain CNS stimulants, certain anabolic agents) may be useful in some patients. In addition, it is possible that many of the reported cognitive improvements seen in selected individuals are entirely secondary to improvements in mood and overall well-being, rather than to any specific effect on cognitive performance.

REFERENCES

1. Abudzzahab, F. S., Merwin, G. E., Zimmerman, R. L., and Sherman, B. A. (1978): *Psychopharmacol. Bull.,* 14:23–25.
2. Aderman, M., Giardina, W. J., and Koreniowski, S. (1972): *J. Am. Geriatr. Soc.,* 20:268–271.
3. Affleck, D. C., Treptow, K. R., and Herrick, H. D. (1961): *J. Nerv. Ment. Dis.,* 132:335–338.
4. Arrigo, A., Brown, P., Kauchtschischwili, G. M., Moglia, A., and Tartara, A. (1973): *Curr. Ther. Res.,* 15:417–420.
5. Aslan, A. (1974): In: *Theoretical Aspects of Aging,* edited by M. Rockstein, M. L. Sussman, and J. Chesky, pp. 145–155. Academic Press, New York.
6. Ball, J. A. C., and Taylor, A. R. (1967): *Br. Med. J.,* 3:525–528.
7. Ban, T. A. (1978): In: *Psychopharmacology: A Generation of Progress,* edited by M. A. Lipton, A. DiMascio, and K. F. Killam, pp. 1525–1535. Raven Press, New York.
8. Banen, D. M. (1972): *J. Am. Geriatr. Soc.,* 20:22–24.
9. Bazo, A. J. (1973): *J. Am. Geriatr. Soc.,* 21:63–71.
10. Billiottet, T., and Ferrand, J. (1958): *Semin. Med.,* 34:635–637.
11. Bondareff, W. (1959): In: *Handbook of Aging and the Individual,* edited by J. E. Birren, pp. 136–172. University of Chicago Press, Chicago.
12. Botwinick, J. (1977): In: *Handbook of the Psychology of Aging,* edited by J. E. Birren and K. W. Schare, pp. 580–605. Van Nostrand Reinhold, New York.
13. Bouvier, J. B., Passeron, O., and Chupin, M. P. (1974): *J. Int. Med. Res.,* 2:59–65.
14. Boyd, W. D., Grahm-White, J., Blackwood, G., Glenn, I., and McQueen, J. (1977): *Lancet,* 2:711.
15. Bromley, D. B. (1974): *The Psychology of Human Aging.* Penguin, Baltimore.
16. Canestari, R. E., Jr. (1963): *J. Gerontol.,* 18:165–168.
17. Cerletti, A. (1974): *Arch. Neurobiol. (Madrid),* 37 (Suppl.): 3–8.
18. Cole, J. O., and Branconnier, J. D. (1977): *McLean Hosp. J.,* 2:210–221.
19. Crapper, D. R., Krishman, S. S., and Quittkat, S. (1976): *Brain,* 99:67–80.
20. Critchley, M. (1956): *J. Chronic Dis.,* 3:459–477.
21. Davies, P., and Maloney, A. J. F. (1976): *Lancet,* 2:1403.
22. Davis, K. L., Mohs, R. C., Tinklenberg, J. R., Pfefferbaum, A., Hollister, L. E., and Kepell, B. S. (1978): *Science,* 201:272–274.
23. Dhrymiotis, A. D., and Whittier, J. R. (1962): *Curr. Ther. Res.,* 4:124–129.
24. Ditch, M., Kelly, F. J., and Resnick, O. (1971): *J. Am. Geriatr. Soc.,* 19:208–217.
25. Domino, E. F., Dren, A. T., and Giardina, W. J. (1978): In: *Psychopharmacology: A Generation of Progress,* edited by M. A. Lipton, A. D. DiMascio, and K. F. Killam, pp. 1507–1515. Raven Press, New York.
26. Dorken, H. (1954): *Can. J. Psychol.,* 8:187–194.
27. Duvoisin, R. C. (1975): *JAMA,* 231:845–897.
28. Drachman, D. A. (1977): *Neurology,* 27:783–790.
29. Drachman, D. A., and Leavitt, J. (1972): *J. Exp. Psychol.,* 93:302–308.
30. Drachman, D. A., and Leavitt, J. (1974): *Arch. Neurol.,* 30:113–121.
31. Droller, H., Bevans, H. S., and Jayaram, V. K. (1971): *Gerontol. Clin.,* 13:269–276.
32. Dunlop, E. (1968): *J. Am. Geriatr. Soc.,* 16:343–349.
33. Dysken, M., Evans, M. E., Chan, C. H., and Davis, J. M. (1976): *Neuropsychobiology,* 2:81–86.
34. Eisdorfer, C., Nowlin, J., and Wilkie, J. (1970): *Science,* 170:1327–1329.
35. Etienne, P., Gauthier, S., Dastoor, D., Collier, B., and Ratner, U. (1978): Lecithin in Alzheimer's disease. *Lancet,* 2:1206.
36. Etienne, P., Gauthier, S., Johnson, G., Collier, B., Mendis, T., Dastoor, D., Cole, M., and Muller, H. (1978): *Lancet,* 2:508–509.
37. Emmeneger, H., and Meier-Ruge, W. (1968): *Pharmacology,* 1:65–78.
38. Fine, E. W. (1971): *Curr. Ther. Res.,* 13:568–574.
39. Fine, E. W., Lewis, D., Villa-Landa, I., and Blackmore, C. B. *Br. J. Psychiatry,* 117:157–161.
40. Forster, W., Schultz, S., and Henderson, A. L. (1955): *Geriatrics,* 10:26–30.
41. Fremont, R. E. (1964): *Am. J. Med. Sci.,* 247:182–194.

42. Gardos, G., Cole, J. O., and Suiffin, C. (1976): *J. Clin. Pharmacol.,* 16:304–310.
43. Gaitz, C. M., Varner, R. V., and Overall, J. E. (1977): *Arch. Gen. Psychiatry,* 34:839–845.
44. Gerin, J. (1968): *Curr. Ther. Res.,* 11:609–620.
45. Gerin, J. (1974): *Br. J. Clin. Pract.,* 28:177–178.
46. Goldfarb, A. I., Hoschstadt, N. J., Jacobson, J. H., and Weinstein, E. T. (1972): *J. Gerontol.,* 27:212–217.
47. Greenblatt, M., Grosser, G. H., and Wechsler, H. (1962): *Am. J. Psychiatry,* 119:144–153.
48. Greenblatt, D. J., and Koch-Weser, J. (1974): *Drugs,* 1:118–129.
49. Grill, P., and Broicher, H. (1969): *Dtsch. Med. Wochenschr.,* 94:2429–2433.
50. Gustafson, L., Risberg, J., Johanson, M., Frannson, M., and Maximilian, V. A. (1978): *Psychopharmacology,* 56:115–117.
51. Hall, P. (1976): *J. Am. Geriatr. Soc.,* 24:41–45.
52. Hamonz, W. (1977): *Pharmacotherapeutica,* 1:398–404.
53. Hanna, P. E., O'Dea, R. F., and Goldberg, V. D. (1972): *Biochem. Pharmacol.,* 21:2266–2268.
54. Hicks, R., and Davis, J. M. (1980): *J. Clin. Psychiatry (in press).*
55. Hofman, G., and Salvendy, J. T. (1968): *Wein Z. Nervenheilk.,* 26:279–284.
56. Hofstatter, L., Ossorio, A., Mandl, B., Kohler, L. H., Busch, A. K., and Nyman, A. (1955): Pharmaceutical treatment of patients with senile brain changes. Scientific Exhibit, Section on Nervous and Mental Disease, 104th Annual Meeting of the American Medical Association, Atlantic City.
57. Hollister, L. E. (1955): *Dis. Nerv. Syst.,* 15:259–262.
58. Hollister, L. E. (1975): In: *Progress in Psychiatric Drug Treatment,* Vol. 2, edited by D. F. Klein and R. Gittelman-Klein, pp. 531–539. Brunner/Mazel, New York.
59. Jacobs, E. T., Winter, P. M., Alvis, H. T., and Small, H. M. (1969): *N. Engl. J. Med.,* 281:753–757.
60. Jarvik, M. E., Gritz, E. R., and Schneider, N. G. (1972): *Behav. Biol.,* 7:643–668.
61. Jarvik, L. F., and Milne, J. F. (1975): In: *Aging,* Vol. 2, edited by S. Gershon and A. Raskin, pp. 203–227. Raven Press, New York.
62. Jennings, W. G. (1972): *J. Am. Geriatr. Soc.,* 20:407–412.
63. Judge, T. G., Urquhart, P., and Blakemore, C. B. (1973): *Age Ageing,* 2:121–124.
64. Karlsberg, P., Elliott, H. W., and Adams, J. E. (1963): *Neurology,* 13:772–778.
65. Kastenbaum, T., Slater, P. E., and Aisenberg, R. (1964): *Gerontologist,* 4:68–71.
66. Katzman, R., and Karasu, T. B. (1975): In: *Neurological and Sensory Disorders in the Elderly,* edited by W. S. Fields, pp. 101–132. Grune & Stratton, New York.
67. Kay, D. W. K., Foster, D. M., McKechnie, A. A., and Roth, M. (1970): *Compr. Psychiatry,* 11:26–35.
68. Kent, S. (1976): *Geriatrics,* 31:105–111.
69. Kety, S. S. (1956): *Proc. Assoc. Res. Nerv. Ment. Dis.,* 35:31–45.
70. Kinsbourne, M. (1977): In: *Aging and Dementia,* edited by W. Smith and M. Kinsbourne, pp. 217–236. Spectrum, New York.
71. Kral, V. A., Cahn, C., Deutsch, M., Mueller, H., and Solyom, L. (1962): *Can. Med. Assoc. J.,* 87:1109–1113.
72. Kral, V. A., and Mueller, H. (1966): *Can. Psychiatr. Assoc. J.,* 11:343–349.
73. Kral, V. A., and Wigdor, B. T. (1961): *Can. Psychiatr. Assoc. J.,* 6:345–352.
74. LaBrecque, D. C. (1966): *Curr. Ther. Res.,* 8:106–109.
75. Lagergren, K., and Levander, S. E. (1974): *Psychopharmacologia,* 34:96–104.
76. Leckman, T., Ananth, T. V., Ban, T. A., and Lehmann, H. E. (1971): *J. Clin. Pharmacol.,* 11:301–303.
77. Lehmann, H. E., and Ban, T. A. (1969): *Can. Psychiatr. Assoc. J.,* 14:361–369.
78. Lehmann, H. E., and Ban, T. A. (1970): In: *Psychopharmacology and the Individual Patient,* edited by J. R. Wittenborn, S. C. Goldberg, and P. R. A. May, pp. 32–54. Raven Press, New York.
79. Lehmann, H. E. and Ban, T. A. (1975): In: *Aging,* Vol. 2, edited by S. Gershon and A. Raskin, pp. 179–202. Raven Press, New York.
80. Lehmann, H. E., Ban, T. A., and Saxena, B. M. (1972): *Can. Psychiatr. Assoc. J.,* 17:315–320.
81. Lu, L., Stotsky, B. A., and Cole, J. O. (1971): *Arch. Gen. Psychiatry,* 25:284–288.

82. Lukas, E. R., Hanbacher, W. D., and Fullica, A. J. (1973): *J. Am. Geriatr. Soc.*, 21:224–225.
83. MacFarlane, M. D., and Baskris, H. (1974): *J. Am. Geriatr. Soc.*, 22:365–371.
84. McConnachie, R. W. (1973): *Curr. Med. Res. Opinion,* 1:463–468.
85. McQuillan, L. M., Loped, C. A., and Vibal, J. R. (1974): *Curr. Ther. Res.,* 16:49–58.
86. Miller, E. (1977): *Abnormal Aging.* Wiley, London.
87. Mindus, P., Crouholm, B., and Levander, S. E. (1975): *Acta Psychiatr. Scand.,* 51:319–326.
88. Moskowitz, M. A., Chiel, H. J., and Lytle, L. D. (1978): In: *Current Neurology,* Vol. 1, edited by H. R. Tyler and D. M. Dawson, pp. 390–436. Houghton-Mifflin, New York.
89. Nickerson, M. (1975): In: *The Pharmacological Basis of Therapeutics,* 5th ed., edited by L. S. Goodman and A. Goodman, pp. 727–743. Macmillan, New York.
90. Muramoto, O., Sugishita, M., Sugita, M., and Toyakura, Y. (1979): *Arch. Neurol.,* 36:501–503.
91. O'Brien, M. C. (1977): In: *Aging and Dementia,* edited by L. W. Smith and M. Kinsbourne, pp. 77–90. Spectrum, New York.
92. O'Brien, M. D., and Veall, N. (1966): *Lancet,* 2:729–730.
93. Pacha, W., and Salzman, R. (1970): *Br. J. Pharmacol.,* 38:439–440.
94. Palmore, E. R. (1970): *Normal Aging: Reports from the Duke Longitudinal Study, 1955–1969.* Duke University Press, Durham, N.C.
95. Palmore, E. R. (1974): *Normal Aging II: Reports from the Duke Longitudinal Study, 1970–1973.* Duke University Press, Durham, N.C.
96. Plotnikoff, N. (1968): *Recent Adv. Biol. Psychiatry,* 10:102–120.
97. Rao, D. B., and Norris, J. R. (1971): *Johns Hopkins Med. J.,* 130:317–324.
98. Raskin, A., Gershon, S., Crook, T. H., Sathananthan, G., and Ferris, S. (1978): *Arch. Gen. Psychiatry,* 35:50–56.
99. Ratner, T., Rosenberg, G., Vojtech, A. K., and Engelmann, F. (1972): *J. Am. Geriatr. Soc.,* 21:556–559.
100. Rehman, S. A. (1973): *Curr. Med. Res. Opinion,* 1:456–468.
101. Renvoise, D. G., and Jerram, T. (1979): *N. Engl. J. Med.,* 301:330.
102. Ritter, R. H., Mail, H. R., Tatum, P., and Blazi, M. (1971): The effect of papaverine on patients with cerebral arteriosclerosis. *Clin. Med.,* 78:18–22.
103. Robinson, D. S., Davis, J. M., Nies, A., Colburn, R. W., Davis, J. N., Bourne, H. R., Bunney, W. E., Shaw, D. M., and Coppen, A. J. (1972): *Lancet,* 1:290–291.
104. Rosen, H. T. (1975): *J. Am. Geriatr. Soc.,* 23:169–174.
105. Roth, M., Tomlinson, B. E., and Blessed, G. (1967): *Proc. R. Soc. Med.,* 60:254–258.
106. Roubicek, M. D., Geiger, C., and Abt, K. (1972): *J. Am. Geriatr. Soc.,* 20:222–229.
107. Royal College of Psychiatrists (1977): *Br. J. Psychiatry,* 131:261–272.
108. Sakalis, G., Gershon, D., Oh, S., and Shopsin, B. (1974): *Curr. Ther. Res.,* 16:59–63.
109. Salzman, C., and Shader, R. I. (1973): In: *Psychopharmacology and Aging,* edited by C. Eisdorfer and W. E. Fann, pp. 159–168. Plenum Press, New York.
110. Samorajski, J. (1976): *J. Am. Geriatr. Soc.,* 24:4–11.
111. Sathananthan, G. L., and Gershon, S. (1975): In: *Aging,* Vol. 2, edited by S. Gershon and A. Raskin, pp. 155–168. Raven Press, New York.
112. Savage, R. D., Britton, P. G., Bolton, N., and Hall, E. H. (1973): *Intellectual Functioning in the Aged.* Methuen, London.
113. Selkoe, D. S. (1978): In: *Current Neurology,* edited by H. R. Tyler and D. M. Dawson, pp. 360–387. Houghton-Mifflin, New York.
114. Shader, R. I. (1979): Personal communication.
115. Shader, R. I., and Goldsmith, G. N. (1976): In: *Progress in Psychiatric Drug Treatment,* Vol. 2, edited by D. F. Klein and R. Gittelman-Klein, pp. 540–554. Brunner/Mazel, New York.
116. Shmavonian, B. M., and Busse, E. W. (1963): In: *Process of Aging—Social and Psychological Prospectives,* edited by R. H. Williams, C. Tibbetts, and W. Donahue, pp. 235–258. Atherton Press, New York.
117. Signoret, J., Whitely, A., and Lhermitte, F. (1978): *Lancet,* 2:837.
118. Sitaran, N., Weingartner, H., and Gillin, J. C. (1978): *Science,* 201:274–276.
119. Smith, W., Lowrey, J. B., and Davis, J. A. (1968): *Curr. Ther. Res.,* 10:613–618.
120. Smith, C. N., and Swash, M. (1978): *Ann. Neurol.,* 3:471–473.

121. Smith, C. M., and Swash, M. (1979): *Lancet,* 1:42.
122. Smith, C. M., Swash, M., Exton-Smith, A. N., Phillips, M. J., Overstall, P. W., Piper, M. E., and Bailey, M. R. (1978): *Lancet,* 2:318.
123. Sokoloff, L. (1976): In: *Basic Neurochemistry,* 2nd ed., edited by G. Seigel, R. W. Albers, R. Katzman, and B. W. Agranoff, pp. 388–413. Little Brown, Boston.
124. Steglink, A. J. (1972): *Arzneim. Forsch.,* 22:975–977.
125. Stern, F. H. (1970): *J. Am. Geriatr. Soc.,* 18:507–512.
126. Stoica, E., Meyer, J. S., Kawamura, Y., Hiromoto, H., Hachi, K., Aoyagi, M., and Pascu, I. (1973): *Neurology,* 23:687–698.
127. Talland, G. A., Hogan, D. Q., and James, M. (1967): *J. Nerv. Ment. Dis.,* 144:421–429.
128. Thibault, A. (1974): *Curr. Med. Res. Opinion,* 2:482–486.
129. Tomlinson, B. E., Blessed, G., and Roth, M. (1970): *J. Neurol. Sci.,* 11:205–243.
130. Triboletti, F., and Ferri, A. (1969): *Curr. Ther. Res.,* 11:609–620.
131. Turek, I. S., and Harlon, T. E. (1977): *J. Nerv. Ment. Dis.,* 164:419–431.
132. Van der Drift, J. H. A. (1961): *Angiology,* 12:401–418.
133. Walsh, A. C. (1969): *J. Am. Geriatr. Soc.,* 17:447–487.
134. Walsh, A. C., and Walsh, B. H. (1972): *J. Am. Geriatr. Soc.,* 20:127–131.
135. Westreich, G., Alter, M., and Lundgren, S. (1975): *Stroke,* 6:535–538.
136. White, P., Hiley, C. R., Goodhardt, M. J., Carrasco, L. H., Keet, J. P., Williams, I. E. I., and Bowen, D. M. (1977): *Lancet,* 1:668–670.
137. Whittier, J. R. (1964): *Angiology,* 15:82–86.
138. Young, T., Hall, P., and Blakemore, C. (1974): *Br. J. Psychiatry,* 124:177–180.

DISCUSSION

Dr. N. Miller: I would like to ask Dr. Davis or Dr. Gaitz about the specific measure used in many of the Hydergine studies to measure intellectual impairment. The instrument most commonly used, the Sandoz Clinical Assessment-Geriatric (SCAG) Rating scale, although designed for assessing multiple psychopathology in older persons, is not in any sense a reliable, systematic measure of cognitive function. Accordingly, I am wondering whether the conclusions regarding reported changes, or reversals, in cognitive function based on data collected with this measure are really valid. Do you have any systematic information regarding this?

Dr. Davis: I think the distinction would be that in objective psychometric tests, a cognitive test is actually administered to the patient, whereas in the Sandoz scale, patients are rated according to whether the *observer* thinks they are confused, and capable of self care.

These two functions, memory function and capacity for self care, might be entirely different. It would be extremely helpful for workers designing protocols to evaluate the correlation between different scales to see if different sources of information agree, or if two different raters agree on which patient improved or did not. Do objective systematic tests and rating scales both agree on improvement? If so, this suggests the change is really a reliable improvement, and not just a random or spurious result.

Dr. Epstein: There is an additional issue in the study protocol, namely an attempt to evolve better standardization as to how the different investigators are using the same scales. It is of interest that even after meeting several times for this purpose, I have found that a standard deviation of approximately 1.0 continues to exist on certain of the items on a seven or eight-point scale. There is also some difficulty in the consistency of measurement of baseline and endpoint status, and attempts are currently being made to better standardize such assessment. In any event, it is most important to recognize these issues, if we are to adequately interpret research findings.

Dr. Solomon: My question is addressed to Dr. Davis. It seems to me that in the published Hydergine studies, the diagnostic criteria used for dementia are not at all clear. I am wondering whether we are actually dealing with a homogeneous population or a heterogeneous one, and whether this inconsistency in selection of a subject sample may result in inconsistent research findings. Also, some of the early studies did not use the double placebo method.

Dr. Davis: Well, there is no doubt that the patients in all the drug trials were a miscellaneous group of patients, and the more homogeneous they could be made, the better.

There are economic factors involved in protocol design. There are also scientific factors: For example, it would be better to have CT scans.

Properly done, double-blind studies should have identical placebos, so that there is no way to determine the code. Without this, it is really no longer a double-blind study. Sometimes some biasing factors can creep into studies, even if it is ostensibly double-blind, and obviously, double-blind studies are never completely perfect, but there is a consistent body of evidence suggesting that there may be something to investigate with Hydergine.

Dr. Gaitz: We have no perfect methodology for the clinical evaluation of drug treatment of Alzheimer's disease. The SCAG, as a behavioral rating scale, is an example of one technique. Other techniques can be used both separately or in combination; they are not perfect, and can be criticized. I believe clinicians have the responsibility to examine results of drug studies in the light of the sampling and methodology that was used. I would like now to address myself not so much to the Hydergine studies per se, but more to the whole problem of studying and treating patients with organic brain syndrome, how we go about doing this, and the problems we encounter.

I am the last person in the world to defend our own study. We reported the results as they came out. It is up to the reader. We didn't push the idea that Hydergine is a magic drug, that it will do anything and everything that we would all like for it to do.

Physicians have to read these reports, whether it is a report of our study or somebody else's, and understand the limitations of the study and its applications. Investigators have a responsibility to report honestly and in detail about sampling techniques, the methodology used for evaluation, and that sort of thing, but a reader of the reports must draw his own conclusion about efficacy and applicability in treating patients.

All kinds of problems are encountered in doing research with demented patients. These are getting more serious as time goes on and it is increasingly difficult to find a patient population you can study freely.

I would like to have a very careful, detailed, prestudy evaluation as much as every other researcher. Ideally, this would include everything one can think of as part of baseline data. However, I have a certain pessimism or cynicism, whatever you want to call it, in terms of where we are and where we are going.

We keep hoping that advances in theory and technology will simplify our tasks. Two years ago, when Gene Cohen started looking into research, education, and training, and how NIMH might get involved, it was very clear that we needed a more perfect way to classify patients.

In those days, just 2 years ago, the hope was that the CT scan was going to be the answer. Today Carl Eisdorfer tells us that he really is not too impressed with this technique, and that we should get on with more thorough investigation of psychological aspects! Yet, as we have just heard, there are enormous problems in psychological measurements.

Positron emission is the newest catchword, so now I am hopeful that positron emission is going to be the answer 2 years from now. We still do not have the techniques necessary to achieve a full understanding of the nature of organic brain disorders and to evaluate treatment of such conditions. We simply don't have the technology.

Still another critical issue has to do with the rights of the subjects who are going to be studied. The more demanding a research protocol is, the less likely you are to recruit patients who will participate.

So there is a paradox. We would like to have a lot of things done, but you approach someone, say, a resident in a nursing home "who doesn't have anything else to do," and you tell him that you want him to take a battery of psychological tests; it is going to take 2 days, and then you want him to have a spinal fluid examination, and you want this and you want that. The more things you add the less likely you are to have a subject!

The resistance is not only for baseline studies, but we are forced to compromise when deciding how much data can be obtained in follow-up observations, not only because of cost considerations, but by limits imposed by the subjects of the research.

So, you get into difficulty in these situations. It is easy to jump on someone—the panel has already defended the institutions; I can defend the drug companies. There are few other sources supporting clinical drug trials. There is comparatively little interest in finding new agents, or evaluating agents already used, to help patients with dementia.

Granted, drug companies have a vested interest. But again, this is a capitalistic society in which they are entitled to have their vested interest. Unless this overall situation changes, and it's not clear to me what might change, researchers must report fully and conscientiously what they have done, and clinicians must do their own evaluations of research reports *and* advertisements by drug companies.

We also should focus more attention on the person who is administering the treatment. We haven't spent much time considering the role of therapists, and yet, with a little bit of reflection, one clearly recognizes that attitudes of therapists are very important factors in any therapeutic intervention. The orientation—be it psychologic or biologic— and the biases and opinions of therapists determine the type of treatment prescribed. But perhaps an attitude of therapeutic hopefulness is more important than the specific therapeutic modality. If I attempt to do what somebody else does, and I really don't have my heart in it, it is not going to work. This may explain why certain techniques such as behavior modification and reality orientation work for some people but not for others. Attitudes, qualifications, and characteristics of the person doing the therapy may be very important in evaluating outcome of a therapeutic intervention.

*Clinical Aspects of Alzheimer's Disease and
Senile Dementia*, (Aging, Vol. 15), edited by
Nancy E. Miller and Gene D. Cohen.
Raven Press, New York 1981.

Treatment and Amelioration of Psychopathologic Affective States in the Dementias of Late Life

William E. Fann and Jeanine C. Wheless

Departments of Psychiatry and Pharmacology, Baylor College of Medicine; and Psychiatry Service, Veterans Administration Hospital, Houston, Texas 77030

The notion that mental illness is a natural concomitant of aging has often prevented elderly patients from receiving effective treatment. Until recently precise psychiatric diagnoses were rare, and the wastebasket diagnosis "senility" implied no hope for improvement and resulted in little being done to ameliorate treatable conditions. Negative staff attitudes contributed to the further deterioration of the psychogeriatric patient (9,62). Even when elderly persons presented with predominantly depressive, anxious, or paranoid symptoms, these symptoms were frequently assumed to be merely prodromal to the emergence of underlying cerebral disease; the possibility of neuroses or psychoses other than those related to senility or arteriosclerosis was often not considered (25,26,59). However, as Pearce (51) noted, "Age alone is no guarantee that dementia is caused by irrevocable cerebral degenerative pathology." He further reported that, with adequate investigation, reversible causes for dementia occur in about 10 to 20% of referrals to hospitals or psychogeriatric units. Even when present, chronic brain syndrome is not always the predominating psychiatric condition.

To date, pharmacological intervention in the senile dementing process has not succeeded in reversing the syndrome. However, a complicating depression, anxiety, agitation, or other psychiatric disorder may accelerate deterioration due to dementia; and many of the symptoms of these conditions which occur concurrently with or as a result of organic brain syndrome (OBS) are treatable (25,26,59,66). Adaptive behavior generally improves when the affective state is improved. For example, reduction of anxiety and depression appears to enhance attention; thought processes may become more orderly once suspiciousness and bewilderment diminish (11).

The pessimism which has surrounded prognoses for elderly demented patients is unwarranted; many of their psychiatric symptoms are amenable to treatment. With expeditious institution of therapy, the patient with senile dementia can live in greater comfort, independence, and dignity.

LITERATURE REVIEW

Interest in the pharmacological management of the symptoms of senile dementias has increased during recent years. Several classes of drugs have been proclaimed as beneficial and clinical trials undertaken to assess efficacy. Many reports in the literature deal with the effect of drugs on cognitive function (mental alertness, recent memory, disorientation) with no mention of effectiveness on the numerous affective and interpersonal symptoms (anxiety, depression, irritability, agitation, uncooperativeness) which are frequent concomitants of chronic brain syndrome. There is a paucity of solid empirical data on somatic interventions of these affective components of OBS. We review studies of the past decade which address themselves either partially or entirely to the efficacy of various drugs on affective states of individuals with diagnoses of senile dementia or cerebral arteriosclerosis. In articles which document cognitive and affective effects, only the latter type of changes are discussed.

Investigators have used widely varying methods, populations, assessment measures, and drug classes. Although many trials were double-blind, some were not blind (6,13,17,28,31,63,71,74), and an additional number, although double-blind, included non placebo-control group (12,49,61). Patient samples included chronically hospitalized (2 years or more) geriatric patients (12,49,56,63,72,78), short-term hospitalized patients (13,71) and outpatients (28,42,49,61,67). Average age of the samples ranged from younger geriatrics in their sixties (7,61) to older geriatrics in their mid-seventies through eighties (12,31,39,56). In addition to formulating a diagnosis of senile dementia, some authors also differentiated psychotic (56,72) from nonpsychotic (12,56,72) samples. Drug trials were conducted with antipsychotics (12,13,17,31,56,63,71), anxiolytics (12), anticoagulants (58,74,75), MAO inhibitors (78), ergot alkaloids (39,49,61), vasodilators (42,49,57,61,68), stimulants (13,42,72), cholinergic agents (6,28), hormones (7,17), enzymes (34), vitamins (2), and nootropic drugs (67). Many investigators report beneficial effects on the affective concomitants of the senile dementias.

Rigorous research techniques must be applied in order for reliable data on the behavioral effects of psychoactive drugs to be collected. Methodological shortcomings of most trials make it difficult to accurately assess the specific drug effects reported. Some of the studies which are neither blind nor controlled are intended to be clinical rather than experimental trials and consequently do not adhere to strict research principles. Although many investigators used a double-blind protocol, only three (7,34,68) used the more sophisticated crossover paradigm. These studies are reviewed in ascending order of methodological rigor.

Not Blind, No Placebo-Control Group

For the past decade, Walsh has treated senile and presenile dementia with an anticoagulant or anticoagulant/psychotherapy regimen. Routine treatment begins with an extensive 2-month trial of bishydroxycoumarin (Dicumarol). Dosage is adjusted individually, and the patient's prothrombin time is regulated at 2 to 2.5 times the control value. If improvement occurs, the patient is referred to his own physician for maintenance therapy, the usual daily dosage being 25 to 75 mg. Twenty-two consecutively admitted patients aged 50 to 89 with varying degrees of organic brain disease completed a 2-month trial of an anticoagulant/psychotherapy regimen. Patients manifested cognitive and emotional concomitants of OBS, including symptoms of anxiety, depression, paranoid ideation, aggressiveness, and hostility. At completion of the drug trial, Walsh and Walsh rated all patients as improved and 8 patients as markedly improved. Each of 8 patients in whom anticoagulant therapy was discontinued suffered a recurrence of original symptoms (74). Case histories of 10 patients with cognitive and emotional components of presenile dementia who responded well to treatment are also reported (75). These authors state that the earlier the treatment is begun, the more effective it is; and that when no significant improvement occurs, further deterioration is prevented. They remark on the difficulty of conducting controlled trials of anticoagulant therapy because treatment must be individualized (74,75).

Ratner et al. (58), however, conducted a double-blind, placebo-controlled year-long study of the efficacy of anticoagulant therapy in senile and/or arteriosclerotic dementia. Seven subjects participated in each group and were assessed prior to treatment and after 6 and 12 months. The drug group showed no significant difference during the year. The control group displayed no significant difference after 6 months but had deteriorated significantly in 4 of 25 variables tested after a year, with a trend toward deterioration in most of the other variables. The authors concluded that the anticoagulant group appeared to deteriorate less than the control group, and they agreed with Walsh and Walsh that the greatest benefit probably occurs in the least deteriorated patients (58). Although the improvement following anticoagulant therapy noted by Walsh and Walsh is difficult to evaluate (patients were also given intensive psychotherapy, which could account for improvement in symptomatology), it is plausible that the regimen prevents further deterioration.

Tobin et al. (71) reported the results of haloperidol for treating 18 hospitalized geriatric patients, each carrying a diagnosis of senile mental syndrome and displaying various affective characteristics. The principal target symptom was psychomotor agitation; other symptoms included anxiety, depression, withdrawal, delusions, and hallucinations. Haloperidol was prescribed for 7 to 40 days with an average period of 18.9 days, and dose was adjusted according to individual response. Symptoms were rated (0 = absent to 3 = severe) at baseline, approximately every 5 days and at the end of treatment. Haloperidol was effective in reducing all symptoms, with an impressive reduction in agitation. Global response values indicated that 11 patients (61.1%) had an excellent or good response, 6 (33.3%) had a fair response, and only one patient responded poorly. Twelve of the 18 were discharged after 12 to 34 days of treatment. Subjects in the study varied widely in terms of length of illness (1 month to 20 years), age (66 to 84 years), dose of medication, and treatment period. Statistical analysis was elementary (71). The study was of benefit only as a clinical trial.

Sixty-six severely agitated psychotic females in a state mental hospital were prescribed promazine HC1. Forty patients diagnosed as schizophrenic reaction had been hospitalized 24 to 34 years; and 26 patients, who had been hospitalized 2 to 3 years, carried a diagnosis of chronic brain syndrome. Agitation often resulted in complete exhaustion. Patients were used as their own controls— behavior patterns established prior to promazine administration were used as baseline and the subsequent response evaluated by comparison. Only objective, observable behavioral changes (which were not specified) were accepted. Agitation was controlled markedly in 25 (38%), moderately in 31 (47%), and slightly or none in only 10; in these 10 patients, however, no incidence or agitation-induced exhaustion occurred after promazine was begun. Agitation associated with chronic brain syndrome was less responsive to the medication than that of chronic schizophrenia. However, in both types of patients, the drug was generally effective in improving behavior and maintaining emotional stability such that custodial care could be replaced by individualized treatment (63). Although the trial did not adhere to rigid research protocol, the behavioral change in these long-term severely agitated patients was dramatic, lessening the likelihood of placebo effect or rater bias.

Goldstein (31) conducted a 6-week trial of mesoridazine in 43 geriatric patients, 36 of whom were diagnosed with OBS. Global evaluation at the end of the study rated 31 patients as much improved, 9 as better, 1 as unchanged, and 2 as worse. On the Psychogeriatric Rating Scale completed at baseline and weeks 1 and 6, significant improvement occurred in numerous symptoms, e.g., agitation, suspiciousness, disturbed sleep, uncooperativeness, irritability, hostility, anxiety, restlessness, nervous tension, violent outburst, persecutory ideas, poor impulse control, and destructive behavior. Nurses' Observation Scale for Inpatient Evaluation (NOSIE) results were similar, with significant reduction in symptoms of agitation, aggression, and overt depressive signs. Mesoridazine produced good results in these patients in whom other drugs had been ineffective (31).

Danto (13) compared the effectiveness of triflupromazine (Vesprin) and pentyl-enetetrazol nicotinic acid (Nico-Metrazol) in 118 patients with senile brain disease (99 patients) or cerebral arteriosclerosis (19 subjects) admitted to psychiatric wards of general hospitals because of the acute onset of unmanageable behavior. Discharge placement followed a 15-day evaluation. During the 2-week trial, 63 patients were prescribed Nico-Metrazol and 55 were administered Vesprin in relatively low doses. Patients were rated on days 1, 8, and 15 on a rating scale concerning general ward behavior and symptomatic behavior (aggression, affect, regressive signs, etc.). Over 90% of the total sample was unchanged, and fewer than 5% were improved. Most patients had to be discharged to state mental hospitals. The findings confirm the observations that change generally does not occur earlier than 4 to 6 weeks.

In a 12-week uncontrolled study, Deutsch et al. (17) prescribed thioridazine–fluoxymesterone combination to 15 female chronic geriatric patients. One-third of the subjects (Ss) were diagnosed as OBS and two-thirds as mixed functional. Progress was assessed using the Brief Psychiatric Rating Scale (BPRS) and the Verdun Geriatric (Target Symptom) Rating Scale (VGRS) at the end of a 2-week washout and following 1, 4, 8, and 12 weeks of medication. A statistically significant improvement in global scales of the BPRS occurred during the fourth week, and improvement was maintained throughout the remainder of the trial. On total BPRS scores, 9 patients improved, 5 were unchanged, and 1 deteriorated. Specific items which improved significantly included anxiety, hostility, suspiciousness, and hallucinatory behavior. Similar significant improvement was noted in the VGRS beginning with the end of the eighth week and continuing through completion of the trial. On total scores, 8 patients were improved, 6 unchanged, and 1 became worse. Significant improvement occurred in symptoms of irritability, hostility, fatiguability, suspiciousness, and anxiety. The authors conclude that "the range of therapeutic activity was pronounced in the symptoms related to arousal, affectivity, and perceptual disturbance" (17). The sample was small—only six OBS patients—and improvement was not classified according to diagnosis; it is possible that the response of the group varied by diagnosis.

It has been suggested that an acetylcholine (ACh) deficiency may underlie memory impairment in senile dementia. Deanol is a drug which is assumed to increase brain ACh. Fourteen geriatric outpatients with very mild to moderately severe OBS (measured by cognitive testing and interview) were treated with deanol for 4 weeks. The initial dose was 100 to 200 mg t.i.d., which was gradually increased to 600 mg t.i.d. A Global Deterioration Scale was given at baseline and after 4 weeks; Sandoz Clinical Assessment-Geriatric (SCAG) was administered at baseline and weekly thereafter. Global behavioral assessment indicated significant improvement: 10 patients improved, and 4 were rated as unchanged. By the third week there was significant improvement in the total SCAG score with nonsignificant trends toward decreases in anxiety, depression, and irritability. Even some patients whose baseline depression rating was "normal" exhibited a reduction in depression or an increase in happiness scores with deanol (28). The trial was an initial study to establish a safe dosage range for geriatrics and was not intended to be a strictly controlled experimental design. Because the trial period was so short, only 4 weeks, and there was no control group, one would have to speculate about the possibility of the occurrence of placebo effect, which is known to be quite strong in geriatric patients.

Boyd et al. (6) reported the results of an uncontrolled pilot study of choline prescription to patients with Alzheimer's syndrome. All seven Ss were severely demented. Although there were no significant differences in cognitive function, the staff noted behavior changes; patients became less irritable and more interested in their surroundings. Improvement in behavior occurred within the first day or two of treatment and at a low dose of choline. The authors speculate that a more favorable response would be possible in less demented patients (6).

Double-Blind, No Placebo-Control Group

Nelson (49) reported a double-blind comparison of Hydergine and papaverine in 45 outpatient and hospitalized geriatric patients. Subjects were selected according to the occurrence of certain symptoms which occur in elderly ("senile") patients; in most of the sample symptomatology was considered to be moderately abnormal. The drug trial, a double-placebo, blind method, lasted 12 weeks and followed a 3-week washout period. Evaluation of change was made at baseline and every 3 weeks thereafter, and was based on the symptoms of the Clinical Status Form (CSF) (which includes such symptoms as anxiety-fears, depression, emotional lability, appetite, sociability, fatigue, self-care) plus two global ratings. Final global ratings showed improvement in both groups—in 86% of Hydergine patients and 55% of papaverine patients. CSF results were similar, with 91% of Hydergine and 57% of papaverine patients exhibiting improvement. Although patients in both groups improved in certain symptoms, the Hydergine group improved significantly more and continued to improve for a longer period of time than the papaverine group. When the difference between the percentage of patients improving in the two groups was compared, Hydergine was significantly superior to papaverine for treatment of affective-type symptoms and overall improvement. The author concludes that Hydergine is efficacious in anxiety, depression, excessive emotional lability, and other distressing symptoms that are commonly encountered in senile patients (49).

Rosen (61) conducted a double-placebo, blind, 12-week study of papaverine and Hydergine in 53 geriatric outpatients with a mean age in the mid-sixties. Patients were carefully selected according to the presence of certain symptoms. The two statistically comparable groups were randomly assigned to treatment. All medication, except for chloral hydrate for occasional nighttime sedation, was discontinued. Evaluation techniques included three measures of affective change: Overall Clinical Impression, Global Change Rating, and Assessment of Clinical States (includes the symptoms depression, anxiety-fears, emotional lability, motivation-initiative, cooperation, sociability, self-care). By the end of the study, patients prescribed Hydergine had improved significantly more (in global changes and overall clinical impressions) than those administered papaverine. The Hydergine group also displayed a significant favorable response in the symptoms of anxiety, depression, emotional lability, motivation, cooperation, and sociability.

Forty senile nonpsychotic patients in a nursing home were randomly assigned to treatment with either thioridazine or diazepam in a 4-week double-blind trial. Average age was about 80, and the two groups were essentially homogeneous. Patients exhibited affective components of OBS, e.g., anxiety, tension, agitation, depressed mood, apprehension, or sleep disturbances. Hamilton Anxiety Rating Scale (HARS), a Modified NOSIE, and global rating of degree of illness and overall change were completed at baseline and weekly. Although none of the items of the HARS changed significantly from baseline in the diazepam group, four items (agitation, anxious mood, fears, and interview behavior) showed significant reduction in severity from baseline in the thioridazine group; comparing the two drugs, thiordiazine was significantly superior to diazepam in reduction of anxiety and depression. NOSIE results indicated that thioridazine patients improved more than diazepam patients for every factor and significantly more for social competence, retardation, depressive manifestations, total positive factors, and total patient assets. Global ratings were significantly favorable for the thioridazine group and indicated a worsening in the diazepam group. Overall, the antipsychotic medication tended to improve the condition of the patients throughout the trial, whereas the anxiolytic patients tended to worsen steadily (12).

Double-Blind, Placebo-Controlled

Rada and Kellner (56) prescribed thiothixene or placebo to 42 hospitalized psychogeriatric patients in a 4-week double-blind trial. All patients had previously been diagnosed as OBS, and 18 Ss also carried a diagnosis of psychotic OBS. Most patients were considered to be "markedly" or "moderately" ill. The mean age was 75.5 years, and the average duration of illness was more than 5 years. Two groups of 21 Ss each were randomly assigned to treatment; there were no significant differences between groups. Following a 1-week placebo washout, a thiothixene starting dose of 2 mg t.i.d. was prescribed which could be raised to 5 mg t.i.d. after 2 weeks; placebo was identical in appearance. Assessments were made following the washout (baseline) and after 2 and 4 weeks of medication. Rating scales included BPRS, NOSIE, and global ratings by psychiatrists. A little more than half of the patients showed improvement. Although there was a slight trend for thiothixene patients to show a greater degree of improvement, the difference between drug and placebo groups was not significant. The only significant difference occurred in the manifest psychosis factor of the NOSIE in which thiothixene produced a slight improvement whereas placebo resulted in exacerbation of symptoms. The authors conclude that thiothixene is no more effective than placebo in the treatment of OBS (56). Although the study was well designed, the severity and chronicity of illness of the Ss may have prevented any appreciable improvement.

Fifty geriatric patients (average age 80) with longstanding symptoms of cerebrovascular insufficiency were randomly assigned in a double-blind comparison of Hydergine or placebo. Twenty-four patients received Hydergine; 26 were given placebo. Changes in clinical status were rated by the symptoms of the Clinical Status Check List (CSCL) and an overall rating. Patients were evaluated at baseline and every 3 weeks thereafter. Patients treated with Hydergine improved significantly compared to baseline for all items except "irritability" and "bothersome," and had a significantly superior response to placebo in all items except irritability, hostility, indifference to surroundings, and self-care. Attitude and behavior improved, with less depression and greater sociability, cooperation, and emotional stability. Overall ratings indicated significant improvement in Hydergine patients. Changes which occurred were dramatic owing to the fact that the Ss were very elderly and were physically and mentally deteriorated (39).

In a 12-week double-blind study 58 hospitalized geriatric patients with symptoms of senility were prescribed either cyclandelate (33 Ss) or placebo (26 Ss). At baseline and weeks 4, 8, and 12, SCAG and NOSIE assessments were completed; and a final global assessment was made at the end of the trial. As early as week 8 the positive effect of the drug on mood depression, irritability, anxiety, hostility, and indifference to surroundings was significantly superior to placebo. By the conclusion of the study, cyclandelate was significantly superior to placebo in all mood/affect and interpersonal relationship factors of the SCAG. NOSIE variables showed no difference between groups of slight favorable effect of placebo; however, drug and placebo groups were not always comparable at baseline. The authors maintain that NOSIE may not be particularly useful in senile populations because of its focus on behavior rather than symptoms (57).

LaBrecque and Goldberg (42) postulated that the mild stimulant effects of pentylenetetrazol and the peripheral vasodilating effect of niacin would be appropriate for use in senile patients. In a double-blind 1-month study, 50 geriatric outpatients with manifestations of senility were randomly divided into two groups of 25. One group was prescribed pentylenetetrazol-niacin combination (Metalex), and the other group received an identical placebo. Weekly assessments were made of 13 behavior characteristics (Malamud-Sands Worchester Rating Scale plus an incontinence item), and these were rated as improved (+1), unchanged (0), or worse (−1); assessment appeared to be somewhat subjective. At the close of the study, the behavioral characteristics were ranked in the order in which active medication demonstrated greatest superiority over placebo in bringing about improvement. In 9 of the 12 items, the drug combination was two to eight times as effective as placebo based on the percentage of patients in whom beneficial results occurred. In descending order, the most improvement occurred in speech, sociability, sleep, mood, eating habits, feeling, appearance, general activity, and interest in work. Difference between average scores of the two groups indicated a statistically favorable response of active drug. The authors conclude that the drug combination alleviates many of the behavior disorders and affective components which frequently accompany senile mental changes (42).

Because pipradol (Meratran) has a stimulating action on the CNS (with comparatively few effects on blood pressure, appetite, and sleep), it is possible that it might alleviate some of the behavioral concomitants of chronic brain syndrome. Turek et al. (72) studied 68 hospitalized psychogeriatric patients with chronic brain syndrome. Ss were divided into three groups: pipradrol HCl (2 mg/day), pipradrol HCl (5 mg/day), and placebo. Medication was given for 6 weeks, after which patients were observed for an additional 3 weeks. Clinical assessments were performed prior to treatment and after 3, 6, and 9 weeks. A psychiatrist rated Impaired Functioning and Retardation and at the end of the trial completed a Final Improvement rating. Nursing personnel completed NOSIE, an Activity Withdrawal Scale, and a Ward Behavior Rating Scale. No statistically significant differences occurred. When psychotic and non-psychotic subsamples were scored separately, a nonsignificant trend was noted. The higher dose of medication appeared to increase positive ward behavior in nonpsychotic Ss by improving social competence, interest, and personal neatness, whereas in psychotic patients it tended to diminish negative ward behavior by favorable effect on psychosis, irritability, and retardation (72). Flaws in the experimental design of the study included a short trial period, no increases in dosage of medication to meet individual needs, and a fairly deteriorated sample of patients, many of whom required uninterrupted neuroleptic treatment and deteriorated further when this medication was discontinued.

The MAO inhibitor effects of Gerovital have been proclaimed as useful in alleviating depression (79) and beneficial in the aging process itself (46,47). Zwerling et al. (78) administered Gerovital in a double-blind study of hospitalized psychogeriatric patients with organic brain syndromes. Although the original protocol called for 60 patients, only 19 (9 drug, 10 control) patients completed the first 6 weeks of the trial, and only 13 (6 drug, 7 control) Ss completed the entire 12 weeks. Several objective rating scales were used to measure drug effects on psychiatric symptoms and interpersonal functioning. Assessment was made at baseline, 6 weeks, and 12 weeks. Seven items on the BPRS relevant to depression were studied separately in order to evaluate the drug's antidepressant properties, and neither the overall depression index based on the sum of the seven items nor each item individually discriminated significantly between drug and placebo Ss. In the overall trial variability between patients was quite large, and the few differences which occurred appeared to reflect random variation rather than true drug effect. The authors concluded that Gerovital had no ameliorative effect on psychologic functioning (78). However, the sample of Ss was small, and all patients had been hospitalized for 2 years or more such that lack of improvement might be due to the deteriorated condition of the Ss.

In a double-blind study Altman et al. (2) treated 132 psychogeriatric patients for 6 weeks with a B-complex and C vitamin preparation or placebo. Patients were rated on an inpatient behavior form (MIBS) that involved 11 factored scales. With one exception, there were no significant results with either vitamins or placebo. The one exception was striking: OBS patients treated with the vitamin complex showed a dramatic and significant decrease in scores on the Excitement Scale as compared to the placebo group; i.e., vitamins had a good effect on excited or agitated behavior of patients with OBS (2).

Stegink (67) reported the results of an 8-week double-blind comparison of piracetam and placebo in 191 patients with chronic brain disease. Patients were assessed weekly, and each week's assessment was compared to the previous week. A statistically significant response in favor of piracetam occurred. Improvement was rated as excellent in 15.3% and good in 25.5%. Piracetam patients improved significantly in symptoms of psychomotor agitation; the drug had a slightly more favorable but nonsignificant response than placebo in symptoms of depressive states and disorders of sleep (67).

Double-Blind, Placebo-Controlled, Crossover

Stern (68) conducted a double-blind crossover study of papaverine HCl (sustained-release form) in 30 hospitalized geriatric patients with chronic brain syndrome. Following a 1-week washout period, patients were divided into two groups and prescribed either active medication or placebo for 8 weeks. After another 1-week washout, the opposite preparation was administered to the groups for 8 weeks. Patients were rated on three categories of symptoms—anxiety, behavioral disorders, associated depression—and each category had five subdivisions. One week before treatment and at weekly intervals patients were rated by six persons, and the weekly scores were consolidated. Papaverine was significantly superior to placebo in 13 of 15 subcategories, with no significant difference in anorexia and sighing, two depressive equivalents. The drug was considered to be a valuable adjunct in the subjective relief of symptoms of chronic brain syndrome secondary to cerebral arteriosclerosis (68).

A double-blind crossover controlled study of Vasolastine, a complex of lipotropic enzymes, was conducted in 48 patients with arteriosclerotic dementia. Patients were treated for a total of 12 months with a crossover at 6 months between placebo and active medication. Complete assessments were made pre- and posttrial and at crossover, and brief assessments were made monthly. Although favorable response to Vasolastine did not reach statistical significance, one surprising result occurred. The active medication group needed concomitant antidepressants far less than the placebo group, and the difference reached a high degree of discrimination during the first and sixth months. Because the placebo group often required the additional administration of antidepressants, the trial was to some extent a comparison of Vasolastine and antidepressants. Vasolastine appears to have a statistically significant effect on subjective complaints of depression and lack of energy (34).

Branconnier et al. (7) undertook a study to ascertain the efficacy of $ACTH_{4-10}$ in modifying the psychological performance deficits associated with senile organic brain syndrome. Eighteen physically healthy Ss with significant impairment due to senile brain disease participated in a double-blind crossover evaluation. Drug or placebo was administered subcutaneously. Each subject was tested twice—once with each preparation—with 14 days elapsing between trials. Results of the Profile of Mood States (POMS) indicate that confusion, anger, and depression showed significant reduction, whereas vigor increased significantly with active medication. The authors conclude that the drug is "capable of improving affective state in patients with mild to moderate senile organic brain syndrome" (7).

Reliability and validity of some of the studies reviewed are questionable owing to several methodological problems.

1. Too small a sample size. Although the original protocol of the study by Zwerling et al. (78) called for 60 Ss, fewer than one-third completed the first 6 weeks and about one-fifth completed the entire 12-week trial; of the Ss in treatment for 12 weeks, only six had been administered active medication. The studies by Deutsch et al. (17) and Tobin et al. (71) also suffer from small sample size such that definitive conclusions about drug effectiveness are impossible to make.

2. Deterioration of the Ss. Geriatric patients with senile dementia vary greatly in their abilities and disabilities. Some of the patients were possibly so deteriorated that appreciable improvement would be unlikely (56,72,78).

3. Use of other drugs. The use of other drugs during an experimental trial presents a dichotomy because the additional medication can either contaminate or stabilize results. Hall and Harcup (34) reported that concomitant prescription of antidepressant agents to their placebo group resulted virtually in a trial between active medication and antidepressants rather than active medication and placebo. In this instance the use of additional drugs contaminated results of the drug trial. Turek et al. (72), however, considered the opposite side of the issue. Some of their Ss who required uninterrupted treatment with neuroleptics regressed from a baseline state as a consequence of the discontinuation of their maintenance medication.

4. Too short a trial period. Danto (13) remarked that drug effect is not likely to occur before 4 to 6 weeks of treatment. Because of the efficacy of triflupromazine in managing agitation is well documented, he chose this agent as "control" and compared pentylenetetrazol nicotinic acid to it; neither drug, however, produced improvement during the short trial period. The results of investigators who used a 4-week period (12,28,42,56) may be inconclusive as a result of the short trial period and the possibility of a placebo effect.

5. Placebo effect. The positive effect of a stimulating environment and extra attention on cognitive and affective components of senile dementia is well known. Much can be done to bring out the potential in elderly patients, even those with OBS. The literature is replete with examples of the beneficial effects of such programs as reality orientation (8,10,15,35,52,69), remotivation (16,29), groups (1,43,48), individual psychotherapy (33), and combination programs using several of these techniques (37,41) on patients with senile mental changes. As Powell (54) stated, "appropriate management of the patient's environment

may completely avert the need for drugs." One study reports, however, that mere exposure to a more stimulating environment is insufficient and that patients also require positive reinforcement from family and/or staff (8). Positive effects resulting from the extra attention experimental subjects are given, termed a "placebo effect," is a plausible explanation in short-term studies which find no difference between placebo and drug groups or in short-term uncontrolled trials which report favorable results.

Although positive attention seems to improve social functioning, elderly patients who receive the usual hospital treatment are likely to deteriorate in overall social adjustment (45). Turek et al. (72) reported that interest in surroundings was increased by medication prescribed to senile patients. Lack of environmental stimulation sufficient to sustain this interest, however, resulted in regression. Frequently, modification of the environment is needed to bring about or maintain drug effectiveness.

Stern's (68) double-blind crossover study was controlled for the variable "placebo effect." Prior to the onset of the drug trial, all Ss had been exposed to an optimal environment—including psychiatric evaluation, psychotherapy, physical therapy, vocational and recreational guidance, and home visits—such that the attention resulting from the prescribing of medication and the assessment procedures used did not ameliorate a deficiency in the environment.

GERIATRIC PHARMACOLOGY

Aging per se is an important variable when prescribing therapeutic agents. Numerous endogenous and exogenous changes in the body occurring with age impair the predictability of drug effects. Not only do drug effects alter senescent functions, but simultaneously senescence alters drug effects. Evidence accumulated over the past decade supports the generally accepted view that the probability of a patient sustaining an adverse reaction increases with age; adverse reactions occurring in the elderly increase in number and severity (4,24,30,64,73).

Several general principles should serve as guidelines for geriatric drug prescription. The frequent concurrent presence of several physical and psychiatric disorders and consequent polypharmacy make it difficult to distinguish among the intended effects of the drugs, side effects, placebo effect, and manifestations of the patient's initial symptoms. The discontinuation of all medication in order to evaluate the patient's drug-free baseline is often a beneficial diagnostic and therapeutic tool. Polypharmacy should be limited as much as possible, and patients treated with multiple drugs warrant continual close observation.

Enormous variations exist in the response of the elderly to medications. Generally the aged have reduced tolerance to psychotropics and require lower doses to reach a desired therapeutic effect. The safest course, therefore, is to prescribe low doses initially (one-fourth to one-half the recommended adult dose) and increase dosage gradually in small increments until therapeutic efficacy is achieved. Because of variations in the homeostatic mechanisms of the aged, adverse side effects can occur at essentially therapeutic doses and can be quite frequent and severe. Consequently, the geriatric patient's condition should be monitored carefully for the advent of untoward reactions (24,73).

PHARMACOLOGICAL MANAGEMENT OF THE AFFECTIVE COMPONENTS OF THE SENILE DEMENTIAS

Efforts to deal with biological causes (arteriosclerosis, circulatory disorders, etc.) of senile dementia have been largely inconclusive. However, disability due to dementia is often accelerated by coexisting physical and mental disorders, and many of these complications are treatable. Drug therapy is directed toward relief of target symptoms, e.g., anxiety, depression, agitation, or psychotic behavior (66,76). Hollister et al. (36) suggested that most of the agents used in the management of senile dementias can be classified as "antianxiety, antidepressant, and antipsychotic" (36).

Antianxiety Agents

Antianxiety agents include a broad range of chemically heterogeneous compounds which have similar clinical effects; these drugs can be sedatives, muscle relaxants, or anticonvulsants. Anxiolytics are indicated for allaying anxiety and reducing its unpleasant somatic components. All of these drugs have a narrow therapeutic range between the dosage that relieves symptoms and one that produces severe decrements in performance. Individual susceptibility to the sedative effects of these drugs varies greatly, and the cautious prescription of lower-than-normal doses with slower increases is recommended. Some elderly patients are quite intolerant to chlordiazepoxide (Librium), although this is generally the drug of choice because of its comparative safety; the initial dose should be 5 mg t.i.d. Reed reported that one organically brain-damaged patient slept for 2 days following the discontinuation of diazepam (Valium) 2 mg t.i.d. (59).

Anxiolytics have also been reported as helpful in alleviating symptoms of depression. These agents are most beneficial in treating agitated or anxious depressed patients (36).

Certain antihistamines, especially diphenhydramine (Benadryl) and hydroxyzine (Atarax, Vistaril), are used as anxiolytics because of their sedative properties. Diphenhydramine has no addiction potential; it is useful for inducing sleep without side effects (73) but has limited value for treating anxiety. Hydroxyzine is efficacious in senile agitation and is especially useful if cardiovascular problems prevent the use of phenothiazines (59). However, these agents have anticholinergic properties and carry the hazard of anticholinergic toxicity, particularly in the elderly.

Although the minor tranquilizers have a low addiction potential, habituation and addiction can occur. Withdrawal symptoms following abrupt cessation of prolonged use have sometimes been mistaken for the onset of psychosis (25,

26,59,76). Anxiolytics occasionally cause paradoxical reactions (e.g., agitation and confusion), but these reactions occur less frequently than with barbiturates (26,73). These agents potentiate the effect of other central nervous system (CNS) depressants, including alcohol, sedatives, hypnotics, neuroleptics, and the sedative effect of tricyclic antidepressants. Patients who are prescribed these drugs concomitantly should be carefully monitored.

Antidepressants

Depression is particularly prevalent in the elderly and can be readily mistaken for OBS (40,70). The depressed geriatric may be incontinent, confused, disoriented, and agitated rather than exhibit overt symptoms of depression (23). In patients with senile dementia, coexistent depression may accelerate progression to total disability. Correct diagnosis is extremely important, and depression should be diagnosed independently of dementia (66). Major depression is the psychiatric illness which most often responds favorably to pharmacotherapy. Antidepressant agents most commonly used are the tricyclic antidepressants and the monoamine oxidase (MAO) inhibitors.

Tricyclics include nonsedative (protriptyline, imipramine) and sedative (amitriptyline, doxepin) agents, the former drugs being indicated for treatment of retarded depression characterized by hypoactivity and hypomentation and the latter types for depressed patients who are agitated and restless. Patients who appear senile, confused, and depressed often respond dramatically to tricyclic antidepressants with improvement in cognitive function and depressive symptomatology (23). These medications are most efficacious in mild to moderate depression; the long lag time (2 to 4 weeks) before the onset of therapeutic action may be a contraindication when depression is unusually pronounced. Patients who are excessively anxious and agitated may require the addition of a more quickly acting substance (e.g., diazepam), but additional medication should be withdrawn as soon as possible (53).

When tricyclics are administered to aged patients, the clinician can expect therapeutic efficacy at lower doses and a greater incidence of unpleasant side effects than when these drugs are prescribed to younger individuals. An initial dose of amitriptyline (Elavil) or imipramine (Tofranil) of 10 mg twice a day with slow increases over a period of 1 to 2 weeks to 50 mg twice a day or less would be prudent. Certain elderly patients, however, may require higher doses (200 mg or more) before beneficial effects are evident.

Hader and Madonick (32) reported their experience with amitriptyline in 21 patients over a period of 13 months. Patients ranged in age from 72 to 94, and 18 of them carried a diagnosis of some type of brain syndrome with depressive reaction. Dosage ranged from 10 to 275 mg/day, and phenothiazines were concomitantly prescribed to 7 patients. Eleven of the 21 patients were clinically improved with no evidence of depression; 7 were slightly improved but required continued medication; 3 were unimproved. Side effects were minimal and relatively innocuous. The authors concluded that amitriptyline is essentially safe for use in the elderly patient and efficacious in relieving depression (32).

Reed reported that endogenous depression occurring concurrently with brain syndrome responds well to treatment with imipramine, whereas tricyclics are not effective in depression due to senile dementia or arteriosclerosis. Mellaril tends to lessen depression and consequently is her drug of choice for the latter group. In cases of severe or agitated depression, concomitant prescription of Mellaril and Tofranil (75 mg/day) or Vivactil (10 to 20 mg/day) is efficacious. Patients who are anxious and depressed often respond best to Elavil (59).

The biology of aging predisposes the geriatric patient to an aggravation of problems related to the anticholinergic side effects of the tricyclics. Dry mouth can cause substantial discomfort to the denture wearer. Blurred vision and confusion can be particularly distressing to patients who are alert to real and imagined perceptual or intellectual decrements. Elderly patients have a lowered threshold for toxic confusion, glaucoma, urinary retention, constipation, cardiovascular embarrassment, and parkinsonism and should be carefully monitored while receiving tricyclics (55).

Although the general effect of the tricyclics is to lower blood pressure, these agents block the effects of the antihypertensive agent guanethidine (Ismelin). When a hypertensive, depressed patient whose blood pressure is controlled by guanethidine is given a tricyclic, blood pressure may return to hypertensive levels. Consequently, blood pressure should be monitored weekly and the dosage of guanethidine adjusted accordingly, or another hypertensive agent should be prescribed when a tricyclic is used concurrently (18,19).

Since the introduction of the tricyclics, which are at least equally effective and less toxic than the MAO inhibitors, the latter have been relegated to a relatively minor role in the treatment of depression. However, the correlation between a decrease in MAO levels and antidepressant effects and the recent finding that there may be an age-related increase in brain MAO activity (50) suggest that MAO inhibitors may be effective in alleviating depression in certain elderly persons (18). Cerebrovascular defect, cardiovascular disease, hypertension, and history of severe headache are contraindications for the use of MAO inhibitors; these drugs would also rarely be used in patients with senile dementia.

Stimulant compounds include amphetamine and its congeners, e.g., methylphenidate. These agents sometimes are efficacious in the apathetic, hypoactive senile patient, but they cannot be recommended for long-term therapy because of their pressor effects on the fragile and partially decompensated cardiovascular system of the elderly. Because they have a high potential for causing dependency, stimulants should be administered to the elderly in low doses (5 to 10 mg amphetamine/day) for a very brief period (1 to 7 days). The therapeutic value of the stimulants appears to be quite limited in geriatric patients with senile dementia.

When depression reaches psychotic proportion, electroconvulsive therapy (ECT) may be indicated (77). Although age per se is no contraindication to

ECT, the seizure can be dangerous to the fragile and partially decompensated organ systems of aged patients. Expanding intracranial growth, cor pulmonale, and hepatic and renal failure are contraindications to ECT. Furthermore, the aged patient's reduced ability to metabolize succinylcholine and barbiturates (the neuromuscular blocking agent and sedative premedications used with ECT) and propensity for cardiovascular and pulmonary illness make careful screenings before such procedures mandatory (20). Although the side effects of ECT are few and relate mainly to problems of memory retention and recall, reduction in cognitive function can be crippling to patients with senile dementia.

Antipsychotics

Antipsychotic agents include the phenothiazines, thioxanthenes, butyrophenones, and rauwolfia alkaloids. These drugs are prescribed to patients with severe anxiety and agitation, delusions, hallucinations, and assaultive or destructive behavior, and are often effective in reducing the symptomatic intensity of a core psychotic process. Dosage must be determined individually in the elderly. Some aged persons are highly intolerant to the effects of the neuroleptics, and an extremely low dose is sufficient to control symptoms. The major tranquilizers can be roughly divided into two categories: those which are strong sedative and hypotension-inducing agents (e.g., chlorpromazine and thioridazine) and those which are less sedating but more readily cause extrapyramidal symptoms (e.g., trifluoperazine, perphenazine, and haloperidol).

Chlorpromazine (Thorazine) is beneficial in agitated, restless, noisy, and aggressive patients. Because of its strong sedative properties it can be oversedating in geriatric patients, and the use of another agent is generally recommended once target symptoms are controlled (59).

Many clinicians list thioridazine (Mellaril) as the drug of choice in geriatric patients. Some investigators report that confused patients treated with Mellaril seem to organize their thoughts better and become more cooperative (59,60). Others point out that in addition to calming effects which lessen agitation, nervousness, combativeness, and hostility, thioridazine has beneficial effects on depression (27,59,60). Depression is a frequent concomitant of senile dementia, and the antidepressant action of the neuroleptic combats depressive manifestations without additional medication.

Trifluoperazine (Stelazine) is beneficial in the aged patient who is very paranoid. Administration of 2 mg b.i.d. is generally adequate; higher doses are likely to cause extrapyramidal symptoms. The combined prescription of trifluoperazine and chlorpromazine may be useful in agitated depressed patients. Stelazine is an activator and can be prescribed in the morning, whereas chlorpromazine (Thorazine) could be used to control nighttime agitation (59).

Perphenazine (Trilafon) is efficacious in aggressive, assaultive, and paranoid patients. Dosages of 8 to 48 mg/day are recommended, but even at therapeutic doses extrapyramidal reactions are often a problem (59).

Haloperidol (Haldol) has been used effectively in senile patients. The drug is less hypotension-inducing than the phenothiazines, and if the dose is kept low (less than 4 mg/daily) extrapyramidal symptoms usually do not occur (59,65).

In a recent study thiothixene, a thioxanthene, produced notable improvement in psychiatrists' and nurses' rating scales as well as global assessments of 26 patients with a diagnosis of senile or arteriosclerotic psychosis. Side effects did not interfere with treatment (5).

Rauwolfia alkaloids appear to be of some value in treating symptoms of anxiety, agitation, and inappropriate aggressiveness in the elderly. These agents are particularly useful when a lowering of blood pressure or pulse rate is desirable. When taken orally, however, there is a delay in onset of action, and occasionally an initial period of excitement precedes improvement. Other adverse effects are a lowering of the convulsive threshold and a decreased possibility of gastrointestinal (GI) bleeding. Increased GI activity may be detrimental to patients with peptic ulcer and ulcerative colitis (44). In addition, there is a very real risk of clinical depression secondary to use of rauwolfia alkaloids, and the clinician should be alert to such an occurrence.

Choosing the most appropriate antipsychotic agent for the individual psychogeriatric patient is difficult. Conservative use of one of the less sedating, less hypotension-inducing agents (e.g., haloperidol or perphenazine) is usually a prudent initial treatment with a switch to thioridazine or chlorpromazine if extrapyramidal reactions develop. Of course the need for a neuroleptic must be demonstrated. Barton and Hurst (3) conducted a double-blind study of chlorpromazine and placebo in 50 demented geriatric patients. All Ss were hospitalized and had been administered the antipsychotic agent for a long period of time. The final week of chlorpromazine administration was compared to the third week of placebo. Although scales measuring agitation, overactivity, restiveness, and noisiness revealed significant but slight deterioration, the staff was unable to differentiate the drug and placebo groups. The authors concluded that about 80% of elderly demented patients receive major tranquilizers unnecessarily (3).

The patient who is over 65 years of age has a greatly reduced ability to metabolize and hence to tolerate the antipsychotic medications. At a given dose, the clinical responses they evoke, therapeutically and toxically, are of greater magnitude than in younger patients. Adverse reactions can occur at essentially therapeutic doses. Possible side effects include dry mouth, urinary retention, constipation, nasal congestion, aggravation of glaucoma, drowsiness, lethargy, hypotension, and extrapyramidal symptoms. In high doses the neuroleptics, especially those with strong atropine-like properties, often exacerbate psychotic symptoms associated with anticholinergic toxicity. The common practice of increasing dosage when confronted with persistent or worsening psychotic symptomatology would be particularly unfortunate in these cases and would aggravate the problem.

Movement disorders secondary to administration of neuroleptics are quite common and range from mild tremors to gross, choreoathetoid, disabling symptoms. Geriatric patients are particularly susceptible to the development of these side effects, which can appear secondary to even moderate doses of neuroleptics in aged individuals. The symptoms of the Parkinson-like syndrome include rigidity, slowing of movement (bradykinesia), pill-rolling tremor salivation, masklike facies, and a gait characterized by short, fast steps (marche a petits pas). The drug-induced parkinsonism is symptomatically similar to idiopathic or postencephalitic Parkinson's disease and responds similarly to treatment with anti-Parkinson agents (14).

Antipsychotic drugs, administered chronically in high doses, also can cause disfiguring, often irreversible, extrapyramidal symptoms known collectively as tardive dyskinesia. These disorders consist of involuntary, gross, choreoathetotic movements of the extremities, face, and tongue. Withdrawal of antipsychotic medication tends to increase the frequency and intensity of the extrapyramidal symptoms. Increasing the dosage of the neuroleptic temporarily suppresses the symptoms but probably increases the underlying neuropathology. Although the hyperkinetic state sometimes remits spontaneously, tardive dyskinesia tends to be irreversible, and attempts at controlling the disorder pharmacologically have been disappointing (22,38). Tardive dyskinesia can occur in up to 60% of patients in psychogeriatric wards (21).

Certain phenothiazines, especially chlorpromazine, block activity of the adrenergic membrane transport system, which actively takes up, in addition to norepinephrine (NE), a variety of ring-substituted bases, including the antihypertensive agent guanethidine. When guanethidine and chlorpromazine are prescribed concurrently, the latter blocks activity of the "norepinephrine pump," thereby preventing accumulation of guanethidine and antagonizing its antihypertensive effects (14,18,19,38).

Recent studies indicate that antacid gels containing hydroxides and silicates of magnesium or aluminum interfere with the absorption of a variety of drugs from the gastrointestinal tract, including chlorpromazine and other neuroleptics. Concomitant administration of an antacid and a major tranquilizer may reduce the effectiveness of the antipsychotic by impairing its absorption (18,19,38).

CONCLUSION

Because it was assumed that mental illness was concomitant with aging, a shocking variety of physical and mental illnesses were collectively misdiagnosed as "senility" or "hardening of the arteries." Even today a predisposition toward the diagnosis of senility in psychiatrically compromised geriatric patients may prejudice accurate assessment and treatment within this population. Geriatrics may present with the entire range of psychopathological symptoms in either the absence or presence of actual senile symptomatology. Although there is no known "cure" for the senile dementias, much can be done to ameliorate coexistent anxiety, depression, agitation, or paranoia. When accompanying symptoms are treated, the senile patient often reacts with an improvement in cognitive function. Psychotropic agents can be useful in treating the senile patient. The elderly patient should be started at a lower dosage of medication and monitored very carefully for side effects. Adverse reactions occur with greater frequency and severity in the aged. However, senile patients generally respond favorably to drug therapy, with improvement in mood, affect, and psychotic symptoms. The elderly deserve the best possible life during their remaining years; pharmacotherapy of the affective components of the senile dementias can improve the quality of these years.

ACKNOWLEDGMENTS

The authors gratefully acknowledge the editorial assistance of Bruce W. Richman and Nancy L. Berry of Baylor College of Medicine and the Houston Veterans Administration Hospital.

REFERENCES

1. Allen, K. S. (1976): *Health Soc. Work,* 1:61–69.
2. Altman, H., Mehta, D., Evenson, R. C., and Sletten, I. W. (1973): *J. Am. Geriatr. Soc.,* 21:249–252.
3. Barton, R., and Hurst L. (1976): *Br. J. Psychiatry,* 112:989–990.
4. Bender, A. D. (1974): *J. Am. Geriatr. Soc.,* 22:296–303.
5. Birkett, D. P., Hirschfield, W., and Simpson, G. M. (1972): *Curr. Ther. Res.,* 14:775–779.
6. Boyd, W. E., Graham-White, J., Blackwood, G., et al. (1977): *Lancet,* 2:711.
7. Branconnier, R. J., Cole, J. O., and Cardos, G. (1978): *Psychopharmacol. Bull.,* 14:27–30.
8. Brook, P., Degun, G., and Mather, M. (1975): *Br. J. Psychiatry,* 127:42–45.
9. Carver, E. J. (1974): In: *Drug Issues in Geropsychiatry,* edited by W. E. Fann and G. L. Maddox. Williams & Wilkins, Baltimore.
10. Citrin, R. S., and Dixon, D. N. (1977): *Gerontologist,* 17:39–43.
11. Cohen, S. (1967): *J. Rehabil.,* 33:16–18.
12. Covington, J. S. (1975): *South. Med. J.,* 68:719–724.
13. Danto, B. L. (1969): *J. Am. Geriatr. Soc.,* 17:414–420.
14. Davis, J. M., Fann, W. E., El-Yousef, M. K., and Janowsky, D. (1973): In: *Psychopharmacology and Aging,* edited by C. Eisdorfer and W. E. Fann. Plenum Press, New York.
15. Degun, G. (1976): *Nurs. Times* 72(Suppl.):117–120.
16. Dennis, H. (1976): *J. Gerontol. Nurs.,* 2:28–30.
17. Deutsch, M., Saxena, B. M., Lehmann, H. E., and Ban, T. A. (1970): *Curr. Ther. Res.,* 12:805–809.
18. Fann, W. E. (1973): *Postgrad. Med.,* 53:183–186.
19. Fann, W. E. (1973): *South. Med. J.,* 66:661–665.
20. Fann, W. E. (1976): *J. Gerontol.,* 31:304–310.
21. Fann, W. E., Davis, J. M., and Janowsky, D. S. (1972): *Dis. Nerv. Syst.,* 33:182–186.
22. Fann, W. E., Davis, J. M., and Lake, C. R. (1973): In: *Psychopharmacology and Aging,* edited by C. Eisdorfer and W. E. Fann. Plenum Press, New York.
23. Fann, W. E., and Wheless, J. C. (1975): *South. Med. J.,* 68:468–473.
24. Fann, W. E., and Wheless, J. C. (1976): In: *Psychotherapeutic Drugs,* Part I, edited by E. Usdin and I. Forrest. Marcel Dekker, New York.
25. Fann, W. E., Wheless, J. C., and Richman, B. W. (1974): *N.C. Med. J.,* 35:672–677.
26. Fann, W. E., Wheless, J. C., and Richman, B. W. (1976): *Gerontologist,* 16:322–328.
27. Felger, H. L. (1966): *Dis. Nerv. Syst.,* 27:537–538.
28. Ferris, S. H., Sathananthan, G., Gershon, S., and Clark, C. (1977): *J. Am. Geriatr. Soc.,* 25:241–244.

29. Fields, G. J. (1976): *J. Long Term Care Admin.,* 4:1–9.
30. Freeman, J. T. (1974): *J. Am. Geriatr. Soc.,* 22:289–295.
31. Goldstein, S. E. (1974): *Curr. Ther. Res.,* 16:316–322.
32. Hader, M., and Madonick, J. J. (1966): *Am. J. Psychiatry,* 122:1289–1291.
33. Hader, M., and Schulmann, P. M. (1966): *Geriatrics,* 21:226–230.
34. Hall, P., and Harcup, M. (1969): *Angiology,* 20:287–300.
35. Harris, C. S., and Ivory, P. B. C. B. (1976): *Gerontologist,* 16:496–503.
36. Hollister, L. E., et al. (1969): *Clin. Pharmacol. Ther.,* 10:170–198.
37. Isler, C. (1975): *RN* 39:50.
38. Janowsky, D., El-Yousef, M. K., and Davis, J. M. (1974): In: *Drug Issues in Geropsychiatry,* edited by W. E. Fann and G. L. Maddox. Williams & Wilkins, Baltimore.
39. Jennings, W. G. (1972): *J. Am. Geriatr. Soc.,* 22:407–412.
40. Judge, T. G. (1977): *Age Ageing,* 6(Suppl.):70–72.
41. Katz, M. M. (1976): *J. Am. Geriatr. Soc.,* 24:522–528.
42. LaBrecque, D. C., and Goldberg, R. I. (1967): *Curr. Ther. Res.,* 9:611–617.
43. Lazarus, L. W. (1976): *Gerontologist,* 16:129–131.
44. Lifshitz, K., and Kline, N. (1963): In: *Clinical Principles and Drugs in the Aged,* edited by J. T. Freeman. Thomas, Springfield, Ill.
45. Linn, M. W., and Caffey, E. M. (1977): *J. Gerontol.,* 32:340–345.
46. MacFarlane, M. D. (1973): *J. Am. Geriatr. Soc.,* 21:414–418.
47. MacFarlane, M. D. (1975): *Fed. Proc.,* 34.
48. Manaster, A. (1972): *Int. J. Group Psychother.,* 22:250–257.
49. Nelson, J. J. (1975): *Geriatrics,* 30:113–142.
50. Nies, A., Robinson, D. S., Davis, J. M., and Ravaris, L. (1973): In: *Psychopharmacology and Aging,* edited by C. Eisdorfer and W. E. Fann. Plenum Press, New York.
51. Pearce, J. M. S. (1977): *Br. Med. J.,* 1:1661–1662.
52. Phillips, D. F. (1968): *Hospitals,* 47:47–49.
53. Post, F. (1968): *Br. Med. J.,* 4:627–630.
54. Powell, C. (1977): *Age Ageing,* 6(Suppl.):83–89.
55. Prange, A. J. (1973): In: *Psychopharmacology and Aging,* edited by C. Eisdorfer and W. E. Fann. Plenum Press, New York.
56. Rada, R. T., and Kellner, R. (1976): *Psychopharmacol. Bull.,* 12:30–32.
57. Rao, D. B., Georgiev, E. L., Paul, P. D., and Guzman, A. B. (1977): *J. Am. Geriatr. Soc.,* 25:548–551.
58. Ratner, J., Rosenberg, G., Kral, V. A., and Engelsmann, F. (1972): *J. Am. Geriatr. Soc.,* 22:556–559.
59. Reed, M. (1971): *Rocky Mt. Med. J.,* 68:44–48.
60. Reedy, W. J. (1967): *J. Am. Geriatr. Soc.,* 15:587–592.
61. Rosen, H. J. (1975): *J. Am. Geriatr. Soc.,* 2394:169–174.
62. Rosenberg, G. (1973): *Can. Med. Assoc. J.,* 108:547–549.
63. Salzberger, G. J. (1966): *Dis. Nerv. Syst.,* 27:57–59.
64. Seidl, L. G., Thornton, G. F., Smith, J. W., et al. (1966): *Bull. Johns Hopkins Hosp.,* 119:229.
65. Silverman, G. (1977): *Br. Med. J.,* 2:318–319.
66. Snyder, B. D., and Harris, S. (1976): *J. Amer. Geriatr. Soc.,* 24:179–184.
67. Stegink, A. J. (1972): *Arzneim. Forsch.,* 22:975–977.
68. Stern, F. H. (1970): *J. Am. Geriatr. Soc.,* 18:507–512.
69. Taulbee, L. R., and Folsom, J. C. (1966): *Hosp. Community Psychiatry,* 17:133–135.
70. Ter Harr, H. W. (1977): *Age Ageing,* (Suppl.):73–77.
71. Tobin, J. M., Brousseau, E. R., and Lorenz, A. A. (1970): *Geriatrics,* 25:119–122.
72. Turek, I., Kurland, A. A., Ata, K. Y., and Hanlon, T. E. (1969): *J. Am. Geriatr. Soc.,* 17:408–413.
73. Verwoerdt, A. (1976): *Clinical Geropsychiatry.* Williams & Wilkins, Baltimore.
74. Walsh, A. C., and Walsh, B. H. (1972): *J. Am. Geriatr. Soc.,* 20:127–131.
75. Walsh, A. C., and Walsh, B. H. (1974): *J. Am. Geriatr. Soc.,* 22:467–472.
76. Webb, W. L. (1971): *Geriatrics,* 26:94–103.
77. Wilson, W. P., and Majors, L. F. (1973): In: *Psychopharmacology and Aging,* edited by C. Eisdorfer and W. E. Fann. Plenum Press, New York.

78. Zwerling, I., Plutchik, R., Hotz, M., et al. (1975): *J. Am. Geriatr. Soc.*, 23:355–359.
79. Zung, W. W. K., Gianturco, D., Pfeiffer, E., et al. (1974): *Psychosomatics*, 15:127–131.

DISCUSSION

Dr. Lippman: The subject has been brought up of using the least anticholinergic drug you can with older people. Yet in the literature, there's much talk about the use of doxepin for the affectively impaired patient, and about the use of thioridazine for the elderly as well. I would like to hear some comment on those two agents in particular.

Dr. Wyatt: It has always surprised me that textbooks of psychiatry and neurology recommend amitriptyline, benadryl, and thioridazine for use in older patients. They have very potent anticholinergic side effects and in older people these side effects limit the drugs' utility.

I suppose the clinicians who use them want primarily to sedate their patients without necessarily easing specific target symptoms. For example, you may never get an antidepressant effect with amitriptyline because the anticholinergic effects prevent ever reaching adequate blood levels. It is a little bit of a mystery as to why these drugs have become the favorites in geriatric psychiatry.

Dr. Gershon: Just to add to that, not only are the elderly sensitive in some way to the anticholinergic effects, but they also seem to demonstrate a real receptor supersensitivity that we don't really understand.

There have been some studies to demonstrate in comparison groups that they respond quite remarkably, in that they develop an organic-like toxic delirious state, and I think the point Dr. Wyatt has raised is quite important.

The problem of course is that there needs to be a treatment of depression in the elderly. It's a necessary thing, because in many cases, some of the features of so-called organicity in pseudodementia are treatable. The availability of such an agent would avoid older depressives being put in a chronic care facility, if in fact they were responsive. Consideration therefore should be given to MAO inhibitors—which most clinicians are scared to death of using. I think that a reeducation program for physicians regarding MAO inhibitors is necessary. Also, there are new antidepressants being tested that are claimed to have minimal or no anticholingeric activity. So in both these areas, there is a promise of a way out of this dilemma.

Dr. Kermin: Just a brief question to Dr. Gaitz regarding the differential use of tricyclics or electroconvulsive therapy (ECT) in older people with dementia: Do you consider senile dementia to have an endogenous depression component, or to be associated more often with exogenous depression, caused by difficulties in environmental adaptation to the problem?

Dr. Gaitz: I would like to talk about these matters in more general terms. My concern is with the issues in making a diagnosis of mental illness, with a lowercase "m" and a lowercase "i," in older people. Diagnosis is complicated because one must take into account "normal aging" and physical disorders mimicking mental illness. To answer one of Dr. Kermin's questions, I do not believe categorically that every patient with dementia also has a depression.

I think we have had a kind of artificial constraint placed on us here in trying to talk about Alzheimer's disease as if it were a very specific disorder and overlooking, or at least minimizing, some of the other very real clinical difficulties.

I think we have some very serious problems in trying to distinguish between a diagnosis of senile dementia, or Alzheimer's disease, and what we might call normal aging. Hardly anybody has spoken about how difficult it is, at times, to differentiate physical illness and its manifestations from mental illness. Trying to make a diagnosis that should be the rationale for treatment can be very challenging. Multiple diagnoses may be necessary and the interactions must be understood.

Theoretical considerations, e.g., neurochemical theories of depression, are of some interest, but as a clinician, I am concerned primarily with what works and whether I can provide symptom relief. Consequently, I don't get caught up too seriously in considerations that may seem paradoxical to the theoretician, but may satisfy a clinician. I keep waiting for my friends in the basic sciences to really be able to give me precise and absolute information that is useful, but until this can be done, clinicians must rely on clinical observations.

In terms of what I prescribe, I prescribe what I am familiar with. If I have been prescribing thorazine and mellaril for a long, long time, as I have, and finding these drugs useful, I am inclined to just go right on using them, even if theoretically they shouldn't work. Reports of dangerous side effects deserve attention, but practicing physicians are likely to go right on doing what they have found works.

I think John Davis referred to this in discussing what clinicians know about shock therapy, and bilateral as opposed to unilateral placement of the electrodes. Clinicians generally are slow to accept changes and tend to do what they have done habitually. When you translate what researchers uncover and try to teach practitioners about these matters, you are into a different ball game.

Now, this doesn't really answer your question, but I believe we must address the issue of diagnosis, not just in terms of nosology and what we are going to call it, but with reference to the specificity of the diagnosis. Is what we have called senile dementia a unique disorder, a precise diagnosis, or condition, in the same way that you can speak precisely of a specific type fracture of a wrist as a diagnosis?

It seems to me that senile dementia as a diagnosis is much more complicated, with less precision and specificity regarding etiology, treatment, and prognosis. This may explain partially why we get into difficulty when we try to understand affective and paranoid components and the other features that we discussed earlier.

Dr. Kermin: Dr. Verwoerdt has referred to the agitated depressive organic patient who becomes a management problem on the ward. What are the drugs of choice in treating this kind of problem?

Dr. Epstein: To begin with, one has to look holistically at the patient and carefully examine each patient's total situation for the purposes of outlining an approach to care and treatment.

The question has been raised about depression in a patient with Alzheimer's disease. Here again, one has to take a complete history and attempt to place the depressive episode in the context of the life history of that patient. For example, have there been previous depressive episodes, and if so, how have such episodes been treated in the past? It is important to differentiate whether the patient has a history of repeated similar episodes or whether one is encountering a depressive episode that may be interpreted as a response to increasing deficit. This difference is important with respect to the therapeutic modalities to be used, ranging from psychotherapy alone to the addition of antidepressant or antipsychotic agents, with careful attention to the potentially serious sequelae associated with these compounds for the elderly.

Dr. Kermin: But with its delayed action, would a tricyclic be the drug of choice in treatment of a ward management problem in an organically impaired agitated depressed patient?

Dr. Epstein: Controlled studies have not found too great a difference in effectiveness between tricyclics and phenothiazines in the treatment of agitated depression. Where serious management issues are present with very agitated patients, I might choose a phenothiazine instead of a tricyclic agent.

Dr. Farell: The question of electric shock treatment in the presence of organicity is an open question and I wonder if the panel members would care to discuss this issue.

In the management of many affectively distressed elderly people with organic brain disorders, electric shock treatment is often not even considered as a potential treatment of choice. This might not necessarily have to be so. I wonder what others would have to say about that?

Dr. Kahn: I would like to comment, particularly bearing in mind the issue raised by Dr. Davis earlier in referring to the work of Squire purporting to show that there was long-term memory impairment following ECT. There appears to be a misconception.

Actually, Squire has shown that although there is some memory impairment following bilateral ECT for events that had occurred within the previous 1 to 3 years, there is return to normal function 1 to 2 weeks after the termination of treatment (1). In patients who were treated with right unilateral ECT, which is now the most commonly recommended technique, no memory deficits were observed at all.

Now, the reason I stress this point is that the elderly appear to be doubly deprived. They are consistently undertreated, partly because of general negative therapeutic expectations toward old people, on the one hand, and partly because of negative stereotypes about certain treatment procedures on the other. There is a tendency for some professionals to be reluctant to use ECT because of exaggerated notions of such undesirable consequences as memory impairment. Yet, ECT may, in fact, be empirically an extremely effective method for treating many cases of depression in the elderly. We must be very careful to consider all the relevant data in determining the real merits of such procedures.

Dr. Epstein: This is a highly emotionally charged issue in which factors other than clinical judgment may influence the determination of therapeutic modality. A specific situation may serve as a case in point. A patient in her early 70s had experienced an involutional depression about 10 years previously. She did not respond to antidepressant drugs at that time, but responded favorably to ECT. A similar depressive episode recently recurred wherein again she responded with profound side effects to a relatively low dosage of an antidepressant, and I experienced difficulty finding someone who would administer ECT in view of clouded medicolegal issues.

It proved as difficult (although certainly not impossible) to secure what was probably the most appropriate treatment for her as someone might have encountered 30 years ago who attempted to secure an illegal abortion.

Dr. Nathan: I wonder if any of the panel are aware of studies done specifically, not necessarily with demented patients, but with elderly patients, utilizing plasma levels of tricyclics against effectiveness of drug usage, against the amount of side effects?

Although we have seen a lot of literature recently on these levels in general populations, I am unaware of any specific studies of the elderly.

Dr. Gershon: I think the question you are raising is a valid one, but I am not aware either of any studies that have looked at this question specifically in an elderly population, or even more relevantly, in an elderly group with cognitive deficit.

This issue is a crucial one to relate to the issue of anticholinergic side effects. There is a recent paper, again not in the elderly, but overall, looking at side effects and not clinical response, suggesting that the level of the parent compound alone isn't the factor that relates to side effects, but rather it is a ratio of the compound with a metabolite which appears to be implicated.

The question you are raising is an important one; it hasn't been done, and additionally, it may require a more complicated way of approaching the problem.

Dr. Epstein: There is another factor possibly related to this, namely the recently discussed concept of a therapeutic window. If this proves to be the case, and it is far too early to be certain, the current practice of increasing dosage until either amelioration of the depression or the appearance of side effects which are too profound may be totally inappropriate. This is especially true for the elderly, and there are absolutely no data yet on any such possible window with respect to the elderly.

In Dr. Fann's presentation, he discussed the particular use of certain psychoactive agents in the aged. I want to ask a question that goes in another direction, which is, are there specific psychotropic drugs that should be avoided in the aged, as we think particularly of the three large groups of antianxiety, antipsychotic, and antidepressant agents? That is, are there particular drugs that you would caution the clinician to avoid in each of these groups when treating patients in the geriatric age range?

The second question that I want to ask Dr. Davis has to do with the studies on hydergine. Is there evidence from his study of the basic data from the Sandoz studies that hydergine ever brings about striking improvement in any individual patient? Is there evidence that it is more effective perhaps in milder than in more severely demented patients?

Dr. Davis: The question about toxicity is a good question. Unfortunately I don't have an answer for it. There is not much evidence from double-blind studies on differential effects of the antipsychotics or antidepressants in the elderly. The tricyclics cause a quinidine-like effect on the heart and so would be particularly contraindicated in patients with preexisting conduction defects, and, hence, it is sometimes appropriate to monitor conduction defects.

It is sometimes said that doxepin might be safer than imipramine (Trofranil) or amitriptyline (Elavil). In certain studies, on which this assertion is based, doxepin was used in a much lower dose than the comparable tricyclics. For valid data, comparable doses should be used.

The second question was about hydergine, both in Dr. Gaitz's study and in the Sandoz collaborative study: In my review, I was impressed that the hydergine effect was small, but reliable. That is, a fair number of patients do a slight bit better on hydergine than they did before on a number of different dimensions. This would be in contrast with the work on choline, where there is a hint that there may be a large effect on some patients. However, those were open studies, so that one would want to be very cautious in drawing conclusions. Perhaps if the effects could be determined, maybe a drug could be developed that would produce a more pronounced effect.

Dr. Epstein: The question of the effectiveness of hydergine is somewhat muddied by the issue of dosage. It has been approved by the FDA at a level of 3 mg per day. One hears, however, that it is being used in practice in daily dosages ranging from 5 and 6 to 10 to 12 mg for short periods. Several practitioners in this country have told me that they prescribe 6, 8, and as high as 10 mg for short periods and have found lower dosage schedules to be ineffective.

The reported studies, and they are few indeed, have used rather low dosages. Your study, Dr. Gaitz, had a 3 or 4 mg daily dosage.

There is also the question of the severity of the dementia and the point at which treatment might not be expected to be effective. We are all in agreement that there is a level in the dementing process where the loss is such that one might not anticipate improvement from any therapeutic modality. Until there has been further elucidation of these issues one can say very little about the effectiveness of hydergine, although Dr. Gaitz's results are certainly provocative.

Dr. Wyatt: There is another class of drugs that we have not talked about which is probably the most commonly used class of drugs in the elderly, the sleep-inducing agents.

One of the most commonly used, of course, is flurazepam, or Dalmane. One of the very disturbing things about this agent that we are just beginning to learn is that it works better on the second night than it does on the first. The reason is that a long-acting metabolite of flurazepam builds up in the body. Not only does flurazepam work better on the second night, it may work better on the third night and so on; after a week people may start to get into serious problems during the daytime with the drug.

There are some studies from Finland that are not widely known here indicating that people have trouble on simulated driving tests after taking flurazepam for a week. You would think that these drugs would be even more disruptive to the behavior of older folks than to that of the young people in the Finnish sample, and especially to those with some form of dementia.

Dr. Gershon: This, of course, is a very significant issue because in many nursing homes the goal is to produce cooperative, agreeable patients, so that there is the phenomenon of using nighttime sedation, daytime control, with consequent drug interaction effects and problems of long-term medication, all of which culminates in producing drunk, somewhat incapacitated individuals.

In Dr. Fann's presentation, he gave examples of patients getting 10, 15, and 20 medications at one time. The issue raised by Dr. Wyatt is therefore a very significant one.

REFERENCES

1. Squire, L. R., Slater, P. C., and Chace, P. M. (1975): Retrograde amnesia: Temporal gradient in very long-term memory following electroconvulsive therapy. *Science,* 187:77–79.

Clinical Aspects of Alzheimer's Disease and Senile Dementia, (Aging, Vol. 15), edited by Nancy E. Miller and Gene D. Cohen. Raven Press, New York 1981.

Individual Psychotherapy in Senile Dementia

Adrian Verwoerdt

Geropsychiatry Training Program, Duke University Medical Center, Durham, North Carolina 27710; and John Umstead Hospital, Butner, North Carolina 27509

Despite increasing interest in psychotherapy with the elderly, there are few if any attempts to explore the feasibility of individual psychotherapy with patients suffering from senile dementia. Systematic research in the aims and efficacy of psychotherapy in general remains difficult, limited as it is by the constraints inherent in putting in operation theoretical concepts and thereby making them objective measures. A review of the literature reveals agreement that (a) psychotherapy with older patients is not conducted often enough in view of the apparent need for it; (b) psychotherapy with older patients can be emotionally and professionally taxing, but also rewarding; (c) there is no basis for therapeutic nihilism; and (d) there is no systematized body of theoretical knowledge about the psychopathology of late life that would provide a scientific basis for rational treatment planning (5,8,18).

When exploring a particular therapeutic approach, we concern ourselves with the following parameters: The *topographical factor,* which refers to the structural aspects and answers the question "Where is something wrong?" This locus may or may not be the target for therapeutic intervention. The *nature of the pathology:* What went wrong in that specific locus or elsewhere and why? The *goal of therapy* is to intervene so that the structural or functional impairment in the topographical locus is alleviated. The *methodological* aspect refers to "know-how": how to implement therapeutic objectives through specific techniques.

DYNAMIC PSYCHOPATHOLOGY

Sociopsychosomatic Framework

The view of senile dementia as a *sociopsychosomatic* disorder was proposed by Wang and Busse (17). The clinical picture of dementia depends not only on the nature and extent of the brain damage but also on the individual's educational level, emotional maturity, socioeconomic factors, and so on. Elderly persons of low socioeconomic status tend to have more physical illness, which is associated with inadequate housing, nutrition, and medical care, as well as lack of social contacts. Social isolation, commonly associated with chronic illness, facilitates regression and withdrawal, which in turn contributes to the development of intellectual deterioration.

In dynamic approaches to psychopathology, we differentiate between the stress itself (e.g., loss of cognitive abilities) and the immediate emotional distress caused by it (e.g., anxiety), the defense mechanisms employed to deal with the stress and its associated distress (e.g., denial), and the psychological and behavioral phenomena associated with the defenses (e.g., denial associated with grandiosity and hyperactivity). In the case of dementia, we also need to take into account the consequences of the impaired autonomous ego functions (mental faculties).

Following a cybernetic schema, we discern three basic groups of mental functions: (a) perception of incoming stimuli; (b) an adaptational function, which includes the autonomous and defensive ego functions; and (c) response patterns involving motor activity or behavioral patterns. Certain stimuli due to quantitative or qualitative factors acquire the nature of stress; they cause tension which demands a solution, e.g., removal of the stress. Motor activity aimed at removing (the source of) stress is a corrective feedback; on the psychodynamic level, we speak of adaptive coping. In maladaptive behavior the output has the effect of amplifying the input and increasing the stress. Defenses can be adaptive (stress-reducing) or maladaptive (stress-amplifying). Intact ego function depends on intact brain functioning. Injury to the cerebral cortex means injury also to the ego functions (2,3). When the cortex is impaired, the ego's defensive (conflict-solving) capacity and the autonomous (conflict-free) functions (thought, memory, speech, perception, neuromuscular control, etc.) are affected.

Effects of Aging on Coping

Age-related changes affect the ego's autonomous functions and defense mechanisms. The autonomous ego functions may be affected by neuronal impairments, when insufficient energy is available to them, or when there is a withdrawal (decathexis) of the energy normally invested in the operation of these capacities. The latter is seen in various psychopathological conditions: Decathexis of perception may lead to hysterical conversion symptoms (e.g., hysterical blindness) and decathexis of memory may cause amnesia.

With aging, the physical and mental energy needed for effective coping is decreasing. As a result, the usual ways of coping, especially the high-energy defenses, may have to be replaced by new techniques of adaptation. Aggressive mastery, for example, may be replaced by acceptance and the capacity to accommodate to the inevitable without self-reproach or bitterness. High-energy defense patterns (the "fight" response) include counterphobic defenses, overcompensation, obsessive–compulsive defenses, the manic cluster (denial, hyperactivity, and suppression through diversion), and the paranoid cluster (projection, hostile aggression against the externalized problem, or repeatedly fleeing from the externalized threat). On the other hand, regressive defenses (the "flight" patterns, e.g., withdrawal) require less energy (20).

Premorbid Personality Factors

A possible link between certain premorbid personality traits (compulsiveness, aggressiveness, rigidity) and an increased vulnerability to dementia is mentioned by several authors (7,11). The patient whose premorbid personality is characterized by versatility in adaptation tends to have relatively less intellectual impairment in association with a certain amount of cerebral neuronal loss. A premorbid behavioral style involving aggressive and high-energy defenses may be especially vulnerable to the psychotrauma of loss of mastery (resulting from organic brain changes). Compulsive, rigid individuals are prone to react with profound anxiety when faced with the necessity of changing their habitual style and accomodating themselves to ego-alien constraints.

Interactional Effects

The awareness of intellectual decline produces the immediate response of anxiety and mobilizes specific defenses, often precisely those whose continued operation is being threatened. An aggressive, ambitious person may try to defend against the threat of loss of control by becoming even more aggressive and controlling. The compulsive person may become more rigid and set in his usual ways. Inasmuch as the patient tries to meet the threat headon, there will be more opportunities to experience failure, compounded by more anxiety, helplessness, and feelings of shame and anger. A second vicious circle is set in motion when auxiliary defenses (e.g., projection) are called into action. When this entails accusatory behavior, the patient may alienate the very persons whose support is vital. If he tries to cope by withdrawal, the net effect is similar: again the loss of external support. Still other vicious circles may be set in motion, linking with those already there and adding to their momentum. The combination of persisting high-energy defenses, intensifying negative emotions, and weakening environmental support sets the stage for another systems breakdown, e.g., a new physical illness. In other patients the course of events is less stormy because they use defenses that are less harmful, e.g., mild degrees of regression or denial.

SYMPTOMS AND SYNDROMES

The signs and symptoms of dementia are determined by the impairments of the autonomous ego functions and the type of defenses selected.

Changes in Autonomous Ego Functions

One of the earliest functions of the ego is to interpose a time lag between stimulus and response, providing an opportunity for selecting effective behavioral responses. Thus the mature ego (secondary process) stands in opposition to the pleasure principle (primary process). The latter is characterized by a tendency to immediate discharge of drive energy; an absence of negatives, conditionals, and time sense; and the use of allusions, analogies, displacements, and condensation. The secondary process (the reality principle) involves the delay of immediate gratification, the use of logic, the presence of the time sense, awareness of alternative modes of action, and decision-making ability. Regression of this ego function may result in "the geriatric delinquent" dominated by the pleasure principle and oriented toward immediate gratification (19).

When the *time perspective* breaks down, confusion between past, present, and future results, with disorientation for time and a tendency for the memory to become the real thing; "living in the past" is for the patient a new present.

Part of the abstract capacity is the ability to voluntarily evoke previous experiences. In addition to *memory* impairments per se, there is a disturbed relationship between the person (ego) and the stored memories. "Living in the past" is a form of autism, of living inside oneself with one's thoughts and memories.

Apperception, a mental scanning process of comparing incoming stimuli and images with those already stored in memory is impaired as well. The capacity to evaluate the significance of afferent stimuli by comparing them with past experience implies the crucial conceptual element of the "as if."

Essential features of a *thought disorder* include the presence of paleologic thought, concretization and perceptualization of concepts, and other impairments of abstraction. In paleologic thought, a common predicate leads to the establishment of an identity of two nouns (6).

> An 80-year-old woman with dementia and without a history of schizophrenia complained "I have stones inside, and it is hard for them to come out." She had fecal impaction and her stools were hard, like stones. She could not conceptualize the "as if" and make proper use of a metaphor. An associative link becomes an identifying link; the attribute: hard, common to both feces and stones, leads to the identity: feces = stones.

Perceptualization of the concept may play a role in the pathogenesis of hallucinations. A patient who had a problem with itching from very dry skin complained that "ants are crawling over my skin." The metaphor—itching is like crawling ants—had become the real thing. The figurative had become literal.

Primary process phenomena such as the use of allusions, displacement, representation by opposites, projection, and condensation are illustrated by the following case.

> A 91-year-old woman talked constantly about death, was suspicious that her family was too interested in her will, and was calling various relatives "Peter" or "Judas." She expressed fear that death would come by way of electric shock treatment. During the interview, she suddenly said that "Jesus comes as a thief in the night" (reference to biblical metaphor—Jesus comes unexpectedly).

The thought of her own death is concretely personified and externalized as a thief in the night. The externalized threat is not only disarmed but changed into its opposite, Jesus the Savior. The original notion of thief meanwhile finds its way toward her relatives: Judas was a thief who betrayed Jesus for some money. Even Peter disowned, betrayed Jesus—and that, just before his death. Likewise, her own offspring might abandon or betray her for money.

The cognitive deficits can be viewed as the principal stress to which the patient responds. What is unique is that the cognitive impairment corresponds with the ego impairment so that the stress has a "pre-empting" effect: healthy, adaptive types of coping (e.g., mastery mechanisms) are being pre-empted by the stress. An impaired abstract attitude is manifested by an inability to assume a definite mental set, account to oneself for certain acts, keep in mind different aspects of a task simultaneously, abstract common properties reflectively, voluntarily evoke previous experiences, imagine that what is merely possible, and detach the ego from the outer world or from inner experiences (observing ego). In the concrete attitude the person is bound to the immediate experience of the very things or situations in their uniqueness. Thinking and acting are determined by the immediate claims made by the particular aspect of the situation. The emotional attitude is not a more primitive attitude than the abstract one but normally exists alongside the abstract attitude. Because the emotional attitude is more closely related to the personality, it is more resistant to brain damage and may remain undisturbed when the abstract attitude is disturbed (9).

Type of Defenses Selected

The selection of a particular defense results in certain characteristic behaviors. This has implications for the individual's adjustment or lack thereof and for clinical management (13). The defense techniques and the behavioral patterns commonly associated with them can be grouped into three categories.

1. *Defenses aimed at mastery and control* include certain obsessive–compulsive mechanisms, overcompensation, and counterphobic defenses. (a) Obsessive doubting and compulsive rituals may serve to avoid decisive action. Obsessive–compulsive mechanisms also may occur in aged persons caught in a regressive drift. Compulsive rituals may emerge in a last effort to prevent the life space from decaying into a "microslum." In such cases we see the evidence of breakdown scattered, with the individual concentrating on keeping one tiny detail straightened out. (b) Overcompensation refers to behavioral patterns aimed at overcoming shortcomings, real or imagined. (c) Counterphobic mechanisms are a response to a challenge outside. However, the external challenge may have come into being through projection (of an inner sense of deficiency). Thus counterphobic defenses tend to be associated with paranoid behavior. Overcompensation or aggressive moves against an externalized threat require much psychic energy and become increasingly maladaptive in the course of aging.

2. Defenses aimed at *excluding the threat or its significance from awareness* include suppression and denial, rationalization, and projection. Denial and suppression are mental mechanisms by which an observation, fact, or its significance are disregarded, dismissed from awareness, or not recognized. Diversionary activ-

ities frequently facilitate denial (getting busy with something else), but these become more difficult as a result of disabling illness or idleness inherent in being isolated. Nighttime is especially difficult because of the lack of social and sensory input. Mild forms of denial are often conducive to good adjustment, but extreme denial, frequently coupled with rebellious protest, is self-destructive, since the person tends to neglect appropriate help.

In projection, the fact of a loss or illness cannot be ascribed to others unless mental disorganization is of psychotic proportion. Much more common is the projection of the *cause* of one's condition onto somebody or something external.

> An 86-year-old man, living with his 84-year-old wife in a rest home had been preoccupied with his loss of manhood. Contributing to his general sense of loss were his children's lack of interest, the sale of his home, and the loss of other belongings in a fire. He resented his financial dependency and required his wife to pin their spending money to her underwear. All expenditures needed his authorization. All the losses, however, converged into the overriding concern of losing his sexual potency. He then used projection to deal with this specific concern; he accused his wife of an affair with the rest home operator.

Typical for the paranoid phenomena in confused patients is the variability and lack of sophistication. A male patient in his 70s had the delusion that he was being poisoned and the "uranium in his blood" was sinking down into the veins of his legs. In actuality, his legs were swollen because of cardiac–renal failure, and attempts were underway to treat his uremia. The idea of something toxic became the focal point of a delusional elaboration. The transformation of urea into uranium, which is poisonous and heavily toxic, served to explain his state of being poisoned and the heaviness in the legs. A few days later, he casually changed his delusion into another one: that his heart was to be cut out.

3. Defenses aimed at *retreat from the threat and at conservation of energy* include regression and withdrawal. Regression is characterized by restriction of interest in the external world, self-centeredness, bodily overconcern, and increased dependency. Regression commensurate with the severity of illness is useful because it enables the patient to accept help in a dependent relationship. Excessive regression backfires because others view the patient as "bad and uncooperative." Because of the reduced scope of the patient's world, he is less able to form reliable judgments about what happens around him. The need for continuous reality testing arises; the resulting disturbing behavior represents attempts to find out where he stands with other people. As regression deepens, dependence on the familiar extends to routines and to inanimate objects. Patients find small disruptions of daily routine upsetting; they need to have their activities fall into a stable pattern. Some consequences of this are the inability to wait, a frustrating sense of impatience, and the occurrence of rage attacks.

Whereas regression is a moving away from adult role responsibilities, withdrawal is a moving away from people; it is a more serious development than regression. The response of withdrawal is often based on feelings of inadequacy or shame.

Signs and symptoms (i.e., the items of the mental status examination) in certain combinations produce characteristic clusters called *syndromes*. Applying the above described psychodynamic concepts, we can propose the following clinical entities within the boundaries of the syndrome of senile dementia. The *anxious–depressed* type is seen more often in the early phases of senile dementia, when there is "free floating" distress. The *obsessive–compulsive* type with rigidity and occasional counterphobic patterns reflects the operation of (high-energy) mastery defenses, and it also occurs during the early phases. When the mastery defenses become untenable, anxiety and depression return compounded by confusion in thinking and orientation. The condition is not yet irreversible. In the *manic type,* denial mechanisms are the line of defense. The affective distress disappears from the surface but at the cost of a break with reality. Psychotic restitution fantasies and a sense of solemn grandiosity may occur. Hyperactivity, often associated with denial patterns, tends to make it a high-energy defense: "economically" feasible in the early phases but not later on. Related to the manic type is the *paranoid type;* there may be an overlap. Some grandiose ideas have a paranoid core ("I am persecuted, therefore I must be special"); or paranoid ideas have a grandiose nucleus ("I am so special that people envy me and try to get my things").

The more advanced phases are characterized by the predominance of *regressive* defenses and phenomena. The thought disorder (with its accompanying impairment of time perspective, memory, and apperception) may be the dominant feature. There is increasing withdrawal into fantasy life, with weakening of behavioral controls. Logical thought and the ability to cope with novel situations progressively decline. The combination of decreased impulse control and the realization of failure results in periodic rage. The environment is interpreted as hostile or protective depending on intrapsychic processes rather than on reality testing. Other regressive phenomena include the abandonment of the upright position. When the patient "goes horizontal," sphincter control is usually lost. At this point, therapeutic intervention is by and large no longer able to reverse the process.

During the early phases, the episodes of living in the past are transient and characterized by hallucinatory experiences involving people of the past who are now dead. Through the patient's living in the past, there is a resurrection of the dead. By observing which people are resurrected, we estimate the depth of the regression into the past. For example, it is one thing to hear the voice of the father who died when the patient was 30 years old but another to hear the mother who died when the patient was 13. During the early phases of senile regression, appropriate treatment can retrieve the patient from his drift into the past. During the intermediate stage, the episodes of living in the past become more frequent and extended. Finally, they coalesce into a continuous existence of living in the past, and this is usually irreversible (15).

TREATMENT GOALS

Treatment efforts can be categorized under three headings. Therapy aimed at adjusting the input to the capacity of the brain comes under the heading of environmental support. Improving the functioning of the brain itself comprises psychotherapy and psychopharmacology. This "through-put therapy" includes two subgroups: treatment aimed at the cognitive deficit and that aimed at the response to this stress (emotional distress and maladaptive coping). Improving activity and action patterns comes under the rubric of behavior therapy or behavior modification. It is theoretically inaccurate and clinically unwise to select one treatment modality to the exclusion of others. Individual treatment is a necessary element in the total spectrum of a comprehensive approach.

The conceptual framework of dynamic psychopathology forms a basis for a rational approach to treatment goals: *where* to intervene and the *direction* and *degree* of our intervention. The overall objective is to re-establish in the patient a homeostatic equilibrium by implementing the following goals: (a) Break up any vicious circle of interacting social, psychological, and somatic factors. (b) Adjust the environment to the patient rather than vice versa. (c) Reduce the patient's need for those capacities that are impaired. (d) Effect restitution and replacement of impaired functions. (e) Maintain residual functions. (f) Treat the distress to forestall further maladaptive defenses. (g) Replace maladaptive defenses with those relatively less harmful. (h) Slow down clinical deterioration by counteracting undue regression. (i) Provide protective intervention.

TREATMENT METHODS

Psychotherapy can be defined as the planned application by a professional therapist of specific psychological techniques to help the patient by decreasing or removing psychological disability or misery and facilitating optimal functioning. The basic skills involved include the ability to: (a) make accurate observations of behavior and draw proper inferences from these; (b) synthesize the inferences in a tentative formulation which serves as a theoretical model and has implications for drawing up the treatment plan; (c) observe the effects of implementing the treatment plan; (d) use this feedback information for testing (confirming, refining, rejecting, etc.) the adequacy of the initial psychodynamic formulation. The goal of the therapist is, first of all, understanding. Whether he communicates his insights to the patient is a separate issue (14).

There are unique difficulties in applying the criteria inherent in this definition when working with patients with dementia. The "application of psychological techniques" is based on the premise that there is a suitable medium for transmitting therapeutic information. In dementia, however, this very medium (the communicative channels) is impaired. Secondly, the target toward which psychological techniques are directed to "decrease or remove psychological disability" (the brain) is afflicted with permanent damage. To deal with these difficulties, it is necessary to view psychotherapy as *therapeutic communication.* Moreover, when we speak of individual psychotherapy with senile dementia, it is more useful to think of it as how to be psychotherapeutic with the individual dementia patient.

Treatment goals with dementia patients are limited in scope. Once this has been realized and accepted, the physician may find that therapy can indeed be rewarding in terms of obtaining improvements in the patient and professional satisfaction for himself (16). It is essential to continue the therapy indefinitely. Clinical improvement should not lead to the conclusion that since the patient is better it is all right to stop therapy. Rather, its success implies the very opposite: to go on with it. By the same token, one would not stop insulin because the diabetic patient has benefited from it.

Therapist–Patient Relationship: Obstacles

Patient Factors

Because of sensory and intellectual impairments the patient has difficulty communicating and cooperating with the physician. It takes him longer to respond to questions, and he is more likely to forget treatment instructions. Therefore one needs to talk more slowly (not necessarily louder), repeat questions and instructions, and write down advice.

Transference

When entering into the doctor–patient relationship, the patient takes with him characteristic attitudes and ways of relating to others derived from early family experiences. *Transference phenomena* also vary depending on the type of clinical setting and personality of the therapist. The latter may be seen as a parental figure, regardless of age differences. The concept of transference has practical implications, especially when negative feelings (hostility, guilt, envy) are being transferred. If one is alert to such transference distortions and tries to understand them, it becomes easier to tolerate and manage difficult behavior. During psychotherapy with dementia patients, transference is not interpreted as in insight-oriented therapy.

Transference usually goes along with an observing ego capable of discerning the "as if" element when comparing a person in the present with one in the past. The dementia patient loses the ability to compare; there is an impairment of the observing ego: The ego can no longer detach itself from an experience but becomes an active participant. Transference phenomena in these patients may develop instantaneously.

A 78-year-old woman's first statement to me was: "Your wife has died." There were several levels of meaning to this; at that moment of getting acquainted, the relevant idea was that if my wife was dead, we would be "available" for each other—and that for this to be on her mind, she probably liked me: somebody to be with. She provided further evidence of this, saying: "And she over here [the nurse] is your daughter." Through this concrete transference, she expressed a specific feeling: that it was like a family here, that she felt at home.

Other transference distortions refer to the environment. When patients say that this place is a hotel, school, courthouse, or jail, this is not just "disorientation for place and person"; rather, such a misidentification often is a concretized representation of an inner feeling state. The above-mentioned patient identified the interview setting as a store: "Look there and you can see it; a store is a place to be with people"—again the idea of getting together. Later she stated "Now you and I are married"—ideas of permanence and closeness are expressed through the concept of marriage. Proceeding along her line of thought, I asked if she was going to be in the family way: "Oh, yes. We'll have children but not now, in a few years"—in other words, the closeness between us will not end for quite a while.

Language and communication

Frequently, taking the patient's statements at face value is not conducive to understanding. Yet for these patients, the very existence of any "true" communication would be in and of itself therapeutic: It keeps the patient in touch with reality. The question is: How do we make sense out of the patient's frequently chaotic thoughts, and how can we enter into his world and speak his language? The chaotic thinking in dementia is the result of an impaired abstract capacity (in psychodynamic terms, regression from secondary to primary process thinking). The thought processes are similar to those observed in dreams. The fact that all of us "share" this primary process thinking may be a basis for understanding the patient's thinking. For the actual clinical situation, some practical guidelines are suggested by the very nature of primary process and the consequences of impaired abstract capacity.

In *paleologic thought,* a common predicate leads to the establishment of an identity of two nouns (subjects) (6). The above 78-year-old patient called her ward physician "a preacher." When asked what preachers do: "They preach about heaven—that is nice." That was also the way she saw her physician. Cognitively, she was unable to recognize him as a member of the general category of "physicians," but emotionally she received from him "good feelings" and associated these with the preacher she had known so long. Technically then, the first step is to observe the concrete idea presented (preacher). Next, we obtain the relevant attributes of this subject (preacher = man in authority + nice). Third, we see if this key fits other locks: "Man in authority who is nice" also fits the patient's doctor.

In primary process, ideas can be expressed by their opposite, and *opposite ideas can exist side by side.* For example, birth and death are common delusional themes.

> An 85-year-old woman with dementia filled her shoes with bath powder and shredded paper, and tore up her clothes. She expressed the delusion that she had just given birth to a baby but the baby had died, and now she did not know what to do with the clothing. This is interpreted to mean that her own impending death was no longer in sight since she had regressed to a time when she still could give birth (a psychotic restitution fantasy). At the same time, her own death was represented by the baby's death concretely dramatized by tearing up her clothes.

The primary process does *not know of a negative, a possibility, or conditionals.* The most frequently asked question by patients on a geropsychiatric inpatient unit is: "When can I go home?" Trying to give a logical answer (in keeping with secondary process and reality orientation) often appears to leave the patient distressed. Further inquiry may reveal that he does not even know where his home is; or he talks about a home where he lived long ago. The point is that the question is a statement; the word "when" means "now"; and "home" stands for "at home." Thus the translation produces: "I do not feel at home here"—or "I don't belong here"—"I don't belong, and I feel lost."

In the primary process, there is no *time sense.* In an interview a patient may move back and forth through the time tunnel without constraints. To tell him that "Today is (day, month, year) and we are at (institution, city, state)," etc. might not be meaningful because he does not have the temporal structure to fit this information into.

The use of *analogies, allusion, displacement, and condensation* was illustrated by the patient calling relatives "Judas and Peter."

Since impaired abstract capacity leads to inability to *account to oneself for one's acts,* it is not fruitful to ask the patient why he did this or that. One patient, when asked why she kept having trouble with her wheelchair, responded: "I have not had lunch yet." This also illustrates projection and condensation: embedded in her response is the accusation "You don't feed me—that's why I can't do things around here."

Dementia patients have *difficulty getting started* on a task, taking the initiative, or making decisions. Once they are put on the right track, though, they may keep going, sometimes to the point of perseveration. Open-ended questions confuse the patient. It is useful to make contact by focusing on a concrete item (e.g., dress) or physical symptoms. Of all the objects in the patient's world, his body remains the closest to him.

There is an *inability to keep in mind various aspects of a situation simultaneously:* The patient can see the individual tree but cannot conceptualize the forest as an idea. If the nurse gives him a shot, "she hurts me—hurting me is what my enemy does—so she is my enemy."

Another phenomenon relevant to this context is that the patient ends up rambling. When he sets out in a statement to make a point, he cannot allow himself to disgress (e.g., by adding descriptive details) because during the moment of digressing he loses sight of where he was heading. He never gets to the point. To prevent such derailments, the therapist should firmly but gently intervene in the rambling and keep the patient on the right track. It is crucial to do this in a good-natured, noncritical manner lest the patient feel put on the spot and is forced to face his failure.

The patient falls back on the so-called *emotional attitude* (9). He responds to stimuli on the basis of the pleasure principle: either pleasant (good) or unpleasant (bad). Example of dialogue: Who is that person (a nurse)? "She is nice." What kind of things does she do? "She is nice to me." How? "She gives me baths and food." Such a patient can enumerate certain qualities of the nurse but cannot recognize her as a member of a conceptual category ("nurses"). Since the ability to express emotions remains relatively intact, it is a good technique to tune in on the patient's emotional channels, rather than something abstract.

Other patient-related obstacles in therapy are *physical and psychological distress, sociocultural* factors (the cognitive impairment makes it more difficult to bridge any sociocultural gaps between patient and therapist), and *family pathology* (some families may deny the patient's illness and cause the patient to go along with this attitude or rebel against it by becoming unduly regressed; other families tend to infantilize the patient, thereby promoting premature regression).

Physician-Related Obstacles

The counterpart of the patient's transference is countertransference in the physician. It may represent a counter-role to the patient's transference. If the roles are fitting and appropriate, the participants in the relationship have something to offer each other. A countertransference becomes a problem when it contains relatively strong neurotic components. Early emotional conflicts between the physician and his own parents may be reactivated, causing specific countertransference attitudes.

Gerophobic attitudes on the part of the physician or his own unresolved fears of aging and death sometimes make it difficult for him to treat patients with dementia (4). The obvious constraints in having to set limited therapeutic goals and the contemporary cultural emphasis on youth and attractiveness are added burdens.

Therapist–Patient Relationship: Optimal Attitude

It is necessary to view disturbed behavior as a malfunction of the total organism, just as one would regard physical symptomatology as a manifestation of malfunction of a particular organ. It is then easier to preserve an *attitude of detached concern* and to remain objective and helpful. This is especially useful when the patient is irritating or unresponsive to therapeutic efforts. Whereas overinvolvement is an "occupational hazard" in the treatment of children and younger adults, the other extreme, defensive withdrawal, is more likely to occur in clinical work with old patients. An attitude of optimal empathy may be facilitated by keeping in mind that "this old person was once at the same age as I am now."

A *realistic approach* to therapy is based on the recognition that no matter what symptoms the patient presents there is always something the physician can do to give relief. It is important to recognize that attempts to alter longstanding character patterns are not only futile but possibly harmful. The patient's behavior should be met with an attitude of matter-of-fact acceptance; helpful assistance should never be accompanied by undue efforts to correct him or by pointing out his deficiencies.

A *consistent approach* combines gentleness and firmness, and makes it possible to set limits to undesirable behavior (e.g., hyperactivity based on denial). Firm insistence, when used in the framework of a positive transference may be effective, e.g., in certain withdrawn or underactive patients.

Several types of therapist–patient relationships involve *dual roles* on the part of both participants. The patient may be older and may have had superior social or professional status; the therapist may feel constrained by some measure of awe, and the patient hesitates to settle in a dependent position. It is then useful to remember that a patient's wish for support from a competent helper cuts across all ages and classes. Yet some of this should remain tacit. On the surface level of the interaction, social amenities can be carried on in keeping with overt differences in status, class, and seniority. The therapist may comfortably assume a deferential attitude especially at the beginning and the end of the contact; he should not challenge any pronouncements but accept them with a mixture of respect and matter-of-factness. However, somewhere during the interview he shifts his weight (e.g., by giving specific advice or changing medication), easing himself and the patient into the other dimension of their relationship.

Getting and staying in touch is important. Physical touch comes about in the most natural way and reflects a basic way of getting in touch. Tuning in on the patient's emotional wavelength is another way of getting in touch. To stay in touch, one needs to keep the interview situation firmly in hand. There is only a limited place for nondirective interviewing technique and free association. It is necessary to prevent the patient from getting lost in his rambling. The question is: How can we remain in control without causing him to feel that we are "against him"? After all, the patient's ability to accurately interpret reality is impaired, and he may perceive our well-intentioned actions as disagreeable and alien. In fact, patients do get angry, turn away, or get up to leave. Yet there may be a way to reduce the risk of alienating the patient. Goldstein uses the term "communion" to indicate a state of solidarity between therapist and the brain-damaged patient (9). Goldfarb (8) proposes that the patient be permitted to regard the therapist as a parent surrogate. Wells appears to refer to the same phenomenon when he states that sometimes the physician furnishes another essential service: his presence alone may be important (16).

SPECIFIC TECHNIQUES

The overall goal of re-establishing psychological equilibrium and maintaining contact with reality is achieved by implementing the following subsidiary goals.

1. *Early recognition and correction* of the many social and psychological factors that may aggravate the clinical manifestations of intellectual deterioration and the decline of physical health are essential.

2. Since the capacity for homeostasis declines and the range of adaptation narrows, one should not attempt to adjust the patient to the demands of the environment but should *adapt the environment to the patient.* When the environment (physical and social) has been adjusted to meet the needs of the patient, a state of equilibrium and health prevails. Concerning environmental support, abnormal sensory input may be quantitative or qualitative in nature. Quantitative input changes include sensory overload (e.g., chronic overcrowding) and sensory underload. Sensory deprivation or social isolation may be imposed on the individual (e.g., being alone in a hospital room) or may be the outcome of life-long ego-syntonic character traits (e.g., schizoid isolation) or major psychopathology (e.g., depressive self-absorption). Qualitative changes in the input pertain to exposure to unfamiliar stimuli, e.g., sudden transfer to an institution.

3. It is important to *reduce the patient's need for his impaired capacities.* The patient's brain status may decompensate because of quantitative or qualitative changes pertaining to the individual's behavior patterns, changes in the demands of performance and work, and modification in coping techniques (e.g., exhaustion from manic hyperactivity). On the "output side" of our schema, we are concerned with modifying behavior in such a way that it deamplifies vicious circles (i.e., corrective feedback behavior) and therefore becomes more personally satisfying and socially rewarding (10).

4. *Restitution and replacement of impaired function* is a priority. Restitution of lost functions aims first at correcting medical and physical limitations. Since the problems of the bed-ridden or chair-ridden patient with dementia are far greater than those faced by the ambulatory patient, every effort should be made to preserve motility (16). The increasing array of prosthetic devices is one of the exciting developments of modern medicine: glasses, hearing aids, dentures, artificial limbs, cardiac pacemakers, artificial hip joint, devices compensating for loss of spincter control, etc. There are limits to the extent that prostheses can be used, particularly the constraints of the "host" characteristics. Even an ideal prosthesis may no longer fit because the infirmity of the prospective recipient does not provide a support basis for the prosthesis. From a utopian point of view, it is conceivable that almost all organs and body parts can be replaced by a prosthetic device, the exception being the brain. However, in the area of memory, thought, and judgment, the patient may rely on others

for support. These persons must be well acquainted with the patient. This type of support, being an extracorporeal cognitive prosthesis or memory device, cannot be expected from somebody who has known the patient only briefly.

5. *Maintaining and utilizing residual functions* is another important area. For the patient to utilize his remaining functions fully, the physician must assume dual roles: He must be personal physician to the individual patient as well as an organizer of health care functions by various professionals and agencies. Utilization of residual functions is related to preventing regression and maintaining activity, and is discussed below.

6. *Treatment of distress* is important for its own sake as well as to prevent additional maladaptive defenses. Generally speaking, to allay *anxiety* all the therapeutic principles underlying the optimal therapist–patient relationship must be observed. Appropriate dependency in the patient is therapeutically useful because it takes his attention away from anxiety-provoking concerns. Optimal regression, possible only in a firmly established therapist–patient relationship, is an effective antidote against anxiety; and when the motive of anxiety is absent, maladaptive defenses may be prevented from developing. When a positive transference exists, the patient looks forward to contacts with his therapist. Visits can be scheduled at regular intervals so that the patient has something definite to look forward to. In a hospital setting, rapport can be quickly established by frequent, brief visits (e.g., 5 min three times a day, at the same times).

Depletion anxiety refers to insecurity about the loss of external supplies and the possibility of isolation and loneliness. Its nature is not primarily in terms of a danger signal pertaining to unacceptable impulses from within but corresponds with separation anxiety (depressive anxiety). The patient may not always be aware of the source of his anxiety, and therefore careful exploration of his life situation is in order.

Anxiety also may be generated by a shift from a perspective of self-confidence in the direction of *helplessness.* Anxiety pertaining to loss of control and mastery may be the result of decrements in the area of personal competence and autonomy. Since the associated anxiety is in terms of loss of self-confidence and shame, it is more difficult to obtain information than in depletion anxiety (where the patient can simply point his finger to an external problem). The patient is gently but firmly advised and assisted to get whatever medical examinations are in order. It is surprising how often elderly patients resist having their alleged physical or mental defects examined. After the medical evaluation, it is also a frequent problem to get the patient to accept the recommended treatment. Here again, the positive transference in the relationship can serve its purpose.

Generally to reduce helplessness and enhance a sense of control, an "obsessive–compulsive" behavioral style may be encouraged: preference for closure and predictability, avoidance of risks and uncertainty, and emphasis on schemas and schedules. Relatives may be advised that the patient's feelings of helplessness can be alleviated by anticipating some of his needs. This fosters a subjective sense of control and may prevent angry frustration, depression, or shame. Patients handicapped by memory loss often have a relationship with one or more relatives in which the latter serve as an extracorporeal, prosthetic memory device. In contacts with such patients and their relatives, one can observe that whenever the patient's memory fails him he sends out a nonverbal signal (a quick look) toward the relative, who then responds by filling in the necessary details.

Acute traumatic anxiety may develop because of weakening of the ego's stimulus barrier. Normally the ego is able to screen unwanted stimuli through selective inattention, external diversions, etc. In conditions of moderate to severe regression, the ego boundary becomes more penetrable, and the patient is more vulnerable to what may amount to a barrage of unwanted stimuli. This type of anxiety is characteristic of infancy, when the ego is immature, but may occur whenever the ego is relatively weak, as in old age. Patients with mild cases show restless tension; those with more severe disability have outbursts of rage or exhibit defensive attempts to re-establish a stimulus barrier by withdrawal. Clinical management is supportive and includes drug therapy and environmental procedures. Supportive measures pertaining to environmental structuring essentially involve providing an "ego prosthesis." Such an artificial ego implies organizing the patient's environment for him, with the spatiotemporal relations of his milieu kept constant. The principle is that of sameness; by keeping the milieu constant, the sense of loss of mastery in the patient is minimized. Constancy can also be applied to arrangements of furniture, temperature, light, procedural methods, and so on. Temporal constancy pertains to times of visits by the physicians, nurses, relatives, and so on.

During interviews, avoid "conceptual" questions which would put the patient on the spot and cause a catastrophic reaction.

> A 79-year-old man showed clinical evidence of some loss of the capacity for conceptual thinking. When asked about the year of his son's death, he knew that this was twenty years ago, but after repeated questions about what year it actually had been, and after establishing what the present year was, he was not able to subtract 20 years from that. Instead, he added them on to the present year, which brought him close to the end of the twentieth century. At this point, he revealed perplexion and profound anxiety. He then mumbled: "or 2000?" The patient gives a wrong answer, is aware of his inability to perform accurately, develops profound anxiety, and becomes totally unable to perform.

Decrease fear of the unknown by focusing on body sensations and physical symptoms. Many patients start off an interview by presenting physical symptoms that are seemingly bizarre or inappropriate. These should not be dismissed as irrelevant because it may be the patient's only way he can still make contact.

Depression usually has an admixture of anxiety and vice versa. Thus treatment of depression lessens anxiety and vice versa. Depression is one of the causes of pseudodementia, but even if the dementia is organic the admixture of depression aggravates the symptomatology. It has been suggested that, since 25% of all demented patients also have depression and since depression may mimic dementia, all "demented" patients should get a trial therapy with antidepressant medications (16).

Depressive loneliness is extremely common. Everywhere one goes in a chronic care facility the question is heard: "When can I go home?" This reflects the wish to be part of a familial, familiar setting—to belong—to be in touch with one's past and present self. Being uprooted in a strange place and cut loose from his mooring, the patient is as much alienated from his inner world as from the world ourside.

Related to depression is *apathy*. Apathetic *withdrawal* may respond to an approach to appropriate stimulation. Many such patients are apathetic because they prefer the gratifications of their inner fantasy world over those provided by the real world. The treatment approach includes elimination of possible iatrogenic apathy (e.g., excessive tranquilization); remotivation, resocialization, and other group experiences; and auxiliary therapies and appropriate stimulation involving antipsychotics or antidepressants. Apathetic *exhaustion* is treated by intensive support. The principle involved is to nurture and restore an organism whose inner resources and adaptive capacity are critically diminished (anaclitic therapy). This involves adequate treatment of any physiologic disturbance and elimination of emotional insecurity by establishing a firm rapport, and permitting the patient to become dependent on the parental figure of the therapist. Upon the return of emotional responsiveness, one should not withdraw his support but maintain contact with the patient.

Shame and embarrassment is the result of increased helplessness and decreased self-confidence. It especially occurs when dignity is lost. Dignity involves a special type of self-esteem: to be regarded well in the eyes of others. One loses dignity in public, not in private. To protect himself against possible ridicule and disgust from others, the patient may withdraw or defiantly use counterphobic defenses, but the price of intact dignity is loneliness or the alienation of others.

The patient's need to maintain self-esteem requires a certain amount of denial on his part. This should be left intact, as long as it does not provide a serious risk to himself, others, or vital business matters. To protect dignity it is necessary to provide the patient with the essentials of privacy, a space he can call his own, where he feels he belongs and can keep his belongings. Efforts aimed at reducing helplessness and promoting a sense of control also enhance the patient's dignity. By protecting the patient's dignity, we protect his person, his self-image, his image to others, and, in the final analysis, our own dignity.

Anger and aggressiveness, being the result of frustration, occur under many conditions. Defensive hostility may be a cover for anxiety or depression; or, through an aggressive display, the patient may try to refute that he is helpless or shameful. In the wake of anger follows the conviction that the obstacle is out there, a comforting thought since attacking an outside threat is far simpler than coming to grips with the enemy within. The manifestations of hostility include vindictiveness; excessive complaining but recalcitrance in cooperating with corrective intervention; lack of appreciation for what is done in their behalf; blaming others; gossiping, cursing, and arguing; hitting others; spiteful acts (e.g., soiling themselves); etc. Management of these behavior patterns requires an exploration of the role played by the premorbid personality and recent stresses, and a recognition that the hostile behavior patterns are clinical manifestations of regression. The next step is, from a position of neutral objectivity and with an attitude of detached concern, to address oneself to the underlying concern and try to alleviate the stress. This may be a feeling of exasperating helplessness, shameful loss of dignity, bitterness about having been betrayed, or fighting against letting go for fear of being let down. When offering support it is often necessary to use a special form of tact. The giving is not done openly or formally, but tacitly and casually. This makes it possible for the patient to have his cake and eat it: He is receiving the needed supplies and can still have his kicks by indulging in various protestations. By now, the stage for a collaborative relationship has been set, and one may attempt to deal with the disagreeable behavior by setting limits. One method is the approach of conveying to the patient the recognition that he is making some good progress, and that this attests to his strength or courage. Again, the fact that the patient's strength has been "borrowed" from the therapist is left unspoken.

Management of Maladaptive Defenses

Removing or mitigating maladaptive coping can be accomplished by alleviating the underlying anxiety that prompted the particular defense or by replacing that defense with a more appropriate coping technique. A patient's defenses should not be exposed or removed without first ascertaining what he is defending against. A specific form of correcting maladaptive behavior is *behavior modification*. The therapeutic goal is to modify maladaptive behavior by extinction procedures, counterconditioning, desensitization, negative reinforcement, and operant conditioning by token regards. It seems that even in cases of moderate or severe organic mental disorders behavior can be modified, provided the reinforcement is specifically suited to the individual patient (1,12).

Defenses Aimed at Mastery

In cases where the premorbid personality was characterized by *excessive self-reliance* and the patient now has developed actual dependency on others (e.g., for basic support in the areas of memory and conceptual thinking), the stage may be set for undesirable developments. The patient may react to increased dependency by becoming more controlling, defiant, and insisting he can do without help from others. If the supporting persons try to correct him, he may react with anger to the point where he might feel that others are against him. If, on the other hand, the supporting people happen to be absent or unresponsive, he will feel lost, confused, and anxious. When projection is the predominant mechanism, pathological suspiciousness and anger follow, resulting in *paranoid behavior*. Clinical intervention is especially indicated when paranoid thoughts receive a charge of aggressive impulses. This mixture of paranoid suspiciousness and aggressive hostility is highly explosive, and there is a serious risk of violence aimed at disarming or destroying his alleged persecutors. The clinician must maintain an attitude of detached concern. Objectivity and neutrality are called for because of the patient's tendency to draw the therapist into the combat zone. Nothing is gained by trying to contradict the angry or paranoid patient or to correct his views. This would only confirm his belief that he is misunderstood by the physician. Nor is it therapeutically proper to agree with the patient. The correct response is to sidestep his attacks, make clear that you will remain strictly neutral vis-à-vis the accusations, acknowledge that the patient is having a hard time, and indicate a willingness to help in accordance with the best of your abilities.

Denial Mechanisms

When dealing with denial, it is necessary to proceed with caution. One should never try to break through the denial by forcefully uncovering the underlying emotions. Blind adherence to the principle of confronting the patient with his mistakes or trying to "correct" him is a caricature of therapy. Ventilation of concerns, however, is useful for specific emotions lying just below the surface, e.g., grief about loss, anger at medical personnel, or guilt about dependency. In patients with dementia the self is in a state of transition or crisis. Therefore it is not always prudent to probe for thoughts and emotions that do not contribute to the patient's sense of closure, e.g., current failures or past disillusionments. The tendency of many patients to make the best of it is not just a denial of some piece of reality. Rather, the attempt to seek out the sunny side of things in the here and now or, in retrospect, to beautify the past is nothing more than the work of that vital principle hope.

Regressive Mechanisms

Withdrawal is maladaptive because it creates distance between the self and other humans and facilitates a final break with reality. If withdrawal is a lifelong pattern (e.g., in schizoid personalities), little can be done. In contrast to such characterological withdrawal, defensive withdrawal can be managed more successfully. First, sources of potential stress and distress should be eliminated to remove the risk of failure and shame. Second, an approach of "passive friendliness" should be tried in the context of brief, frequent visits. Third, one may try to change the withdrawn person into a hypochondriac; this would also apply to the schizoid cases. Bodily overconcern focuses attention on the real object of the body; the somatic symptoms provide a covenient alibi for mental failures; and the physical symptoms can set the stage for a traditional physician–patient relationship.

Although in most cases hypochondriasis is the consequence of social isolation and self-absorption, in some instances the reverse is true. This happens when a withdrawn or autistic patient begins to turn his attention toward the real world. The first object encountered is his own body, which is a bridge between the inner self and the outer world. The presence of physical complaints sets the stage for contact and interaction between the patient and another person. Hypochondriasis then represents a favorable development which actually may be encouraged.

Optimal *regression* maintains a balance between the reduced assets (mental faculties) and the demand for performing tasks and activities. Therapeutic efforts include maintaining residual functions and preventing further regression through activity programs. Daily activities can be structured according to a regimen that is consistent, predictable, and sufficiently diversified. The activity spectrum should provide diversions and stimulation in keeping with the patient's personal wishes and remaining potentials. Avoid the extremes of overstimulation and social or sensory deprivation as each will exacerbate the symptomatology. Premature or excessive support has an adverse effect by promoting regression. Thus it is often difficult to stay on an intermediate course, avoiding on the one hand the extreme of insufficient support (which would create more anxiety), and on the other hand too much support (which would promote undue regression).

Motivation for activity must include a goal worth the effort. A patient may learn to walk again, but unless he has a motive for walking he will soon abandon the attempt. The milieu of the average institution frequently offers little incentive to activity, thus fostering regression and deterioration. Self-care has appeal only to the extent that there is something to live for. The therapist and other treatment team members can become sources of incentive by appropriately rewarding the patient's efforts. Activity is to be more than passive participation in time-filling work. Therapeutic activity has purpose; the more completely it absorbs the patient's energies, the more beneficial it will be. When activities bring about contacts with other people, isolation is reduced.

When designing an activity program, find out the patient's interests; make a list of potential activities (indoor, outdoor) appropriate for the season; determine the patient's attention span for each of the activities; note the preferred time of the day and preferred sequence of activities; arrive at a mutually agreed regimen of daily activities; have the patient come back to report on the regimen. The need for an individualized approach to the patient is pointed up by the fact that for each individual, sick or healthy, the pattern of age-related decrements is specific and the rate of decline varies from one function to another.

Protective Intervention

Although it is important to convey respect to the patient and allow him to continue in roles and customs in keeping with his self-image, it is also necessary to provide him with the protection that his condition requires. This protection can be given in tacit or direct ways. Tacit protection is called for when it is clear that the inherent demands of a situation would exceed the patient's capacities, e.g., tasks requiring the use of abstract thought, independent initiative, innovative problem-solving, or decisions involving complex issues with far-reaching consequences. Protective support can be given by allowing others to have the information available and providing it to the patient in a matter-of-fact, casual manner. The patient may well accept such help and information without openly acknowledging it, as if he himself accomplished something important.

SUMMARY

It may be emphasized that psychotherapy with patients who have senile dementia is an essential part of a comprehensive treatment approach; the other therapeutic components include somatic treatment, environmental manipulation, and behavior therapy. Psychotherapy with these patients can best be thought of as therapeutic communication with specific goals and methods. These goals and methods follow from our understanding of the structure and function of the mental apparatus and include consideration of the cognitive deficit and the impairment of defensive and autonomous ego functions.

REFERENCES

1. Ankus, M., and Quarrington, B. (1972): *J. Gerontol.,* 27:500–510.
2. Bertalanffy, L. Von (1966): In: *American Handbook of Psychiatry,* Vol. 3, edited by S. Arieti, pp. 705–721. Basic Books, New York.
3. Brosin, H. W., (1952): In: *Dynamic Psychiatry,* edited by F. Alexander and H. Ross. University of Chicago Press, Chicago.
4. Bunzel, J. H. (1973): *J. Am. Geriatr. Soc.,* 21:77–80.
5. Butler, (1975): In: *American Handbook of Psychiatry,* ed. 2, Vol. 5, edited by S. Arieti, pp. 807–828. Basic Books, New York.
6. Domarus, E. Von (1944): In: *Language and Thought in Schizophrenia,* edited by J. S. Kasanin, pp. 104–113. University of California Press, Berkeley.
7. Gianturco, D. T., Breslin, M. S., Heyman, A., Gentry, W. D., Jenkins, C. D., and Kaplan, B. (1974): *Stroke,* 5:454–460.
8. Goldfarb, A. I. (1967): In: *Comprehensive Textbook of Psychiatry,* edited by A. M. Freedman and H. I. Kaplan. pp. 1564–1587. Williams & Wilkins, Baltimore.
9. Goldstein, K. (1959): In: *American Handbook of Psychiatry,* Vol. 1, edited by S. Arieti, pp. 770–793. Basic Books, New York.
10. Katz, L., Neal, M. W., and Simon, A. (1960): In: *Psychopathology of Aging,* edited by American Psychopathological Association.
11. Kiev, A., Chapman, L. F., Guthrie, T. C., and Wolff, G. (1962): *Neurology,* 12:363–385.
12. Mueller, D. J., and Atlas, L. (1972): *J. Gerontol.,* 27:300–392.
13. Verwoerdt, A. (1972): *Adv. Psychosom. Med.,* 8:92–114.
14. Verwoerdt, A. (1976): In: *Clinical Geropsychiatry,* pp. 132–146. Williams & Wilkins, Baltimore.
15. Verwoerdt, A. (1976): In: *Clinical Geropsychiatry,* pp. 185–199. Williams & Wilkins, Baltimore.
16. Wells, E. (1977): *Contemp. Neurol.,* 15:247–276.
17. Wang, H. S., and Busse, E. W. (1971): *Contemp. Neurol.,*
18. Weinberg, J. (1975): In: *Comprehensive Textbook of Psychiatry,* ed. 2, Vol. II, edited by A. M. Freedman, H. I. Kaplan, and B. J. Sadock, pp. 2405–2420. Williams & Wilkins, Baltimore.
19. Wolk, R. L., Rustin, S. L., and Scotti, J. (1963): *J. Am. Geriatr. Soc.,* 11:653–659.

20. Zetzel, E. R. (1965): In: *Geriatric Psychiatry,* edited by M. A. Berezin and S. H. Cath, pp. 109–119. International Univ. Press, New York.

DISCUSSION

Dr. Wyatt: I was extremely interested in Dr. Verwoerdt's presentation of his use of psychodynamic psychotherapy with patients with organic disease or Alzheimer's disease.

A question I would like him to untangle for me is, very crudely, how do you distinguish the defense mechanism of denial that has a psychological basis from the kind of denial that arises from anatomical deficit? How do you disentangle these two so you can deal with them as a psychotherapeutic ally?

Dr. Verwoerdt: You are talking about organic denial versus a psychological denial, is that correct?

Dr. Wyatt: Yes.

Dr. Verwoerdt: It is very hard to differentiate between the two. I think there is an interplay here that is to me very fascinating, but also rather frustrating. Very often, the denial that has an obvious organic component is used in the service of psychological denial.

I have seen over and over again where patients have an actual memory loss, and I seem to be satisfied on that score, and then they make some kind of comment, such as "I forget what I want to forget."

In fact, the whole business of living in the past can be used as a massive form of denial. For example, one organic patient goes around the ward, holding his hand out, asking patients to give him a parking fee of 25 cents, because he thinks he is a parking lot attendant for the ward. The patient is delusional, and his memory is disturbed. He doesn't know that it was 5 years ago that he was a parking lot attendant. But, he feels much better being this parking lot attendant than being a patient in a mental hospital.

So, I think there is a good deal of purpose in what is obviously an organically determined living in the past. It is an adaptive response to loss of function, but I don't know really that you can draw any sharp lines here.

*Clinical Aspects of Alzheimer's Disease and
Senile Dementia,* (Aging, Vol. 15), edited by
Nancy E. Miller and Gene D. Cohen.
Raven Press, New York 1981.

Behavioral and Psychological Therapies for the Older Patient with Cognitive Impairment

Carl Eisdorfer, Donna Cohen, and Caroline Preston

*Department of Psychiatry and Behavioral Sciences, University of Washington School of
Medicine, Seattle, Washington 98195*

The focus of this chapter is primarily on one aspect of treatment in the spectrum of care for older patients with dementing illness, specifically that involving purely behavioral strategies. It should be clear, however, that except for heuristic purposes a focus on any narrow treatment approach, to the exclusion of other possibilities, is inappropriate. Careful diagnostic evaluation by an interdisciplinary health team leading to the provision of a range of alternative health and social services at home, in the community, or in the institution, and a careful ongoing assessment as to the most appropriate array of services and their provision, are (or should be) a minimal standard of clinical care.

Mental health care has traditionally been oriented toward a concern with two classes of illness: (a) the functional or environmentally induced and therefore (believed to be) potentially curable disorder (e.g., neurosis) and (b) the organic diseases or disorders involving structural changes, which are therefore incurable (e.g., the chronic dementing illnesses). Psychotherapy was available to those with "functional" problems, but individuals with organic problems were seen as incurable and therefore not treatable. Since chronic brain syndromes represent the epitome of the "organic" mental illnesses, it is not surprising that in the past mental health professionals felt little or no responsibility for the therapeutic (as contrasted with custodial) care of patients with this disorder. Except for custodial management, it was believed that there was nothing to offer.

When evaluating a given condition of older persons, it is theoretically possible to describe the result of age as contrasted with the effect of accumulated trauma or disease which exaggerates the possible vicissitudes of age per se (18). On a practical level, if a given clinical finding is clearly accepted as the consequence of normal aging, it is unlikely to warrant therapeutic intervention. Alternatively, if other factors are implicated in causing deviation from what is considered normal, the potential for prevention and reversibility is likely to be heightened.

An additional consideration should be recognized. Our federal policy equates "long-term care" with institutional placement and custodial maintenance, and federal reimbursement policies perpetuate this pattern, including stringent limitations on care for mental illness. Thus federal policymakers must also share the responsibility for exacerbating the current nihilistic climate associated with cognitive impairment among older persons. The concept that long-term care involves treatment, management, and rehabilitation of chronically impaired patients who require a range of coordinated strategies, including the introduction of new therapeutic approaches, is absent from federal fiscal policy although the problem is now recognized.

The aforementioned comments take note of a few examples of consequential background issues affecting outcome of patient care. They are included in order to alert the clinician and clinical investigator to the context in which patient care (and thus outcome) may occur at this point in time. The remainder of this chapter presents the nonbiological approaches to the treatment and management of the aging patient with a central nervous system disorder and associated cognitive dysfunction.

GOALS OF TREATMENT

Defining the goals of treatment is a fundamental part of the therapeutic plan. Thus the clinician may treat an individual in a medical emergency to stabilize her/him for further treatment; may treat a terminally ill patient to alleviate pain rather than prolong life; or may use medication to alleviate a disruptive symptom (e.g., high temperature), recognizing that additional or alternative strategies may be necessary for treating the precipitating disorder. Treatment goals can be broad or narrow, encompassing problems ranging from adjustment reactions in living to the behavioral sequelae of irreversible dementing illness.

Psychological therapies may be implemented using similar principles. The therapist may focus on alleviation of a specific phobic symptom, treatment of dysfunctional affective patterns in coping with chronic disease, difficulties in relationships involving authority figures, maladaptive behavior in family or marital crises, problems related to bereavement and loss (including multiple losses), or more general difficulties in understanding the etiology of one's behavior in relationship to life experience. With specific regard to the impaired aged, the focus can be on adaptational problems associated with dementing illness, with crises related to cognitive loss(es), and/or with the existential life situation of this population and their families.

When developing a treatment plan, the goals of the therapist, and if possible of the patient, should be as explicit as possible. Should the focus be on a disruptive behavior to be reduced and/or eliminated (e.g., cursing, urinating on the floor) or on improving social participation and long-term adaptation to the environment?

Outcome is related to the therapeutic model chosen in a given clinical instance. However, the model itself may alter the treatment program chosen for the patient. Thus the assumption that there is a paucity of available psychic energy, or that the aged are too rigid in their traits to undergo major character changes, doubtless were factors in the early reluctance of psychodynamically oriented psychotherapists to accept older patients. Similarly, the belief that cognitively impaired older persons cannot learn leads to exclusive reliance on medications and failure to institute alternative behavioral or environmental therapies.

The physical properties of the environment also play a crucial role in facilitating or inhibiting certain types of behavior and, as uncontrolled variables, may influence outcome of therapy independent of psychosocial interactions and psychological manipulations (9). Indeed morale, social interaction, and other indices of the quality of life may also be related to environmental variables (e.g., community structure, relocation, nearness to facilities, emotional closeness to family and friends), thus affecting the outcome of otherwise salutary programs. In spite of well-meaning psychological interventions, environmental characteristics may continue to be an obstacle to well-being.

Plasticity (i.e., the capacity to adapt or modify behavior in the face of internal or external demands for change) is the essential ingredient in the assumption of psychological interventions. Plasticity has typically been linked with growth and early development, applicable only to formative years. During the past few years, however, plasticity has begun to be accepted as characteristic of the aged as well.

To train and maintain adaptive behavior in the cognitively impaired elderly, stimuli must be defined in the environment, appropriate rewards identified, and devices provided or designed for making responses. Optimally, learning is self-paced, with opportunities for overlearning (85). Woods and Brittin (85) emphasized that little attention has been devoted to designing environments to stimulate appropriate behavior, although laboratory studies confirm that conditioning techniques are effective in elderly brain-damaged patients (3,44,45).

A recent review provides a summary of much of the material on intervention, treatment, and rehabilitation of psychiatric disorders in the elderly patient (30). As a result, this chapter highlights only a limited number of salient issues emerging specifically in the behavioral management of the cognitively impaired individual. A number of other potentially valuable approaches [e.g., music (melodic) therapy, dance (movement) therapy, and art therapy, as well as vocational and rehabilitational approaches] were also omitted in view of the paucity of data applicable to the organically impaired patient. Hopefully, future reviews will include such alternative treatments on the basis of their empirically demonstrated efficacy. The material in this report is organized by major therapeutic approach: contingency strategies, reality orientation and cognitive interventions, psychosocial approaches, family counseling, and institutional and environmental programs. Individual studies may fall in more than one category so that assignment to a given section is not to be construed as rigid.

CONTINGENCY STRATEGIES

Contingency strategies, also called operant techniques, derive from a model of learning developed by Skinner in contrast to the classical conditioning model of Pavlov. In the classical model a neutral environmental event (e.g., a sound) is associated with a somatic process (e.g., salivation) through its association with another environmental event characteristically evocative of the somatic process (e.g., food); the result of this procedure is that the previously neutral event itself evokes the somatic consequences (e.g., the sound of a bell leads to salivation). Operant conditioning, on the other hand, refers to a reward strategy in which a reward is made contingent on certain behaviors, the rewards serving to increase the likelihood that the behaviors in question would continue and/ or increase in frequency.

The operant approach to patient care involves analysis of the functional relationship between current environmental events and the consequences of the patient's behavior. The management of contingencies is the basic tool, and environmental events are delivered or withheld contingent on the behavior in question in order to strengthen, maintain, or weaken the likelihood that the specific behavior will recur.

The behavioral therapies should not be seen as exclusive, alternative, or conflicting approaches to patient care, but rather as adjunctive ones, with the recognition that with our current level of knowledge these may be the most effective strategies available. However, much more research into alternatives and effective strategies is needed. In most of the studies reviewed here, the behaviors were not labeled as secondary to dementing illness. Rather, the etiology of the behaviors was ignored, and the emphasis is on the behavioral changes themselves which happened to occur among patients with identified cognitive impairment. Although the interventions described are limited treatment strategies, they emerge as simple but successful approaches to management. Modification of the more distressing behavioral characteristics of particular patients can also yield positive socialization effects as well (85).

Operant techniques have been used with the elderly to change or moderate a wide variety of behaviors (for review, see refs. 47,75,82), such as speech and verbalization, sensory–motor behaviors, self-care, physical problems, and activities of daily living (e.g., ambulation). Hoyer et al. (49) hypothesized that the absence of verbal communication among elderly mental hospital residents represented operant behavior maintained by existing reinforcement contingencies (as opposed to being due to irreversible disease and aging phenomena). The study demonstrated that verbal communication could be re-established using operant procedures. In a case report, chronic screaming behavior of an 80-year-old nursing home resident was reversed by shaping and strengthening behaviors incompatible with screaming in conjunction with a modified time-out contingency following each screaming episode (6).

A resocialization program was implemented by Mueller and Atlas (72) using operant principles on a ward where prevailing conditions on the ward had fostered withdrawal, nonverbal behavior, and regression. Interactions were increased among the regressed geriatric residents in that institution.

A variety of other studies reported successful results using individual treatment methods to change exercise and eating patterns. Four geriatric residents of a psychiatric hospital were individually reinforced for exercising on a stationary bicycle, and three of the four increased their rate of exercising (61). Malament et al. (65) even facilitated exercise in wheelchair patients using an avoidance conditioning paradigm. An auditory alarm was sounded if the individual did not do an arm–body lift (45 sec duration) during 10-min intervals. Furthermore, the exercises implemented to prevent pressure sores were reported to continue even after the conditioning procedure was stopped. Positive reinforcement procedures were used with six geriatric inpatients who showed markedly low rates of correct eating. The average number of meals eaten correctly increased from 12% to 84% over the duration of the study (36).

Self-injurious behaviors of elderly persons (e.g., failure to eat or dress, or the ingestion of nonfood objects) have been altered using operant procedures (70,71). In one example, the behavior of the geriatric mental hospital resident who had refused to wear clothing for years was changed by gradually requiring the subject to wear additional pieces of clothing for longer periods of time each day, using beer as the reinforcer. Additionally, this resident's verbalizations concerning "voices" that told him not to wear clothes were extinguished after being ignored by the staff. It is noteworthy in this instance that by mediating staff reaction it was deemed unnecessary to use psychotropic medication with its attendant risk for side effects and further cognitive impairment.

Observation of patients to determine specific problem behaviors, as well as the utilization of operant techniques to mediate such behaviors, has been employed for recruiting attendance at nursing home activities (12,24,66). These treatment programs were concerned with the modification of simple operant behaviors. To our knowledge only Berger and Rose have utilized a social learning model to develop complex skills such as social interaction patterns in a group of institutionalized elderly. However, the generalizability of the training remains to be demonstrated.

Reinforcers can, but need not, be external edibles (e.g., candy, food) or tokens. For example, a high probability behavior can be used to reinforce a low probability behavior. This principle has been used with human subjects to strengthen exercising and participation in other activities. For example, in a study reported by Hoyer (48), baseline records of the daily behaviors of an institutionalized 78-year-old woman who refused to attend exercises or any other therapeutic activity were obtained. Over half of her awake time was spent in voluntary, extremely obsessive cleaning of the ward; none of her time was spent in structured ward activities. A program in which cleaning was made contingent on attending exercises for 5 min mornings and afternoons was established. As a result, she began to attend exercises twice a day. An increasing number of structured group activities (i.e., reality orientation, resocialization, work for pay) were required of her, and the time contingency in each was gradually increased over a 5-week period. This patient's behaviors changed in response to this management, and the change persisted over time.

Geriatric milieu programs generally involve the redesign of the institutional environment to be more compatible with the elderly person's functional capacities. Among the most common types of behavior modification program within the milieu approach is the "token economy." A program designed for geriatric patients in which tokens were awarded for engaging in specific social interactions, ward work, personal hygiene, and self-care has been reported (69). Tokens were exchangeable for "back-up" reinforcers, e.g., supplemental food and special privileges. A matched comparison group residing on a separate ward without a token economy received the same positive reinforcement but on a noncontingent basis. Significant behavioral improvement was obtained on both wards, but those individuals on the token economy showed greater participation in work activities and a greater increase in frequency of social interaction.

Similar results were reported in a study of the effects of milieu on disabled elderly men in a Veteran's Administration hospital ward (31). Greater improvement was obtained in the milieu in which the men were rewarded with money, special privileges, and membership in an "exclusive" club contingent on their degree of rehabilitation compared to an identical milieu without this reinforcement contingency.

Bowel and bladder training methods have been applied widely with mixed success (5,43,74,84). Habit training plus rewards appears to yield the best results according to Carpenter and Simon (23). For example, one patient was visited whenever she used the toilet appropriately, and in a week's time the incontinencies were reduced from six to two. Carpenter and Simon (23) also reported that when people were allowed to have personal pajamas, which they selected and bought, the rate of incontinence was reduced by a third. Incontinence is a multifaceted problem, however. Operant techniques may be particularly effective when incontinence is an "attention-getting" behavior, but combining the operant approach with treatment of urinary tract infections, reduction of delirium, and simplifying and teaching bathroom behaviors are probably also necessary.

REALITY ORIENTATION AND COGNITIVE INTERVENTIONS

Reality orientation involves the use of environmental and interpersonal cues to inform the patient about significant factors in his/her environment (4,32,83). Typically, patients are organized in groups of 5 to 10 individuals, and the therapist(s) reviews patient and staff names, the date, the location, and similar information. Based on meager evidence, reality orientation programs have received mixed reviews. Improved behaviors have been reported by independent observers of the subjects, although this improvement has not been documented using geriatric rating scales (7,46). Furthermore, systematic evidence suggests that reality orientation does not generalize to other behaviors, e.g., self-care or social behavior at home or on a hospital ward (25). A study by Brook et al. (17) suggests that if there are beneficial effects from reality orientation they may be the result of the patient–therapist interaction, a confounding variable in many psychotherapy studies.

A pilot study was conducted with cognitively impaired nursing home patients to compare the effects of reality orientation in relation to a program of cognitive training. The training programs required the residents to practice a series of cognitive tasks including receptive and expressive language functions, pattern perception, and Piagetian tasks of conservation of space and volume. The participants of the cognitive training showed significant improvements over the reality orientation subjects on WAIS subtest scores (Cohen, *in preparation*). The preliminary evidence in this study suggests that reality orientation appears to have no lasting effects and may be equivalent to no intervention at all.

Two rigorous studies support the notion that memory dysfunction in nursing home patients can be improved (59). The underlying assumption of this work is that cognition may be enhanced by not only increasing the individual's attention to the environment but also increasing the cognitive demands of the environment. Langer and co-workers (59) hypothesized that active coping with new contingencies in a stimulating environment would increase cognitive activity, and that this would be demonstrated in performance scores. In both studies the cognitive demands of the psychosocial environment were increased by a series of interviews challenging the individual to think and become involved in the discussion. The extent to which residents became involved in attending to and remembering these environmental factors varied by the experimental condition. Involvement was manipulated by varying the degree of reciprocal disclosure (i.e., personal information) offered by the interviewer in a series of dyadic interactions between the patient and the interviewer. Previous work (52) suggested that clients talk more about themselves in situations in which the interviewer offers personal comments in contrast to a standard interview. Thus nursing home patients were assigned to an experimental high self-disclosure condition, a low self-disclosure condition (standard interview), and a no-interaction condition. Individuals in both treatment conditions were visited four times during a 6-week period. All persons were tested for memory functions 1 month prestudy and 1 week poststudy. The results revealed significant improvement in standard short-term memory tests for the high self-disclosure group but not for the low self-disclosure or the no-treatment condition. Furthermore, the group in the no-treatment condition showed a significant decline in test performance. Improvement was also found on nurses' ratings of alertness and mental activity and on staff evaluations of social adjustment.

A second study was implemented to manipulate the involvement variable. Nursing home patients were assigned either to a "contingent" condition in which they were given tokens contingent on remembering information correctly during the interview or a "noncontigent" condition in which they were give tokens simply as a remembrance of the visit. The tokens could be redeemed for a gift at the end of the study. There was also a no-treatment condition in which the patients were visited initially and asked the same questions as the two experimental groups. The patients were told that the experimenter would return within 3 weeks to see them again and that they would receive a gift in appreciation of their participating in the study. The patients in the two treatment conditions were visited a total of nine times during a 3-week period.

Patients assigned to the contingent condition performed consistently better on memory tests regarding medications, nursing home activities, visitors, etc. than individuals assigned to either the noncontigent or no-treatment condition. Both of these studies are strong arguments that restructuring the long-term care environment can have a profound impact on memory functioning and social adjustment. These investigations with older persons in long-term care settings (where diagnostic classification is not explicit) are consistent with other reports evaluating the impact of the environment on intellectual performance in institutionalized older people (56,68,73). Although Langer's studies with impaired elderly did not provide the participants with specific training on cognitive tasks similar to the dependent variables of the study, significant improvement did become evident on those variables. Further research is necessary to document the impact of psychosocial and environmental factors on formal cognitive test performance as well as the motivation to learn and respond to the environment in general.

The development of therapeutic programs to enhance cognitive skills is an important research area. Fozard and Popkin (33) emphasized that any treatment intervention should include enhancement of cognitive skills as well as counseling or psychotherapy. Individual or group supportive psychotherapy may be important to develop the motivation to practice cognitive skill training. Furthermore, specific interventions to treat depression and anxiety may also have the effect of improving cognitive performance (29).

There are several components to effective cognitive enhancement strategies, and each aspect requires an empirical data base. These include: (a) appropriate techniques for identifying and monitoring cognitive skills; (b) appropriate reinforcers for older patients; (c) attention to premorbid level of function and individual differences; (d) the integration of cognitive enhancement strategies into a system of comprehensive care; and (e) the use of environmental contingencies, especially those which sustain the individual's attention to, and interest in, the environment. There is also some speculation suggesting that cognition could be enhanced by encouraging appropriate play activity (86). Play and games may well prove effective when used to develop and exercise sensory–motor, cognitive, and social skills in the impaired elderly.

PSYCHOSOCIAL THERAPIES

The usefulness of conventional individual and group psychotherapy for older people has been reported by many investigators (for review see refs. 30,42). The subjects involved in these interventions are typically described either as nonpsychiatric older people, physically ill geriatric patients with emotional problems, or institutional geriatric patients. However, the presence or degree of cognitive impairment among the subjects of these studies is not identified. The lack of carefully controlled studies to determine the efficacy of the conventional group therapeutic approaches continues to be a conspicuous problem (30).

Although Freud (34) wrote that people in their fifties lacked the mental plasticity necessary to be treated successfully with psychoanalysis, and even declared that older people could not learn, other psychotherapists have generally been more cautious in rejecting the aged as patients. The capacity for changing behavior seems to rest on a variety of personality traits, e.g., flexibility of the person *and* the environment, motivation, intelligence, and the ability to learn (10,20, 22,35). Such traits are indeed present in older persons and make them appropriate candidates for psychological therapy.

Psychotherapy and counseling among the elderly are now practiced in many forms, ranging from crisis-oriented therapy to longer-term insight-oriented and reconstruction therapy (16,21,22,30,42,50). However, despite the probable efficacy of many psychotherapeutic modalities, the aged still are seen infrequently in outpatient psychiatry clinics and mental health centers (55); furthermore, therapists continue to be reluctant to deal with aged patients (19,26).

Psychotherapeutic activity with the nonimpaired aged may now be expanding as a focus of interest (19,30,67); however, there appears to be little activity oriented toward the aged with severe cognitive impairment. Because the aged with dementing illnesses are not usually considered appropriate candidates for individual psychotherapeutic approaches, only a limited discussion of the data on psychotherapeutic intervention is included here.

The selective review of Ingebretsen (50) provides a helpful orientation to the issues in psychotherapy with aged patients and has particular implications for the treatment of patients with dementing illness. She identifies three foci for psychosocial therapy, i.e., neurotic symptoms and character disorders, adjustment reactions to changes and loss, and multiple losses in later life (e.g., retirement, death, isolation, anemia, clinical disease, existential adaptation to life transition, aging, and death).

Goldfarb and his associates (37–41) identified the importance of intrapsychic processes in the impaired older patient and clarified the contribution of dependency and feelings of helplessness to a spiraling of the impairment process. Goldfarb's early emphasis on emotional factors and how they could exacerbate the degree of impairment in central nervous system disorders was an important contribution but unfortunately did not develop into a systematic strategy of patient care. For the patient with serious cognitive difficulties, the potential of such a strategy remains largely unexplored.

Reports primarily limited to group therapy suggest that activity and milieu therapies, for example, may increase even a disoriented individual's control over the environment (53,63,64,77). However, the challenge remains to evaluate those factors which are important in order to effect changes. Furthermore, to the authors' knowledge, not a single study has been done to evaluate the effectiveness of any behavioral or psychosocial therapeutic strategy on a variety of specific emotional symptoms often exhibited by cognitively impaired persons, e.g., depression and anxiety, However, psychosocial strategies have been identified as useful in the treatment of paranoid behavior (27).

A variety of group therapeutic approaches, including remotivation, resocialization, and activity processes, have all been reported to be successful (30), but unfortunately most of these studies have ignored the tedious route of controlled investigation. There seems little doubt that increased attention of whatever nature to the older person does yield positive results, but the scientific significance of these results remains to be explored more rigorously.

FAMILY THERAPY

Personality change is a predictable consequence of the course of brain damage. In view of the impact that families have on their individual members, it is reasonable to believe that a number of treatment and management problems posed by the patient with dementing illness might be appropriately cared for within the family constellation by working directly with the family members. Lezak (60) proposed that counseling of families improves the quality of their adjustment such that the pattern of interaction between family and patient improves. Tobin *(in press)* found a positive relationship between the knowledge of community resources on the part of the family and maintenance of the older impaired relative in the community. Brody (15) and Isaacs (51) also emphasized the central role of the family in patient adaptation. Clearly the family must become a focus for more concern and therapeutic assistance in managing the organically impaired older person. It is hoped that a body of data will emerge in support of this position.

ENVIRONMENTAL AND INSTITUTIONAL STUDIES

In view of the problems which emerge during adaptation of the impaired aged who move from one facility to another (2), it seems important to deal with intervention strategies associated with institutional change as well as with physical environmental factors. Two specific psychological mechanisms have been identified as mediators in the stress response to relocation of the elderly: (a) the perceived controlability and predictability of events surrounding the move; and (b) differences in environmental controlability pre- and postrelocation (79). Although the specific environmental configurations (i.e., age-segregated or age-integrated, high density or low density of old people moving or not moving) are important, change per se seems less significant than whether the individual has a choice in the change. A study cited by Seligman (80) is a prototype of the gathering evidence. He reports as follows: "Ferrari has written a doctoral dissertation on perceived freedom of choice in an old age home. Her main interest was in attitude change in the home, but during the course of writing the dissertation she produced a major finding on survival. Fifty-five females over 65 years of age and with an average age of 82 applied for admission to an old age home in the Middle West. Ferrari asked them on admission how much freedom of choice they felt in moving to the home, how many possibilities had been open to them, and how much pressure their relatives had applied to them to enter the home. Of the 17 women who said they had no alternative but to move to the home, 8 died after 4 weeks in residence and 16 were dead in 10 weeks. Apparently only one person of the 38 who saw an alternative died during the initial period. These deaths were called 'unexpected' by the staff. Another sample of 40 merely applied for admission but never became residents because they died. Of the 22 whose families made application for them, 19 were dead within 1 month after application was received. Of the 18 who applied for themselves, only 4 had died by the end of the month."

It is probable that these data are confounded by a number of uncontrolled variables, including different levels of physical health in the various groups; thus fewer options would be available to the sicker individual or the less affluent, etc. Indeed the failure to control for these and other variables (reflecting data from a number of studies of relocation) significantly compromises the interpretation of the Ferrari study. On the other hand, the results may reflect the profound effect of helplessness in old people. This hypothesis, with its rather profound implications for patient care and the range of human services deserves careful study. We do know from Blenker's (14) study that people who experience "learned" dependence in receiving social services showed higher death rates than those for whom supportive services were not available. This probably resulted from their higher rate of institutionalization.

Seligman (81) makes a case for old age as a period of special vulnerability to loss of controls of one's environment. "If a person or an animal is in a marginal state, weakened by malnutrition or heart disease, a sense of control can mean the difference between living and dying." Helplessness or the absence of response related to control of one's environment has been implicated in the institutionalization and death of humans (80).

Construing many situations in which elderly patients find themselves as reflecting "programmed helplessness" is not unreasonable. One important aspect of contingency programs that may have been overlooked is that in addition to shaping subjects' behavior by a system of reinforcements, such a system also gives individuals greater control over what is going to happen to them, and thus they regain some measure of subjective mastery which, alone, may be a significant reward in these paradigms.

The meaning of the transition from community life to residence in a home for the aged may be viewed by males as a loss of power and by women as being rejected and unwanted (62). An analysis of the personal significance of institutionalization for the aged residents and staff revealed that staff members saw themselves as caretakers for a group of powerless clients in need of services, and residents were seen as passive recipients of care. The residents eventually responded to the perceptions (expectations) of institutional life and accepted the roles assigned to them. In a recent report, Bergman (11) summarized three studies on long-term care, pointing out that medical and nursing staff emphasized "conformity" as the single most important attribute of the "good" patient.

The encouragement of decision-making among elderly nursing home patients, giving them decisions to make and providing them with some living things outside of themselves (a plant) for which to be responsible, resulted in making a group of subjects happier, more alert, and healthier (76). An alternative to viewing the experimental group as "responsibility-induced" as was originally conceived, may be the view of them as a "thought-encouraged" group. This implies that some optimum level of cognitive activity may be necessary for survival. A study is now being conducted to parcel out the utility of perceived control as one explanation of those mortality findings (57).

Studies of the positive effect of increased control in subjects who were retirement home residents have also been reported (78). In one study subjects were assigned to one of four treatment conditions: no treatment, unpredictible visits by an undergraduate student, visits at a time and for a duration known in advance by the resident, and visits controlled by the residents. The combined groups of subjects who could predict and control visits showed a more positive effect than did the combined no-prediction, no-treatment subjects.

Langer and Rodin (58) manipulated perceived control in the verbalizations of a retirement home administrator informing residents about how much choice and responsibility they had in their daily routines. Subjects led to believe that they had considerable control over their lives fared noticeably better than did the comparison subjects. An alternative interpretation of these results is provided by Blaney (13), who states, "It seems likely that the helplessness-reducing communication in both studies constitutes an act of deference and respect; the results may thus reflect the salutary effects of being treated with respect and may not reflect anything about perception of control."

Abramson and co-workers (1) recently reformulated the "learned helplessness' hypothesis and used a revised attribution approach to explain universal versus person helplessness and chronic versus acute problems. According to the authors, when there is no specific contingency for loss of control, people find a cause or contingency. The specific causal agent(s) to which etiology is attributed varies—internal–external, greater or lesser degree of specificity—and is dependent on a number of variables related to personal style of the subject and the nature of the precipitants. Four therapeutic strategies are suggested: (a) reduce the probability that the environment will be aversive and increase desired outcomes; (b) diminish the preferability of the most preferred outcomes by reducing the aversiveness of unmodifiable actions which will certainly occur and reduce the value of unobtainable outcomes; (c) change expectation from uncontrollable to controllable when outcomes are attainable and, if necessary, train in appropriate skills; (d) change unrealistic attribution for failure toward external, unstable, specific factors (i.e., away from oneself) and unrealistic expectations of success to internal, stable, global factors. Therapeutic strategies based on these hypotheses appear to relate directly to the institutionalized elderly patient and to offer an important conceptual approach to the depressive elements in patients with cognitive disorders.

The effects of orienting institutional staff from a patient focus to a *person* orientation was the basis of a series of studies by Kastenbaum and his colleagues (54). The work—best known for its use of wine and beer in a hospital setting—focused on the conflict in models created by giving patients wine rather than pills; i.e., patients get pills, people get wine. Unfortunately, the salutary outcome of the person-oriented strategy has not been extensively followed up in the literature. The value of deinstitutionalizing the institution, moving from an exclusive focus on custodial and health care to a spectrum of therapeutic and social programs maximizing individual options within the communal setting seems to have great promise. This would involve greater personal risk for some patients, perhaps the majority of those who are older and institutionalized but would emphasize nonmedical innovations, e.g., an increased area in which to walk versus pills to sedate. Here the "trade-off" would be on maximizing quality of life rather than protecting and swaddling the older person (Kahn and Tobin, *this volume.*)

In their review of the literature on the impact of physical and social environments on the institutional aged, Bennett and Eisdorfer (8) concluded that behavior was multidetermined, with no one institutional variable playing a clearly dominant role in predicting behavior. The aged appear to be no less sensitive to the impact of the physical environment than is any other group, and perhaps they are more sensitive than other adults (Lawton, *this volume.*) The authors found that more innovative approaches came from large mental institutions than from nursing homes. This may be the result of the size of staff and budget in institutions or because of a therapeutic tradition for younger patients which generalized throughout institutional settings. Of considerable interest too is the finding that advances made during the course of therapy are often lost rapidly when treatment stops. In their final conclusion, Bennett and Eisdorfer (9) state, "There is reason to believe that the aged, at any level of competence, will respond particularly if helped to play an active, participating role in their own care."

CONCLUSIONS

Behavioral approaches to the treatment of the aged have been fraught with numerous difficulties, including therapeutic nihilism, a focus on curative treatment rather than management and maintenance of function (or prevention of decay) in chronic diseases, negative attitudes toward the investment of resources in "the aged" (the most frequent victims of dementing disease), and economic policies mitigating against such therapies while favoring custodial care for "mental illness" in elderly persons. Apart from those problems which relate to propensity to treat are issues related directly to the effectiveness of treatment strategies if applied.

The variables affecting outcome of therapy include diagnosis, goals, expectation of outcome, conceptual model of the disorder and of therapy employed, the nature of co-therapies (if any), the ecosystem in which the treatment is taking place, as well as the system to which the patient must eventually adapt. Although a detailed analysis of all these variables could not be included in this chapter, future studies of these factors could lead to important insights affecting clinical outcome.

A few points are appropriate for final discussion. Diagnosis clearly influences choice of treatment. As indicated, one must be careful to avoid pitfalls of therapeutic nihilism associated with some diagnoses. For that reason, some therapists choose to ignore diagnostic statements. Inappropriate or misdiagnosis, however, can lead to errors in choice of treatment. Thus clinical depression, masquerading as cognitive impairment, once correctly diagnosed is a treatable illness. Because there is evidence that older persons with brain disease are at risk for poorer evaluation (for review, see ref. 30), this problem is worthy of note.

With advances in cognitive therapeutic strategies, greater refinements in the diagnosis of dementing illness must occur. Thus differentiating between cerebrovascular and Alzheimer's variety of dementia is probably not sufficient. Precise delineation of the nature of the cognitive deficit in a given patient could lead to the application of more specific cognitive approaches to help compensate directly for the loss experienced by the individual (28,29).

We may find that we are not able to substantially reduce the perceived helplessness of the elderly patient in the later stages of a dementing illness. However, a therapeutic approach which would decrease the helplessness of the family or staff in the management of these patients could well result in significant improvement in patient care.

Much more needs to be known—not only about behavioral modification among the elderly but about the behavior modifiers themselves, their relationship to stages of dementia, and the specific modes of enhancement of contingency programs. The impact of affective change, environmental mastery, situational anxiety, and a range of associated psychological variables on cognition is not yet well understood, and further study could yield much of clinical value. The range of psychological therapies, even in the presence of cognitive impairment and family-focused care, as well as a greater investment in training and concern for the attitudes of institutional staff, remain important areas for future work.

REFERENCES

1. Abramson, L. Y., Seligman, M. E. P., and Teasdale, J. D. (1978): *J. Abnorm. Psychol.* 87:49–74.
2. Aldrich, C. K., and Mendkoff, E. (1963): *J. Am. Geriatr. Soc.,* 11:185–194.
3. Ankus, M., and Quarrington, B. (1972): *J. Gerontol.,* 27:500–510.
4. Anon. (1969); *Reality Orientation.* American Psychiatry Association, Washington, D.C.

5. Atthome, J. M., Jr. (1972): *Behav. Ther.*, 3:232–239.
6. Baltes, M. M., and Lascomb, S. L. (1975): *Int. J. Nurs. Stud.*, 12:5–12.
7. Barnes, J. A. (1974); *Gerontologist*, 14:138–142.
8. Bennett, R., and Eisdorfer, C. (1975): In: *Long-Term Care: A Handbook for Researchers, Planners, and Providers*, edited by S. Sherwood. Spectrum, New York.
9. Berger, R. M., and Rose, S. D. (1977): *J. Gerontol.*, 32:346–353.
10. Berezin, M. A. (1972): *Am. J. Psychiatry*, 128:1483–1491.
11. Bergman, S. (1978): Studies of adaptation in congregate facilities in Israel. Presented at the Gerontological Society, Dallas.
12. Blackman, D. K., Howe, M., and Pinkston, E. M. (1976): *Gerontologist*, 16:69–76.
13. Blaney, P. H. (1977): *J. Abnorm. Psychol.*, 86:203–223.
14. Blenkner, M. (1967): *Gerontologist*, 1:101–105.
15. Brody, E. M. (1977): *Long-Term Care: A Practical Guide*. Human Science Press, New York.
16. Brody, E. M., Kleban, M. H., Lowton, M. P., and Silverman, H. A. (1971): *Gerontologist*, 2:124–133.
17. Brook, P., Degun, G., and Mether, M. (1975): *Br. J. Psychiatry*, 127:42–45.
18. Busse, E. W., (1969): In: *Behavior and Adaptation in Later Life*, edited by E. W. Busse and E. Pfeiffer. Little Brown, Boston.
19. Butler, R. (1975): *Am. J. Psychiatry*, 132:893–900.
20. Butler, R. N. (1963): *Psychiatry*, 26:65–76.
21. Butler, R. N. (1968): *Psychiatr. Res. Rep.*, 23:233–248.
22. Butler, R. N., and Lewis, M. I. (1977): *Aging and Mental Health*, 2nd ed. Mosby, St. Louis.
23. Carpenter, H. A., and Simon, R. (1960): *Nurs. Res.* 9:17–22.
24. Cautela, J. R. (1966): *J. Geriatr. Psychol.*, 198:9–17.
25. Citrin, R. S., and Dixon, D. N. (1977): *Gerontologist*, 17:39–43.
26. Crisp, A. H. (1977): *Lancet*, 2:1342–1345.
27. Eisdorfer, C. (1980): In: *Handbook of Geriatric Psychiatry*, edited by E. Busse and D. Blazer, pp. 329–337. Van Nostrand Reinhold, New York.
28. Eisdorfer, C., and Cohen, D. (1978): In: *Alzheimer's Disease, Senile Dementia, and Related Disorders*, edited by R. Katzman, R. Terry, and K. Bick. Raven Press, New York.
29. Eisdorfer, C., and Cohen, D. (1978): In: *The Clinical Psychology of Aging*, edited by M. Storandt, Plenum, New York.
30. Eisdorfer, C., and Stotsky, B. A. (1977): In: *Handbook of the Psychology of Aging*, edited by J. Birren and W. Schaie, pp. 724–748. Van Nostrand, New York.
31. Filer, R. N., and O'Connell, D. D. (1964): *J. Gerontol.*, 19:15–22.
32. Folsom, J. C. (1967): In: *Current Psychiatric Therapies*, Vol. 7, edited by J. H. Masserman. Grune & Stratton, New York.
33. Fozard, J. L., and Popkin, S. V. (1978): *Am. Psychologist*, 33:975–989.
34. Freud, S. (1924): In: *Collected Papers*, Vol. 1. Hogarth Press, London.
35. Fromm-Reichman, F. (1950): *Principles of Intensive Psychotherapy*, p. 24. Chicago University Press, Chicago.
36. Geiger, O. G., and Johnson, L. A. (1974): *Gerontologist*, 14:432–436.
37. Goldfarb, A. (1953): *Ment. Hyg.*, 37:76–83.
38. Goldfarb, A. I. (1956): *Am. J. Ment. Sci.* 232:181–185.
39. Goldfarb, A. I., and Sheps, J. (1954): *Psychosom. Med.*, 16:209–219.
40. Goldfarb, A. I., and Turner, H. (1953): *Am. J. Psychiatry*, 109:916–921.
41. Goldfarb, A. I. (1955): *Psychoanal. Rev.*, 42:180–187.
42. Gottesman, L. E., Quarterman, C. E., and Cohn, G. M. (1973): In: *The Psychology of Adult Development and Aging*, edited by C. Eisdorfer and M. P. Lawton. American Psychological Association, Washington, D.C.
43. Grosicki, J. P. (1968): *Nurs. Res.*, 17:304–311.
44. Halberstein, J. L., and Zaretsky, H. H. (1969): *Arch. Phys. Med.*, 50:133–139.
45. Halberstein, J. L., Zaretsky, H. H., Bruckner, B. S., and Guttman, A. R. (1971): *Arch. Phys. Med. Rehabil.* 52:318–336.
46. Harris, C. S., and Ivory, P. B. C. B. (1976): *Gerontologist*, 16:496–503.
47. Harris, S. L., Snyder, B. D., Snyder, R. L., and Magraw, B. (1977): *J. Chronic Dis.* 30:129–134.
48. Hoyer, W. J. (1973): *Gerontologist*, 13:18–22.

49. Hoyer, W. J., Kafer, R. A., Simpson, S. C., and Hoyer, F. W. (1974): *Gerontologist*, 14:149–152.
50. Ingebretsen, R. (1977): *Psychotherapy*, 14:333–314.
51. Isaacs, B. (1971): *Br. Med. J.*, 4:282–286.
52. Janis, I. L. (eds.) (1980): *Counselling on Personal Decisions: Theory and Research on Helping Relationships.* Yale University Press, New Haven *(in press).*
53. Kahana, E. (1971): *Gerontologist*, 1:282–289.
54. Kastenbaum, R. (1965): *J. Hum. Relations*, 13:266–275.
55. Kramer, M., Traube, C. A., and Redick, R. W. (1973): In: *The Psychology of Adult Development and Aging*, edited by C. Eisdorfer and M. P. Lawton. American Psychological Association, Washington, D.C.
56. Labouvie-Vief, G., and Gordon, J. (1976): *J. Gerontol.* 31:327–332.
57. Langer, E. (1978): In: *New Directions in Attribution Research*, Vol. 2, edited by J. Harvery, W. Ickes, and R. Kidd. Lawrence Erlbaum Associates, Hillsdale, New Jersey.
58. Langer, E., and Rodin, J. (1976): *J. Personality Soc. Psychol.* 34:191–198.
59. Langer, E. J., Rodin, J., Beck, P., Weinmer, C., and Spitzer, L. (1980): Environmental determinants of memory improvement in late adulthood. Submitted.
60. Lezak, M. (1978): *J. Clin. Psychiatry*, 39:592–598.
61. Libb, J. W., and Clements, C. B. (1969): *Percep. Motor Skills*, 28:957–958.
62. Lieberman, M., and Lakin, M. (1963): *Processes of Aging*, Vol. 1, edited by C. Tibbetts and W. Donahue. Atherton Press, New York.
63. Linden, M. (1953): *Int. J. Group Ther.* 3:150–170.
64. Maizler, J. S., and Solomon, J. R. (1976): *J. Am. Geriat. South*, 24:543–546.
65. Malament, J. R., Dunn, M. E., and Davis, R. (1975): *Arch. Phys. Med. Rehabil.*, 56:161–164.
66. McClennahan, L. E., and Risley, T. R. (1972): The organization of group care environments: living environment for nursing home residents. Presented at the American Psychological Association, Honolulu.
67. McGee, J., and Lakin, M. (1977): *Psychotherapy*, 14:333–342.
68. Meichenbaum, D. (1974): *Hum. Devel.*, 17:273–280.
69. Mishara, B. L. (1977): Geriatric patients who improve in token economy and general milieu treatment programs: a multivariant analysis. Presented at the meeting of American Psychological Association, San Francisco.
70. Mishara, B. L. (1973): *Int. J. Aging Hum. Devel.*, 4:133:145.
71. Mishara, B. L., Robertson, B., and Kastenbaum, R. (1973): *Gerontologist*, 6:311–314.
72. Mueller, D. J., and Atlas, L. (1972): *J. Gerontol.*, 27:390–392.
73. Plemons, J., Willis, S., and Baltes, P. (1978): *J. Gerontol.*, 33:324–341.
74. Pollock, D. D., and Liberman, R. P. (1973): *Gerontologist*, 13:488–491.
75. Richards, W. S., and Thorpe, G. L. (1978): In: *The Clinical Psychology of Aging*, edited by M. Storandt, I. C. Siegler, and M. F. Elies. Plenum, New York.
76. Rodin, J., and Langer, F. (1977): *J. Personality Soc. Psychol.*, 35:897–902.
77. Saul, S. R., and Saul, S. (1974): *Gerontologist*, 14:446–450.
78. Schulz, R. (1976): *J. Personality Soc. Psychol.* 33:563–573.
79. Schulz, R., and Brenner, G. (1977): *J. Gerontol.*, 32:323–333.
80. Seligman, M. E. (1975): *Helplessness: On Depression, Development and Death.* Freeman, San Francisco.
81. Seligman, M. E. P. (1972): *Annu. Rev. Med.*, 23:407–412.
82. Storandt, M. (1978): In: *The Clinical Psychology of Aging*, edited by M. Storandt, I. C. Siegler, and M. F. Elias. Plenum, New York.
83. Taulbee, L. R., and Folsom, J. C. (1966): *Hosp. Community Psychiatry*, May:22–25.
84. Wagner, B. R., and Paul, G. L. (1973): *J. Behav. Ther. Exp. Psychiatry*, 1:29–38.
85. Woods, R. T., and Brittin, P. G. (1977): *Age Ageing*, 6:104–112.
86. Vandenberg, B. (1978): *Am. Psychologist*, 33:724–737.

DISCUSSION

Dr. Gershon: Dr. Eisdorfer in part of his presentation raised the issue of differential diagnosis and got a very positive response from some members of the audience. Dr. Wells, would you like to elaborate on that issue?

Dr. Wells: Well, I was glad that it was raised again as a matter of fact, because I think while we've talked a great deal about nomenclature, we haven't spent quite so much time on the problems that occur in diagnosis. As I was thinking about Dr. Eisdorfer's statement, about his reasonable questioning of the accuracy and precision of our diagnoses, the thing that was really coming to my mind was the extent to which, despite all our words to the contrary, we persist in making the diagnosis along a single axis. I am not using "axis" in its DSM-III sense, but I mean how we tend to diagnose along a single continuum, without a consideration of multiple diagnoses in most of these people.

For example, the problem always exists of reaching an accurate diagnosis as to which organic disease, if any, is present. That is an admirable aim and one that probably can be attained with considerable certainty, as a lot of different studies over the past several years have shown.

What we are not accustomed to doing, however, is considering that often there should be a second diagnosis, one that falls in the realm of what we usually consider to be functional disorders. That is, to what extent is this person suffering also from the functional psychiatric disorder that may be either exaggerating or emphasizing the organic aspects of the patient's dysfunction?

The possibility that a patient who has minimal or even more severe organicity also suffers from a depression, for example, has been adequately considered. Certainly Dr. Kahn and others have shown the close association between loss of memory or complaints of loss of memory and depression.

On the other hand, I think we have perhaps given too little attention to the possibility that many of these patients with complaints of memory loss actually suffer from rather profound character disturbances that have been present for many years.

In studying some of our patients who appear clinically to be demented, but who show relatively little solid evidence for an organic lesion, I am struck with the frequency with which these persons have been extremely dependent individuals throughout their lives.

In summary, I think it is very important that we reach the correct diagnosis of any organic disease that may be present. I think it is equally important for us to consider other factors and to make multiple diagnoses in many of these patients, and therefore to consider the possibility of multiple treatment modalities even in patients who have very definite organic dysfunction.

Dr. Eisdorfer: Basically, I am contending that a simple atomistic approach to the notion that we can do CT scans and figure out how large the lesion is, or how large the size of the ventricle is, and therefore make a diagnosis, is probably not the best route.

This is not to imply that it is not a valuable route; I just don't think it is the best route. I am going to switch hats and play the psychologist for a while: We have learned a lot about cognitive structure in the last 15 or 20 years that we have not at all applied to functional capacity in later life.

I would contend that specific functions go, and that there are different patterns of functional loss that make up in the aggregate the symptomatology of dementia. I would contend that we need to get about redefining dementia, shifting from simple ideas about the loss of recent and late memory to a conceptualization of the cognitive structure of the individual.

Dr. Weinberg: I would like here to make a plea for the individuation of the person. I feel that I ought to take some sort of issue with Carl Eisdorfer, who tells us we must make a good differential diagnosis, and once we do that, then we label the individual into a patient. And, that we believe that once we have a name for it, we can either treat that name or not. On the other hand, Carl says, treat him/her as a person. My feeling is that what we need to do is to see that the individual is in a state of flux, and that he/she is a person who is in trouble.

Then, Dr. Wells, you say we must make one diagnosis and another type of diagnosis, secondary and tertiary, and it is difficult to make a diagnosis in psychiatry without making a speech. Yet this is really what is required of us. So, I think there is a great need to be able to see that here is an individual in difficulty. Let's try and help that person, and we will arrive at the diagnosis eventually; it will emerge as we review the historical aspects of the problem.

While we are talking about diagnosis, with the issue of pseudodementia, dementia, depression, and so on, we need also to recognize, as you Carl have pointed out more than once, that the greatest anxiety that a human being can experience is the feeling that he is beginning to decompensate, and beginning to experience serious cognitive difficulties and losses.

I believe that Dr. Verwoerdt has really made a plea for the understanding of these patients that I hope is not lost on us. He tried painstakingly to enhance our attempt to understand the behavior of these patients, and to outline the defensive mechanisms involved. My question to Carl is, how will he reconcile the person and patient?

Dr. Eisdorfer: One of the hangups we have is what I would call "the emotional attachment to a diagnosis." Treating an individual as a patient in no way means to me that I shouldn't have a sense of what is wrong or right with that individual. The trap that you lay out so beautifully is that we may make the diagnosis, and then treat the diagnosis, rather than the person. That, of course, is a signal of failure.

On the other hand, just knowing that a patient is depressed is not nearly as valuable to me as a therapist, clinician, psychiatrist, or psychologist, as having an understanding as to whether that person has a bipolar depression, or a unipolar depression, or reactive depression, or what I call existential sadness. The value of diagnosis makes that individual more the individual for me. I have a better understanding of his or her problem in order to help the human being, and I am still treating the person.

I feel that one of the failures of all of us in psychiatry has been to lose sight of the fact that the true purpose of making the diagnosis is to give us greater precision in caring for the individual, rather than treat the pigeonhole.

So, my feeling is that it is not that diagnosis is bad, it is what people do with diagnosis, which is after all a cognitive tool, that can be a problem. I find that for me and the way I teach it, as long as you know that diagnosis gives you a better field in which to work with the individual, you will learn a lot from it.

To ignore the importance of diagnosis is, I think, to really lose the forest and the trees and the human beings in the midst of all of it.

Dr. Solomon: In relation to Dr. Eisdorfer's presentation, I wonder if Bob Kahn would comment on the usefulness of the learned helplessness paradigm as a way to give older institutionalized patients more control.

Dr. Kahn: Well, I think that Dr. Eisdorfer's comment on the learned helplessness paradigm to characterize patients in nursing homes was a very apt one. The kind of withdrawal and helplessness that has been noted repeatedly in such patients does fit the paradigm.

What troubles me in his comments, however, is that psychologically, the tremendous trauma and loss of control over one's own life that follows the enormous dislocation of being put in a nursing home is balanced by giving the person control over some plants or some other trivial aspect of his life. Such substitute controls may be diversionary, at best, but can hardly be considered as a serious psychological compensation for the real losses.

Clinical Aspects of Alzheimer's Disease and Senile Dementia, (Aging, Vol. 15), edited by Nancy E. Miller and Gene D. Cohen. Raven Press, New York 1981.

Sensory Deprivation and the Effect of the Environment on Management of the Patient with Senile Dementia

M. Powell Lawton

Philadelphia Geriatric Center, Philadelphia, Pennsylvania, 19141

The task of writing a chapter on the environment as an aspect of the treatment system is potentially rewarding, since the gains to be derived from concern over our treatment environments are substantial and yet are often unrecognized. On the other hand, the task is frustrating because of the great void in empirical research to guide us in the better use of the environmental component; one cannot at this stage of development, produce a genuine critical review of the research literature. This chapter incorporates such findings wherever possible, leaning heavily on some relevant research done at the Philadelphia Geriatric Center. It also refers to research in related fields, such as that done in mental hospitals, general hospitals, and institutions for the nonimpaired, with the reasoning that some principles derived from other subject populations may be useful when applied to the elderly organic brain syndrome patient. A concluding section will consider unresolved conceptual issues and research needs.

Inevitably, implications for physical design or social organization arise infrequently from empirical data and much more frequently from *a priori* reasoning. While we hope that design decisions would increasingly be based on hard data, the need for improved environments will not await the completion of such research. For those who will design such environments, the first step is sensitization to the characteristics and needs of this specialized user population; the second step is an attempt to apply the relatively general principles to be discussed below. Even in the absence of much other necessary knowledge, accomplishment of these two steps alone can result in a significant improvement in the quality of the treatment environment.

THEORETICAL BACKGROUND

Before considering the substantive areas of concern, it is necessary to discuss some of the concepts around which concern for the environment has developed in gerontology. Over the past decade a general reintroduction of "the environment" into the thinking of social science has occurred. This represents a considerable break with the tradition in psychology whereby explanations for behavior have typically been sought within the individual to the exclusion of what goes on around him. The core problem in environmental psychology is the specification of the conditions under which human behavior may be determined by particular environments and, conversely, those circumstances in which the individual significantly shapes the environment.

Accepting generally the demonstrated salience of the environment to human behavior (for general review, see refs. 1–3), Nahemow and I (4,5) have suggested, based within a more general ecological framework, that the aging are more vulnerable to their environmental context than are younger adults. This vulnerability stems from age-related negative changes such as those in biological health, cognition, sensory-motor behavior, social isolation, and so on. To the extent that these factors are relatively resistant to change and are lodged within the individual, they may be seen as different aspects of "competence." These intrapersonal aspects are contrasted with the context outside the skin of the individual: physical environment; personally relevant individuals and groups; and the larger institutional, social, and cultural milieu in which the individual behaves. While all behavior clearly occurs in an environmental context, our conception suggests a dynamic interplay between the individual and the envionment such that the "demand character" of the environment has an optimal level and range for a person of a given level of competence. I have suggested Henry Murray's (6) concept of "environmental press" to represent the demand character of the world outside the individual.

Figure 1 schematizes personal competence and environmental press as the coordinates of a system where a point represents the outcome of the action of an individual dealing with an environmental situation. The outcome may be behavior, evaluated in terms of its adaptive quality, or affect, evaluated on a positive-to-negative continuum. The diagonal line through the center of the figure, labeled "adaptation level," (7) marks the normal homeostatic points where the demands of the environment are approximately equal to the level of competence of the individual at that time. At adaptation level, awareness of the environment is minimal and the outcome is positive in terms of behavior and affect. This is the normal situation, where we have adapted to the demands and stimulation of the environment so that it is tuned out and we can attend to the focal task of the moment. A shift toward higher press level will result in heightened environmental awareness and should evoke behavior at a still-adaptive level until the press level exceeds a threshold of magnitude varying with the competence of the individual—the threshold marking the onset of "stress." At that point, the behavioral or affective outcome becomes negative. The dynamics of the model imply, however, that successful coping with press moderately stronger than adaptation level may succeed in elevating competence, while a prolonged negative outcome will lower competence. To the left of the central area of

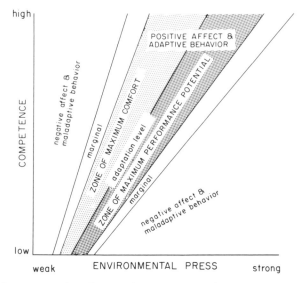

FIG. 1. Schematic representation of personal competence and environmental press as coordinates of a system in which a point represents the outcome of the response to an environmental situation.

Fig. 1, a negative outcome is also indicated for very low press levels, which in the extreme may represent true sensory deprivation.

In general, most people deal adequately with environmental press of a relatively wide range of strength. Figure 1 suggests that within the positive-outcome range, press slightly above the adaptation level is likely to be most successful in elevating competence ("area of maximum performance potential"); press slightly below adaptation level is also apt to be perceived as having a positive affective quality, while behavior is less active ("areas of maximum comfort")— a normal state of relaxation and mild dependence.

It should be noted that regardless of competence level, there is some range of press strength where the behavioral and affective outcomes are positive. On the other hand, this range becomes narrower as competence decreases. Thus, a small absolute amount of change in press strength may make a major difference in the quality of outcome for a person of low competence. This particular principle was stated as the "environmental docility hypothesis" (8): As individual competence decreases, the environment assumes increasing importance in determining well-being. One corollary of this hypothesis is that the low-competent are increasingly sensitive to noxious environments. The opposite and more positive corollary is that a small environmental improvement may produce a disproportionate amount of improvement in affect or behavior in a low-competent individual.

This volume is concerned with individuals of very low competence. The relevance of the theoretical model is obvious: To the extent that the typical environments in which those with senile dementia are either deprived or stressful, behavioral and affective outcomes will be more negative than necessary. Of course the concept of "competence" is not limited in its application to aging. Judiciously applied, some of the principles deducible from the model may be applicable to other low-competent populations, such as the mentally ill, the physically ill, or the mentally retarded. Conversely, some research from these populations may be applied to environments for the OBS patient.

In a more concrete vein, environmental interventions for those of diminished competence may be thought of as "prosthetic environments," a term coined by Lindsley (9), one of the leaders in the development of applied behavioral psychology for environments that would continuously maintain desired behavior. These environments would be for user populations with disabilities expected to be resistant to change. "Therapy" is thus provided for conditions expected to improve, and it can be discontinued as treatment succeeds. Prosthesis, on the other hand, must be applied continuously, since the basic impairment will persist. Theoretically, at least, if an enivironment can be designed and programmed to support positive behavior, efficiency will be high as compared with use of a human staff to provide equivalent support, a much more costly method. In practice, of course, human and nonhuman prostheses need not be seen in such opposing terms. However, Lindsley's concept provides another ideal model to strive for: The design of a physical environment with structural aspects that will counteract known deficits associated with the particular user population.

DESCRIPTIVE ECOLOGY OF SENILE DEMENTIA

Roger Barker, the founder of ecological psychology, has repeatedly called our attention to the lack of information on how people use their environments in ordinary ways. Using the analogy with standardized psychological tests, he argues that we can understand unusual behaviors or uses of the environment only through comparisons with the norm; yet norms are rarely thought of in connection with the way people use space. I shall first present data relating the parameters of the institutional environments inhabited by the OBS and the non-OBS patient, derived from two studies on which I have worked.

In both studies behavior-mapping was the data-gathering method used. In behavior-mapping an observer traverses the entire residential area, noting the position and behavior of each person. Table 1 shows some basic characteristics of five types of residential areas in a long-term care institution and of nine wards in four different types of state mental hospital units. Within each of the two types of institutions, a greater proportion of patients from OBS wards were likely to be observed. The OBS patient was less mobile, less frequently engaged in treatment or recreational activities away from the ward, and less likely to be behind a closed bedroom door, where our observers did not intrude.

TABLE 1. *Ecological characteristics of treatment areas in two types of institution*

Type of unit	Ward	Census	Mean % observed	Observed nursing staff-to-resident ratio	Observed other staff-to-resident ratio
Long-term care institution					
Fully independent floor		74	32	.068	.036
Fully independent floor		54	39	.080	.072
Partially independent floor		74	57	.067	.042
Limited independence floor		74	51	.080	.049
OBS wing		40	83	.157	.083
Mental hospital					
Geriatric infirmary (many	A	74	95	.161	.009
OBS patients)	B	73	99	.097	.008
	C	84	99	.178	.005
	D	81	99	.095	.000
Geriatric active (few OBS)	A	83	82	.087	.002
	B	83	85	.086	.005
Active treatment (younger	A	42	55	.104	.044
patients)	B	28	43	.123	.066
Continued treatment	A	92	50	.057	.015
(younger & middle-aged)	B	73	43	.018	.003

Nursing staff ratios in the nursing home tended to be higher where OBS patients were housed, this ratio being equalled only in the mental hospital active-treatment wards. Non-nursing staff ratios were generally higher in the nursing home than in the mental hospital; in the nursing home the OBS area was particularly well-supplied with other staff, while in the mental hospital the OBS area was as deprived as most other wards in this respect.

Table 2 shows the locations of all residents observed in the nursing home. The bedroom was the usual location for residents on three floors, the lounge for one independent floor, and the hall for the OBS wing. By contrast, Table 3 shows similar data for the mental hospital. Here the primacy of the "dayroom" and some wards' proscription of bedroom use shows up. However, the concentra-

TABLE 2. *Percentages of nursing home residents observed in ward areas*

Type of unit	Nurses' station	Bed-rooms	Lounge	Hall	Not noted	Total
Fully independent floor	9	38	20	26	7	100
Fully independent floor	2	32	47	5	14	100
Partially independent floor	7	41	19	25	8	100
Limited independence floor	5	38	12	36	9	100
OBS wing	3	29	16	52	0	100

TABLE 3. *Percentages of mental hospital residents observed in ward areas*

Type of unit	Ward	Halls	Nurses' station	Day-room	Bed-rooms	Bath-room	Other common spaces
Geriatric infirmary	A	4	1	69	16	9	1
(many OBS)	B	0	0	81	9	9	0
	C	1	0	72	26	0	2
	D	3	0	95	1	0	1
Geriatric active	A	1	0	40	13	3	43
(few OBS)	B	3	0	40	21	3	34
Active treatment	A	18	4	35	22	4	18
(open, younger)	B	30	5	47	3	3	13
Continued treatment	A	11	2	76	4	4	2
(open, younger)	B	13	0	3	41	5	38

tion in the dayroom is far greater for the OBS ward, while in the active geriatric ward patients were frequently found in a lounge or activity space as well.

In Table 4 the behavioral milieux of these different environments is shown as the dominant behaviors observed. Isolated passive behavior (primarily sleeping and sitting) was generally the most frequent behavior, particularly among the geriatric patients. Within the geriatric group, isolated passive behavior constituted over 80% of all behavior in the mental hospital infirmary wards, approximately 67% among non-OBS mental hospital patients, and slightly less among OBS nursing home patients. Notably less behavior of this type was observed in other nursing home areas. Isolated active behavior—including instrumental tasks, walking, and watching TV—was highest among younger mental hospital patients and was lowest in the infirmary of the mental hospital. Social behavior was highest in the active-treatment wards for younger mental hospital patients and next highest in the non- or mild-OBS nursing home areas. Low levels of social behavior were found diversely in the OBS nursing home area and in the mental hospital geriatric infirmary, geriatric active, and younger continuous-treatment wards.

To summarize these findings, important differences were seen between younger and older institutionalized people, between mental hospital and nursing home residents, and between OBS and non-OBS geriatric patients. Each of these contrasts is associated with differences in the behavioral-spatial milieu to which the individuals are exposed. Therefore, we must immediately be cautious about extrapolating findings from one type of institution to another.

Some important inter-area differences included the following:

1. Lesser activity and mobility among the aged, the ill, and those with OBS;
2. Equal nursing staffing patterns, but richer other-staff coverage for older people in the nursing home as compared to those in the mental hospital;

TABLE 4. *Percentages of residents engaged in different behaviors*

Type of unit	Ward	Pathological behavior[a]	Isolated passive	Isolated active	Social	Staff giving nursing care[b]
Long-term care institution						
Fully independent floor		1	51	30	18	11
Fully independent floor		0	52	27	21	6
Partially independent floor		1	53	28	18	8
Limited independence floor		2	50	22	17	6
OBS wing		17	63	27	9	12
Mental hospital						
Geriatric infirmary	A	6	87	9	4	
	B	15	78	18	3	
	C	3	85	6	8	
	D	4	87	7	5	
Geriatric active	A	0	68	24	7	
	B	1	65	29	6	
Active treatment	A	0	34	32	34	
	B	0	29	44	26	
Continued treatment	A	4	52	35	8	
	B	2	49	44	7	

[a] Pathological behavior rated for every patient; isolated-passive, isolated-active, and social total 100%.
[b] Staff nursing care not tallied in mental hospital.

3. Wider diversity of spatial experience for younger mental patients and for non-OBS older patients; and

4. A low absolute level of social behavior, particularly among OBS patients and among all geriatric mental hospital patients.

More emphatically, the poverty of a typical day, both spatially and behaviorally, is starkly portrayed by these findings; if one both is old and suffers from senile dementia, things are at their very worst.

For our present purpose, we should consider these parameters of space occupancy, spatial range, and modal behaviors as constituting a part of the total stimulus environment impinging on a given individual. Of course, these particular parameters consist of observations of individuals, but in the aggregate they constitute an important part of the milieu for all people who inhabit it.

The results described above are indirectly relevant to a major question in the environmental treatment of the OBS patient: Should patients with senile dementia be clustered in a single location or housed in an area together with people who are fully mentally competent? Regrettably, there is not yet strong empirical evidence to answer this question. I am aware of one attempt to test the effect of deliberate mixing of degrees of mental competence in activity groups; given a very small N, no outcome differences were found to be associated with segregation or integration by mental competence (10). The behavior-map data presented above describe residential areas constituted through deliberate grouping by age and physical and mental status; they highlight the depressed level of activity and the impoverishment that result when all residents of an area are severely impaired. One may safely conclude that deliberate mixing would have elevated the lowest level of ward activity; under such conditions, no patient would be without some "role model" of people engaging in social behavior and other enriching activity. The possible aggregate result in terms of the number who would model their behavior after the most competent versus those whose behavior would be depreciated by the least competent cannot be judged; a clear need exists for such an empirical test.

A relevant series of studies on the "sociospatial schema" of OBS residents has been reported by Lipman and Slater (11) and Harris and associates (12) in eight English nursing homes. In these homes a strong tendency toward segregation by mental competence was observed both in room assignment and in occupancy of common spaces. The intact residents were likely to occupy spaces in fullest public view; even within the same social space, confused residents occupied the less desirable seats. Conversational interactions were counted and occurred primarily between people of similar competence, i.e., intact with intact and moderately confused with moderately confused. The severely confused were, as expected, least likely to have any conversations. The data displayed by Harris et al. (12; Table 2) suggest that if the confused resident is to converse at all, the presence of more intact residents is required. These researchers concluded that the spatial segregation was primary and that social integration, with its presumed gains for the more impaired, could not occur within the framework of current institutional practices.

Research done at the Philadelphia Geriatric Center also included a consumer survey of staff and OBS residents' relatives (residents were too impaired to respond to such an inquiry), to be described in more detail below. Responders to the survey were asked their opinion of mixing impaired and nonimpaired patients. In qualitative terms, nursing personnel tell us most vehemently that the more intact become very anxious when forced into close proximity with the OBS patient. Of both relatives and staff, only about 15% approved of having "confused" residents live in the same area with those who are not confused. These two important components of the system—staff and relatives—clearly support the widespread practice of segregation by mental status.

Thus, the issue of segregation by mental status is far from settled. Institutional practice seems almost unanimous in accepting it, but Lipman's studies force us to continue to wonder whether some method can be found of achieving the benefits of integration without its negative effects on the more intact.

A closer look at the spatial distribution of the OBS patients confirms the impression that their institutional milieu verges on sensory deprivation: Very few of the patients appear to leave their residential areas for any reason; within the treatment unit the highly restricted and unvarying environments of the dayroom, the hall, and the bedroom constitute the spatial choices. The implications are clear. First, a deliberate attempt must be made to expose these relatively immobilized people to new physical spaces, through planned walks or wheeling into other areas of the institution or to the outdoors. Second, since diversity of spatial environments is very limited even with such efforts, diversity within the circumscribed treatment area should be emphasized through such means as (a) providing richness and diversity in colors, decor, type of furniture, graphics, etc.; (b) differentiating subspaces in terms of their function, such as, reading corner, game side, TV area, etc.; and (c) insuring that individual patients use different spaces at different times of day rather than occupying the same chair all day every day.

Data that are too complex to display here also showed amazingly little variation in the pattern of behaviors and space occupancy over the course of the day; only meal times differed substantially from other times in the typical patterns. Thus time had little texture in the OBS wards. To the extent that differences did occur, the latter half of the afternoon could be characterized as a time of low activity, lack of staff, and null behavior (13). Ameliorative efforts could therefore be made to produce greater variations in the types of behavior demanded of individuals as the day progresses, e.g., a time of day for self-maintaining activities, another for unstructured time, and so on. Day-to-day variations were not analyzed in our data, but variability among days could also be deliberately introduced as a way of counteracting the overall stimulus deprivation of the institution. The extreme state of deprivation typifying the late afternoon could be reduced by active programming.

Gross behavioral categories and generic types of spaces such as those described in the Philadelphia Geriatric Center studies represent only the most elementary kinds of ecological stimuli. The aspects of environment that are apprehended and perceived by the individual as response-activating are far richer and more complex than the elements discussed thus far. For the present purpose these environmental aspects are difficult to discuss. They have rarely been studied separately, as they vary with the mental status of the individuals who occupy them. For the sake of completeness, however, a brief reference to what is known about the quality of the physical and psychosocial environments of institutions for the aged will be made. Since as many as 60% of nursing home residents are thought to be "confused" (14), our knowledge regarding such institutions in general may, in fact, be relevant to our target group of OBS residents. However, the data presented earlier show that there are great intrainstitutional variations. We must therefore await a specific research effort to characterize OBS and non-OBS areas differentially before claiming firm knowledge about these environmental parameters.

Kleemeier (15) postulated three basic dimensions along which institutions might be arrayed: the segregate, the congregate, and the institutional control. Some years later these were operationalized by Kahana (16), and the effect of matches versus mismatches between residents' needs and these dimensions was tested. Significant increments in morale were found to be associated with person-environment congruence in the congregate and control dimensions. Other empirical work in this area has been reported by Pincus (17), Pincus and Wood (18), Marlowe (19), Slover (20), and Moos et al. (21). This is a rich literature, although there are two major limitations to its usefulness for the present purpose. First, with some exceptions (18,21), social and physical aspects of the environment either are not differentiated or are lumped together in single dimensions or ratings. Second, none of the work deals with the differential mileu dimensions, or the outcome correlates, of environments for the OBS patient as compared to other kinds of institutional residents. At this point one can point only to general evidence that some psychosocial institutional dimensions are associated with different kinds of outcomes; a high payoff may result if such research is extended to the OBS patient.

One set of empirical descriptive data on higher-order physical and psychosocial characteristics of treatment environments for OBS patients is shown in Table 5, from the mental hospital study. In this case, the unit is an entire building. Data from 6 of the 23 buildings assessed is shown for illustrative purposes. Self-maintenance skill was measured by staff ratings of individual patients, and the milieu characteristics of the wards were assessed by the ratings of experts, research workers, and ward staff and by objective counting and observation. Without attempting to discuss the nuances of Table 5, considerably less regularity in these environmental attributes was seen as a function of either age or chronicity than was seen in the behavior-mapping results discussed previously. For example, the self-maintenance skills of the OBS patients in the two infirmary wards were

TABLE 5. *Patient and milieu characteristics of mental hospital buildings*

Characteristic	Admission building	Continued treatment	Geriatric active		Geriatric infirmary	
			A	B	A	B
Patient characteristics						
Age	40	54	67	73	64	72
Length of stay (years)	0.3	20	18	17	21	19
Self-maintenance skill	5.3	4.6	5.0	4.3	—	1.1
Milieu characteristics[a]						
Institutionalism	−0.45	1.06	−0.06	0.67	1.43	1.55
Quality of therapeutic staff	−0.12	0.22	0.61	−0.52	−1.97	0.47
Quality of nursing staff	−0.09	0.49	−0.28	1.10	−1.54	−0.32
Ward cleanliness	0.58	−0.78	0.07	−0.34	−0.05	−0.33
Adequacy of supplies	0.23	−0.95	0.13	0.70	0.31	0.10
Effort to individualize	−0.64	−0.45	−0.56	−0.33	−0.78	−0.93
Homelike	0.46	−0.63	0.60	0.19	−1.19	−0.70
Staff satisfaction with enriching facilities	−0.97	−0.84	0.93	0.35	−1.10	−0.61

[a]Figures are transformed and standardized scores are based on distributions of mean scores of 23 buildings.

extremely low (although the exact value for building A was inadvertently omitted) and their overall "institutional" quality was high. Yet these two buildings differed radically from one another, one having both a staff that was rated very poorly and a less homelike and well-furnished physical aspect than the other. In general, these two buildings emerged as having a less desirable total gestalt than the two active geriatric buildings, which in turn seemed to have more positive environmental qualities in a number of dimensions than did the buildings serving as admissions or continued-treatment units. Focusing on the OBS buildings, it seems that in this particular hospital these patients were housed in buildings with a very strong institutional quality. This was evidenced by there being few personal possessions in evidence, much "state clothing," few homelike furnishings, and little equipment or space for anything other than custodial care. Nonetheless, the difference in staff quality between the two may have been the crucial factor in mitigating the situation in building B as compared to building A.

EVALUATION OF INSTITUTIONAL ENVIRONMENTS

Moving from description to evaluation, the general question to be addressed is whether some institutional environments are superior to others in their effects on the behavior or the psychological well-being of the OBS patient. This general question may be asked with respect to variations in environmental scale, from the macro scale of total environment to the micro level of individual sensory cues such as the color, texture, or form of very minute features of the environment. While the amount of research-based data specific to the OBS patient is minimal, at least partially relevant studies will be discussed in terms of global evaluation, travel time and treatment efficiency, social behavior, and consumer evaluation of environmental specifics.

Global Evaluation

Some light is shed on the issue of global evaluation by two mental hospital studies. One study involved the remodeling of a dayroom to increase its visual appeal and social uses (22). As predicted, the incidence of active and social behavior increased. Fortunately, behavior was measured not only in the redecorated social space, but also in other ward areas. A "hydraulic" effect was found such that the increase in social and active behavior was limited to the dayroom while a corresponding increase in passive behavior was observed elsewhere on the ward. Holahan and Saegert (23) extended the remodeling research paradigm to an entire ward, which they compared to an identical ward that was not altered. With physical changes applied to all ward areas, social behavior increased overall and was distributed over all significant ward areas. Nonetheless, the Ss of these studies were acutely ill mental hospital patients of much younger age than the OBS patient. Thus we gain from these results only generalized encouragement regarding the use of physical intervention rather than knowledge that is necessarily relevant to our present purpose.

Lawton et al. (24) reported an evaluation of a small-scale remodeling effort that changed two large four-bed rooms into six small single bedrooms plus a shared social area set off from the main hallway by a half-wall. Direct behavior observation before and after the change indicated, first, the obvious exercise of the choice of being alone in one's room (about 20% of observation occasions), a choice that was unavailable in the earlier shared-bedroom arrangement. Second, the Ss' spatial ranges increased markedly—the occasions on which they were observed outside the bedroom increased from 7 to 38%. We inferred that their greater visual access to the space beyond the room area (occasioned by the half-wall) led to a greater desire and willingness to explore. Finally, there was a decrease, rather than an increase, in the amount of staff–resident social behavior. This unexpected finding can conceivably be explained by the fact that the remodeled plan allowed staff to monitor residents' behavior from a distance; the original situation required staff to enter the four-bed rooms for general surveillance, bringing them physically close enough to stimulate some social interaction with residents. Thus the new design made it too easy for staff to provide their surveillance function in a manner that defeated their social function. While the amount of patient-to-patient social behavior did not change appreciably, the option to be alone in one's room or out walking in the residential area in effect deducted time that, in the original condition, had been available for social behavior. Thus there may have been a proportionate increase in this desirable form of behavior. There was no change in amount of self-maintaining or recreational-type behavior. This small-scale study had the limitation of a very small N. However, it did have the advantage that the physical changes made were few enough to allow one at least to speculate *post hoc* about the reasons for some of the behavioral changes.

An evaluation of changes introduced into the dayroom of a geriatric mental hospital ward that housed a high proportion of OBS patients was done by Frazer et al. (25) and Frazer (26). Both studies tested the effects of furniture rearrangement (Phase 1) followed by introduction of esthetically pleasing furnishings and materials for recreation and reading (enrichment, Phase 2). Direct behavioral observation before and after the redecorating showed some social gains and decrease in pathological behaviors for experimental groups, together with some effects that appeared to be specific to the level of impairment of the patient. There was also evidence that the environmental intervention may have produced an initial negative reaction, followed by improvement to a point about baseline level.

An unusual opportunity to construct a total prosthetic nursing home environment explicitly for the OBS patient was afforded by the Philadelphia Geriatric Center. The details of the planning effort and the rationale for its design decisions are specified at greater length in Liebowitz et al. (27). Briefly, an attempt was made, largely on *a priori* principles, to incorporate physical designs that could counteract some of the behavioral deficits associated with senile dementia and related conditions. Examples of such physical features are

A very large (40 × 100 feet) open central area with bedrooms on the periphery, with the several purposes of (a) enhancing orientation by allowing a full view of all important areas, (b) stimulating social behavior by providing an attractive social area where there is also high traffic, and (c) encouraging activity participation by locating activities in the high-density social area;
Variations in room decor, furnishings, and bulletin boards, used to individualize personal areas;
Color variations, three-dimensional numbers, large clock face, etc., used to enhance orientation, and
Graphics, textures, and material colors, used to provide sensory stimulus variety.

An even more unusual opportunity to evaluate the milieu was afforded through NIMH and NCHSRD funding. The original plan was for a longitudinal control-group design where patients would be randomly assigned to early- and late-move groups; in actual fact, for administrative and treatment-related reasons, the control-group move could not be delayed as long as planned and the critical tests of the effect of the new milieu had to be performed only directly. Data were gathered by the behavior-mapping described earlier, a form of direct behavior observation that tracked individual residents, and a limited number of staff ratings, all performed on several occasions before and after the move over a period of 18 months; the only data obtained directly from the patient was the Kahn-Goldfarb Mental Status Questionnaire (MSQ).

The experimental effect was measured by the own-control design, with elaborations. The first relevant finding was that the familiar decline over time was observed in comparing the pre-move and the post-move measures of the most basic indicators of competence, i.e., mental status and physical self-maintenance abilities (PSMS); the new environment did not counteract the steady erosion of these skills. The second relevant finding was that the directly observed and rated indicators of competence showed substantial correlations with MSQ and PSMS at the first pre-move occasion. Third, when pre-move and post-move comparisons of these competence indicators were made, the results showed 1 instance of undesirable change, 39 instances of no change, and 14 instances of desirable change. We suggest that the lack of decline in behavioral competence to parallel the decline in more basic (and less amenable to intervention) functions, with which the behavior is correlated, constitutes indirect evidence of a prosthetic effect and, in some instances, a possible positive effect. Specific changes included:

Less time spent in bedrooms in the new building—a desirable change on the theory that time in other spaces is more likely to expose the S to other people and activities;
Less crowding in relationship to other people—a function largely of the lack

of occasion in the new building for having people close to one another in a crowded hallway;

A greater maximum angle of gaze—an observer-estimated index of the amount of visual scanning (as opposed to fixed staring) done by the resident;

An increased frequency of "effectance" behavior—this included reading, TV, recreation, etc.,

A decreased frequency of maintenance activity, including that performed alone and with help—this change is relatively neutral in meaning except to the extent that it was replaced by higher-level behavior; and

An increased rating by the observer of the degree of apparent interest in surroundings displayed by the resident.

Another look at the change is provided by comparing the behavior maps in the old and the new residential areas (see Table 6). Of course, this is only a rough comparison, since all Ss in a physical area were mapped rather than just those who were Ss for this study; some but not all individual residents were observed under both conditions. Table 6 shows significant increases in "therapeutic" effectance and decreases in maintenance behavior (noted above in individual observation data) and pathological behavior. Fewer instances of nursing care being given by staff were observed, in parallel to the decline in self-maintenance behavior on the individual level noted previously. Finally, more instances of visiting were noted in the new environment.

TABLE 6. *Behavior in old (traditional) and new (prosthetic) nursing home*

Observation	Mean percentage[a]		F[b]
	Old	New	
Resident behavior			
Ambulating	3.64	4.88	
Social	5.48	6.85	
Effectance-solitary	0.92	1.84	
Effectance-therapeutic	1.65	6.99	43.4
Self-maintenance	21.65	14.99	9.3
Pathological	16.54	11.26	75.5
Sleeping	15.37	17.05	
Null	38.33	37.49	
Staff behavior			
Ambulating	7.75	6.72	
Social	9.36	9.12	
Patient care	12.07	8.04	22.9
Number nursing staff observed	19.32	16.82	
Other staff observed	10.15	8.33	
Visitors, number observed	3.13	6.31	28.8

[a] Patient figures are standardized in terms of total number of residents observed; staff figures represent adjusted staff-observed patient ratios $\times$ 100.

[b] $p < 0.01$.

Each of the studies reviewed above tested some general hypotheses of the type, "These structures should facilitate social behavior." Few of the studies, if any, proposed a direct one-to-one relationship between a single structural feature and a specific behavior. The fact is that in no case could a single physical stimulus be abstracted from the totality for such study. The experimental variable was not a redecorated ward or a new building, but an entire system composed of countless physical and staff changes, sometimes a new resident mix, different treatment programs, and not least, changed expectations by staff, residents, and administrators (for an analysis of the system aspects of mental hospital change, see ref. 28). In real life treatment environments exist in this complex form; it is appropriate that they be evaluated as such. However, the limitations of such global evaluations must also be recognized, primarily their inability to allow one to draw conclusions about which aspect of the experimental change contributed to which observed changes in the dependent variables.

Travel Time and Treatment Efficiency

Much time and energy of the institutional staff is consumed in going from one place to another. There is a long history of examining general hospital design in terms of required staff travel time. Travel time is evaluated by observing and timing staff travel between pairs of major points on a ward and attempting to express travel time on a ward of any physical configuration as a function of the distance between these critical points. For example, Lippert (29) found that much nurse travel could be accounted for by two important paths: patient room-to-patient room and nurses' station-to-patient room. With such "equations" in hand, one could theoretically take several architectural plans and, using only a few of the standard pathways, calculate the relative gains to be experienced by one ward design as compared to another. McLaughlin (30), for example, compared specific circular versus rectangular and circular versus single-corridor versus double-corridor designs. The circular units did not usually generate less travel according to these formulas. However, several studies compared different shaped hospital designs by directly observing behavior (31–33). With construction that in fact provided shorter travel distances and better visual surveillance capacity for a circular design, as compared to a single-corridor and a double-corridor design, the circular plan generated less staff travel time. Only part of this saved time was devoted to patient care, however; the remainder of the saved time was spent in the nurses' station (33). This greater amount of time spent with patients was the major patient-related gain found among the general hospital studies reviewed.

It must be acknowledged that the needs of people in intensive or intermediate care general hospital wards are very different from those of the elderly OBS patient in a long-term care unit. Referring back to the Philadelphia Geriatric Center remodeling study, one could even assert that more, rather than less, staff travel time might be desirable because such travel removes the nurse from her station and puts her in closer physical proximity to more residents. Thus, one may suggest that staff travel time is a relatively minor criterion for the quality of long-term care institution design.

Social Behavior

Effects on social behavior have been mentioned in connection with all of the global environmental evaluations discussed above. Two relevant mental hospital experiments with older patients offer further information on a smaller scale. A classic experiment by Sommer and Ross (34) and a confirmation and extension by Holahan (35) showed an increase in social behavior consequent to the rearrangement of dayroom seating from the typical perimeter arrangement to that of a number of square tables with a chair placed on each side of each table. As a matter of interest, the main problem in this intervention was insuring that staff and patients did not rearrange the furniture in the old manner every day. Kahana and Kahana (36) controlled the age mix of mental hospital wards so that an age-homogeneous and an age-heterogeneous ward could be compared. A favorable outcome, by pre- and post-measures, was observed in the cognitive performance and social interaction of older patients in the age-integrated ward.

Several recent small-N experiments have been designed to increase the amount of control over their own lives experienced by long-term care institutional residents. For example, the patient is offered a chance to choose whether and when to be visited (37) or which plants to have in his room (38). The largely intact residents observed in these studies were shown to experience favorable health and psychological outcomes as the result of expanded choice.

Several studies by McClannahan (39,40) and McClannahan and Risley (41) have indicated that the overall level of "environmental participation" (i.e., all kinds of engagement with things or people) of nursing home patients may be increased by providing manipulatable objects and materials. Mere presence was not enough, however; active offering of materials by staff was required to increase participation above baseline, while making announcements and offering prizes further potentiated participation. While the finding that use of objects increases if objects are provided carries a hint of tautology, this intervention did in effect reduce the proportion of null behavior. Perhaps the most useful aspect of the findings, however, was their underlining of the idea that staff activity was an essential aspect of the intervention system; presence of objects in and of itself was not sufficient to elicit use.

Consumer Evaluations

The consumer evaluation is perhaps the most primitive method in environmental evaluation, but when used judiciously it can add to knowledge (42). In the case of senile dementia, however, the primary consumer does not usually have the cognitive ability to respond to the typical structured interview. Therefore, secondary consumers such as staff or residents' family members have been sought as "expert" informants. In our Philadelphia Geriatric Center evaluation, for example, staff and families responded to a questionnaire dealing with both specific and global aspects of the traditional and prosthetic environments (43). The general feeling toward the new building was strongly positive, but enough differentiation was present among the specifics to allow the identification of a number of problem areas. Some highly approved features were the amount of activity space in the center, the location and design of the nurses' station, the amount of lighting, the access of residents to staff offices, and the ease of operating lavatory fixture handles. Some problem areas included inaccessibility of closet shelves to residents, internal crowding of the toilet area, lack of bathroom storage, and noise in the center space. Since staff and family are essential components of the treatment system, their pleasure in the institutional environment is clearly desirable. On the other hand, it must be recognized that their evaluations can at best provide only a partial measure of a building's success. While the OBS patient will infrequently be able to share his evaluation of the residential environment with the researcher, there is no guarantee that the preferences of the resident will coincide with those of staff or relative.

The only other relevant consumer evaluation found in the literature appraised the different shaped acute care hospital designs. Staff overwhelmingly preferred the circular design (33), but surprisingly, patients do not appear to have been queried regarding their preferences.

SENILE DEMENTIA AND THE NONINSTITUTIONAL ENVIRONMENT

If we can accept even the most conservative estimate of the population prevalence of OBS (44), a 4% rate means that nearly one million people with OBS are living in noninstitutional situations. We know very little about the environments in which they live. Such people are no doubt over-represented among the segment of the older population living with non-spouse relatives. However, an unknown proportion live alone in older hotels, rooming houses, mobile homes, and all other types of environments that provide no surveillance and no concessions to barrier-free or prosthetic design. A first line of approach to designing for the OBS patient living in the ordinary community is to recognize that good design for people in general may be expected to be good for the OBS patient as well. One specific consideration for our target group is the development of a household design technology for providing within the residential environment relatively simple modifications that could counteract the behavioral deficits associated with OBS. While some of these modifications would be for safety purposes, others could be directed toward orientation and sensory and cognitive stimulation. These services could be incorporated into those delivered by various in-home service agencies. This author is aware of no research in this area, however, and simply calls it to the reader's attention that such a need exists.

RESEARCH NEEDS

Having drawn some relatively pessimistic conclusions regarding the present state of empirical research in the environmental psychology of senile dementia, a virtually limitless panorama of research needs might be discerned. Some way of setting a limit to all that could be done is clearly required. Therefore, before discussing explicit research needs, two fundamental issues will be discussed. The first issue concerns the *a priori* definition of desirable environmental qualities in the absence of research. The second issue asks whether there is a variety of research indigenous to the environmental design area that can provide usable knowledge other than the more expensive traditional social scientific methods.

Inalienable Environmental Rights of the OBS Patient

The inquisitive gerontologist might wish to test the effect of substituting an esthetically pleasing surrounding for one that is dingy and depressing—a difficult feat in operation, but one conceivably within the realm of possibility. This example represents a class of questions that could be asked. My question is, "Should they be asked?" Several considerations argue against doing so, the major one being that the desirability of some environmental qualities should be based on value judgment rather than on empirical test. To insist that their quality be proven on the alien ground of traditional research removes the researcher from more productive work, risks of nonconfirmation, and sets up precedent among those who control design decisions of demanding empirical confirmation of the utility of what are really inalienable rights. Relatively little of theoretical significance seems to be extractable from research on the effects of such attributes as beautiful versus ugly, safe versus unsafe, clean versus dirty, or homelike versus institutional environments. Some of the negative poles of these qualities have been excused in institutional design because they presumably are not salient to the OBS patient. Why should we have to prove that this assertion is false? Other design issues, such as the right to privacy, may fall into the same self-evident category, although in these cases there may be better theoretical reasons for studying them.

Nontraditional Environmental Research

An almost infinite number of design-relevant questions can be asked. One can probably find a dozen generic types of door openers, for example, each of which could conceivably be tested in the framework of the classic experiment. For each type of door opener one might need to represent systematically *S*s with several different types of disabilities. The point is that the number of tightly designed experiments necessary to provide full knowledge about the best designs for each user subpopulation would quickly deplete *S*s, researchers, and funds.

Nonetheless, the alternative is not simply to settle for blind design or its armchair cousin. Systematic observation of people using their environments can be done scientifically without mobilizing the total armamentarium of traditional behavior scientists. The behavior scientist should be in the act, but preferably in the role of consultant or co-observer. The designer and the service professional can be trained to observe objectively, to replicate occasions, and to sample situations and individuals. Those who have developed the art of observation become quite skilled in recognizing the single instance of dysfunction that suggests a potential design defect or a possible improvement. Some rehabilitation professionals have been trained in this skill. An example is the fine-detailed clinical study by Azar and Lawton (45) of gait that allowed conclusions to be drawn about types of pathways that could minimize pedestrian accidents. Nonscientists can also become sensitized to situations where optimizing, or "satisficing," rather than 100% need matching is necessary. The researcher as consultant is also the source of user-specific scientific information without which the designer cannot function. To many designers, old people, or the institutionalized elderly, are a homogeneous group; the consultant's knowledge of the disabilities to be compensated for is essential and in itself will often lead the designer directly to prosthetic innovations.

Traditional Research Needs

Elimination of two areas as targets for research reduces somewhat the scale of the potential research task. However, a bewildering array of possibilities remains.

The most important issue involves the general question relevant to almost every topic pertaining to senile dementia: What is the range of behavioral plasticity of the patient suffering from senile dementia, in this case, plasticity to environmental intervention? The evidence reviewed earlier confirms that space use is clearly amenable to environmental intervention. However, space use is of little intrinsic interest except as it moderates the occurrence or nonoccurrence of other kinds of behavior. Despite the intention that the global treatment environment improvements increase sensory stimulation, orientation, activity, self-maintenance, effectance, and social behavior, only very soft evidence is in hand that any of these results have occurred. At this point, it seems that research should retreat somewhat from the global experiment and approach the single independent variable experiment in order to test the magnitude of improvement that can be expected in response to some innovations. The classic Sommer and Ross (34) experiment, for example, was repeated for younger mental patients (35) and for older OBS patients (25). If other such simple interventions could be demonstrated to change social behavior significantly, then the plasticity of social behavior in spite of basic neural damage would be established. This question is clearly of both theoretical and practical interest.

Despite the many aids to orientation suggested in the literature (9) or incorporated into institutional design (27), no clear empirical evidence exists to suggest whether these aids are effective in helping the patient regain the ability to find his way in space and time. Many orientational aids, such as different colored door jambs, cost little extra and can be placed in the "inalienable-right" category; nonetheless, for theoretical reasons we need to test whether any orientational ability can be regained through such interventions.

There is some knowledge in general psychology regarding the effects of sensory deprivation, sensory overload, stimulus complexity, multisensory stimulation, novel experience, and so on (46–48). Whether there are any differences in response to these conditions as a function of age has hardly been explored, however, and never, to my knowledge, with reference to the elderly OBS patient. It has been asserted that lowered cognitive competence requires simpler environmental stimulus fields if adaptive behavior or a positive mental state is to result (4). Obviously this is a question of great import, leading as it does to very concrete issues regarding the complexity and diversity of colors, forms, textures, sounds, etc. that may be associated with a favorable residential environment. For example, I have heard both sound damping and the importing of white noise suggested as improvements to the auditory environment of the institutional ward. Yet it appears that no small-scale experimental attempt has been made to test the effect of such variations in complexity.

Another general issue concerns the basic notion of the prosthetic environment. Which aspects of the environment (and with which individuals) can elevate behavior in the ideal prosthetic manner, i.e., simply by virtue of their existence? I have many times called attention to the cost savings inherent in the inert object that can orient the patient, funnel traffic into a social area, or entice the individual to participate (49). In how many real-life situations, however, have we seen a brilliant design innovation become incorporated into the undifferentiated background, having become a mystery to both residents and staff? One example is the reality board. Clearly there are some situations where both residents and staff need to be taught to respond to a prosthetic feature; however, no experimental contrast between passive and active prosthesis use has appeared in the literature to date.

Finally, the greatest void of all is in knowledge of how the one million or more mentally impaired community residents cope with the problem of furniture, household pathways, hazards, self-maintaining artifacts, neighborhood resources, transportation, and so on. The need in this area is for really low-level descriptive data to form a basis for more interesting hypothesis generation. Clinical and survey-type interviews with family members plus direct observation of OBS patients behaving within the household will be necessary to gain even the most elementary idea of how these people respond to the barriers and facilitators of the noninstitutional environment.

In conclusion, a backward glance suggests that, at present, not much systematic information is available. The only solace for writer and reader is the hope that some may be stimulated to probe further into the psychology of stimulation as it affects those with senile dementia.

ACKNOWLEDGMENTS

Some of the research described was supported by grants MH 16139 and MH 17473 from the National Institute of Mental Health and grant HS 00100 from the National Center for Health Services, Research and Development.

REFERENCES

1. Proshansky, H. M., Ittelson, W. H., and Rivlin, L. G., eds. (1976): *Environmental Psychology.* Holt, Rinehart, & Winston, New York.
2. Altman, I. (1975): *The Environment and Social Behavior.* Brooks-Cole, Monterey, California.
3. Holahan, C. J. (1978): *Environment and Behavior: A Dynamic Perspective.* Plenum Press, New York.
4. Lawton, M. P., and Nahemow, L. (1973): In: *Psychology of Adult Development and Aging,* edited by C. Eisdorfer and M. P. Lawton, pp. 619–674. American Psychological Association, Washington, D.C.
5. Lawton, M. P. (1980): In: *Theory and the Environmental Context of Aging,* edited by M. P. Lawton, P. G. Windley, and T. O. Byerts. Springer, New York.
6. Murray, H. A. (1938): *Explorations in Personality.* Oxford University Press, New York.
7. Helson, H. (1964): *Adaptation Level Theory.* Harper & Row, New York.
8. Lawton, M. P. (1970): In: *The Spatial Behavior of Older People,* edited by L. A. Pastalan and D. H. Carson, pp. 40–67. University of Michigan Institute of Gerontology, Ann Arbor.
9. Lindsley, O. R. (1964): In: *New Thoughts on Old Age,* edited by R. Kastenbaum, pp. 41–60. Springer, New York.
10. Kahana, E., Kahana, B., and Jacobs, K. (1970): Functionally integrated therapy programs for the elderly. Paper presented at the Annual Meeting of the Gerontological Society, Toronto.
11. Lipman, A., and Slater, R. (1977): Status and spatial appropriation in eight homes for old people. *Gerontologist,* 17:250–255.
12. Harris, H., Lipman, A., and Slater, R. (1977): Architectural design: The spatial location and interactions of old people. *Gerontology,* 23:390–400.
13. Fulcomer, M. C., Frey, R. E., and Lawton, M. P. (1977): Observational differences among treatment environments for the elderly. Paper presented at the Annual Meeting of the Gerontological Society, San Francisco.
14. National Center for Health Statistics (1977): Characteristics, social contacts, and activities of nursing home residents. *Vital Health Stat.,* Ser. 13, No. 27.
15. Kleemeier, R. W. (1959): In: *Handbook of Aging and the Individual,* edited by J. E. Birren, pp. 400–451. University of Chicago Press, Chicago.
16. Kahana, E. (1980): In: *Theory in Environmental Context and Aging,* edited by M. P. Lawton, P. G. Windley, and T. O. Byerts. Springer, New York.
17. Pincus, A. (1968): The definition and measurement of the institutional environment in homes for the aged. *Gerontologist,* 8:207–210.
18. Pincus, A., and Wood, V. (1970): Methodological issues in measuring the environment in institutions for the aged and its impact on residents. *Aging Hum. Devel.,* 1:117–126.
19. Marlowe, R. A. (1973): Effects of environment on elderly state hospital relocatees. Paper presented at the 44th Meeting of the Pacific Sociological Association, Scottsdale, Arizona.
20. Slover, D. (1972): Relocation for therapeutic purposes of aged mental hospital patients. Paper presented at Annual Meeting of the Gerontological Society, San Juan, Puerto Rico.
21. Moos, R. H., Gauvain, M., Lemke, S., Max, W., and Mehren, B. (1979): Assessing the social environments of sheltered care settings. *Gerontologist,* 19:74–82.
22. Proshansky, H. M., Ittelson, W. H., and Rivlin, L. G. (1976): In: *Experimental Psychology,* edited by H. M. Proshansky, W. H. Ittelson, and L. G. Rivlin, pp. 170–180. Holt, Reinhart, & Winston, New York.
23. Holahan, C. J., and Saegert, S. (1973): Behavioral and attitudinal effects of large-scale variation in the physical environment of psychiatric wards. *J. Abnorm. Psychol.,* 82:454–462.
24. Lawton, M. P., Liebowitz, B., and Charon, H. (1970): Physical structure and the behavior of senile patients following ward remodeling. *Aging Hum. Devel.,* 1:231–239.

25. Frazer, D. W., Stahler, G., and Middledorf, J. (1978): Behavioral effects of environmental changes among a psychiatric geriatric population. Pilot Project 1. Norristown State Hospital Psychology Department, Norristown, Pennslyvania.
26. Frazer, D. W. (1978): Behavioral effects of environmental changes among a psychiatric geriatric population. Pilot Project 2. Norristown State Hospital Psychology Department, Norristown, Pennsylvania.
27. Liebowitz, B., Lawton, M. P., and Waldman, A. (1979): *Am. Inst. Architects J.,* 68:59–60.
28. Holahan, C. J. (1976): *Hum. Relations,* 29:153–166.
29. Lippert, S. (1971): *Hum. Factors,* 13:269–282.
30. McLaughlin, H. (1961): *Mod. Hosp.,* 96:81–87.
31. Sturdavant, M. (1960): *Hosp. Monogr.,* No. 8.
32. Jaco, E. G. (1973): Nursing staffing patterns and hospital unit design: An experimental analysis. Research on Nursing Staffing in Hospitals, Final Report to the National Institutes of Health, No. 73–434, pp. 59–76. NIH, Bethesda, Maryland.
33. Trites, D. K. (1970): Influence of nursing unit design on the activities and subjective feelings of nursing personnel. Report to the National Center for Health Statistics NCHS-RD-70-7. NCHS, Washington, D.C.
34. Sommer, R., and Ross, H. (1958): *J. Soc. Psychiatry,* 4:128–133.
35. Holahan, C. J. (1972): *J. Abnorm. Psychol.,* 80:115–124.
36. Kahana, E., and Kahana, B. (1970): *Arch. Gen. Psychiatry,* 23:20–29.
37. Schulz, R. (1976): *J. Pers. Soc. Psychol.,* 33:563–573.
38. Langer, E., and Rodin, J. (1976): *J. Pers. Soc. Psychol.,* 34:191–198.
39. McClannahan, L. E. (1973): *Ther. Recreat. J.,* 26:26–31.
40. McClannahan, L. E. (1973): *Gerontologist,* 13:424–429.
41. McClannahan, L. E., and Risley, T. R. (1974): *Gerontologist,* 14:236–240.
42. Lawton, M. P. (1977): In: *The Behavioral Basis of Design. Book 2,* edited by P. Suedfeld, J. A. Russell, L. M. Ward, F. Szigeti, and C. Davis, pp. 211–216. Dowden, Hutchinson and Ross, Stroudsburg, Pennsylvania.
43. Kleban, M. H., and Agger, S. (1976): Staff and relative evaluation of traditional and prosthetic treatment settings. Paper presented at the 29th Annual Meeting of the Gerontological Society, New York.
44. Gunner-Swenson, F., and Jensen, K. (1976): *Acta Psychiatr. Scand.,* 53:283–297.
45. Azar, G. J., and Lawton, A. H. (1964): *Gerontologist,* 4:83–84.
46. Fiske, D. W., and Maddi, S. R., eds. (1961): *Functions of Varied Experience.* Dorsey Press, Homewood, Illinois.
47. Berlyne, D. E., and Madsen, K. B., eds. (1973): *Pleasure, Reward, Preference.* Academic Press, New York.
48. Wohlwill, J. F. (1972): Behavioral response and adaptation to environmental stimulation. MER Publication Series No. 72-1. Department of Man–Environment Relations, Pennsylvania State University, University Park, Pennsylvania.
49. Lawton, M. P. (1974): *J. Architect. Res.,* 3:51–54.

DISCUSSION

Dr. Kahn: I think that one of the major characteristics of innovative mental health practices since World War II has been in the direction of devising ameliorative measures to compensate for the noxious effects that were created in the first place by our previous methods of care.

Thus, a large part of our current community mental health services are concerned with patients suffering from the deleterious effects of long-term hospitalization. The difficulties of the "deinstitutionalization" program may be as much the product of chronic institutionalization as of chronic schizophrenia.

Today we've heard very fine expositions regarding individual and environmental mental therapeutic approaches, but these were based primarily on chronically institutionalized populations. Such studies have serious limitations because they fail to differentiate primary and secondary pathological behavior patterns—those due to the illness, and those due to the custodial care. To put somebody in a custodial institution and then to try to administer some sort of ameliorative effort is like going after somebody with a bat in one hand while giving him a bandaid with the other.

It is the damage that we have helped create in the first place that is so extensive that even if these other efforts are significant they may, at best, be just partially undoing the very effects we have created initially by our custodial treatment.

My total impression of the kinds of programs that have been described here is that they are, in effect, manifestations of benevolent custodialism. Although different than a condition of neglectful custodialism, these methods are still operating within a matrix of custodial care without challenging the basic issues involved in that care.

These kinds of well-intentioned therapeutic programs seem to trivialize the needs of the elderly. They may aim for superficial amelioration, but operating within a custodial context they are preserving the custodial structure, even while doing it in a more benevolent and humane manner.

To make the point, I would like to emphasize one of the studies mentioned earlier in the presentations but not full described. That was the Kahana and Kahana study, which was a controlled study with a new approach. They worked with newly admitted patients rather than with those who had been chronically hospitalized. Instead of accepting some of the premises of the existing system of care, they investigated one of the most common custodial manifestations, age segregation of psychiatric patients. They studied elderly male patients being admitted to a state mental hospital and randomly distributed to two wards, one a typical age-homogenous geriatric ward, and the other an age-heterogeneous adult ward. At the end of 3 weeks they found significantly greater improvement in the patients on the age-integrated ward, being more responsive and scoring better on cognitive measures (1).

This was a tremendously important study, demonstrating the therapeutic effect of an age-integrated environment on the mentally impaired. It confirmed a principle first shown at the opposite end of the life cycle spectrum in the famous study by Skeels. He found that mentally retarded young children will show considerable improvement in cognitive function if they are placed in an age-heterogeneous setting in an institution for the retarded, an effect that lasted into adulthood (2).

Dr. Lawton: Dr. Kahn identified the *situation* rather than the individual as the beginning point in our chain of problems, here, and I don't think that is fair.

It seems to me that we must acknowledge that the beginning point on the road to an institution is the passing of the family threshold of tolerance for difficult behavior and the precipitous growth of anxiety for the physical safety of the older individual. From the family's point of view, surveillance and relief of burden are the needs that are being served first by the institution.

Thus, it seems to me that we are getting off the hook the easy way by pointing to the institution as the cause of everything. I see our task as one of improving the institution and filtering out those who shouldn't be there, but how are we going to eliminate institutions?

Dr. Kahn: This touches on the very topic we discuss in our paper, where we consider some of the theoretical and programmatic issues. It is a very complex problem that has to be seen in total perspective. It is not simply a dichotomous issue, e.g., of whether institutions per se are good or bad, or are the main source of our troubles. There are in the literature both many descriptions of the deleterious effects of chronic custodial care, and of the benefits of comprehensive programs, using such methods as day hospital or home care, which have drastically reduced the necessity for institutionalization.

REFERENCES

1. Kahana, E., and Kahana, B. (1970): Therapeutic potential of age integrated hospital environments on elderly psychiatric patients. *Arch. Gen. Psychiatry,* 23:20–29.
2. Skeels, H. M. (1966): Adult status of children with contrasting early life experiences. *Monogr. Soc. Res. Child Devel.,* Ser. 31, No. 3.

Clinical Aspects of Alzheimer's Disease and Senile Dementia, (Aging, Vol. 15), edited by Nancy E. Miller and Gene D. Cohen. Raven Press, New York 1981.

Community Treatment for Aged Persons with Altered Brain Function

Robert L. Kahn and *Sheldon S. Tobin

*Departments of Psychiatry and Behavioral Science (Human Development) and *School of Social Service Administration, University of Chicago, Chicago, Illinois 60637*

There is substantial evidence to support the effectiveness of community mental health programs in treating and caring for elderly persons with severe mental disorders, including those with altered brain function. Indeed, the success of past programs with the elderly provided impetus to, as well as theory for, the development of the community mental health movement. Yet today community mental health centers in the United States are neglecting the elderly, not only by providing disproportionately fewer services for old people compared to other age groups but also by providing even less treatment for them with the passage of time (84,92). To understand this paradox, a historical perspective is necessary, after which we review the major contemporary developments in community care, consider the important theoretical issues, and suggest possible future action.

HISTORICAL PERSPECTIVE

The aged have habitually had problems receiving adequate treatment in the mental health system. In 1854 a survey was conducted in Massachusetts to determine the presence of insanity in the general population, and the findings were compared with the proportion of treatment by age in a public and a private mental hospital (94). It was found that although there was an increasing rate of insanity with age, older persons were less likely to be receiving hospital treatment. Of all insane persons in their twenties, 61.1% were in Worcester State Hospital, and of all those in their thirties, 72.3%. Among the insane in their sixties, however, only 35% were hospitalized at Worcester, and for those in their seventies a still lower 28.7%. Decreasing percentages in treatment with age were even more pronounced at the private mental hospital.

The aged continued to be underrepresented in the state hospitals during the period when there was a predominantly positive attitude toward treating the mentally ill. When the character of the patient population changed during the latter part of the nineteenth century following the great waves of immigration and the expansion of the urban, working-class poor, the hospitals were transformed into custodial institutions with minimal therapeutic expectations (41). During the years of custodialism, which continued through World War II, the first-admission rates to mental hospitals showed a constant pattern increasing with age. As Malzberg (74) reported for New York State, the first-admission rates for all age groups between the years 1910 and 1950 remained stable with the exception of the rate for those persons aged 65 and over, which kept increasing precipitously. This led to extreme overcrowding of the state hospitals and resulted in the warehousing of large numbers of elderly patients. The pressure of over-crowding and the economic cost involved were factors that made the custodial mental health system especially receptive to the concepts and practices of community mental health.

ORIGINS

Community mental health is an idea whose time has come and come and come again. The basic philosophy that many symptoms of chronic mental illness are due in part to the effect of the environment and that deterioration is induced by our treatment, has been shown repeatedly throughout psychiatric history in periodic waves of reform and discovery (58). Zusman (115) pointed out that Pinel's great contribution was demonstrating the relationship between symptoms and the hospital environment. He cited John Reid as finding in 1812 that confine-ment in a hospital often led to worsening or perpetuation of mental disorder. During the nineteenth century "moral treatment" sought to eliminate the use of force and restraint, and notable examples of this change in treatment orienta-tion are found in the classic reports of Tuke and Conolly. During this century, a major rediscovery of community mental health occurred in military wartime psychiatry (29,42). Psychiatric battle casualties during the two World Wars were so great that military medical services were compelled to develop new techniques. They found that men were more readily returned to combat by brief treatment close to the front lines instead of extended hospitalization. Al-though this approach was first empirically established during World War I, it was discovered again during World War II and was finally systematically and successfully applied during the Korean War. Of all the United Nations forces in Korea who were given psychiatric care near the front line, 50% were returned to duty within 48 hr (63). Those psychiatric casualties who returned to duty, including 10% who had been recommended for administrative discharge, were compared with four control groups of men who returned to combat after an absence for other causes including hospitalization for disease and injury. It was found that the rating by noncommissioned officers of combat effectiveness was only slightly lower for the former psychiatric casualties (41).

The military experience, although dealing with young, healthy males at war, illustrates some of the basic principles of community mental health which are applicable to all populations. It demonstrates the effectiveness of "minimal inter-vention" (19,51), which is applied as early and with as little dislocation as possible (5). The casualties were treated in the combat zone by a simplified program of rest, food, reassurance, and a prompt return to combat. By keeping them with their units they were enabled to reassert usual adaptive mechanisms and to have the support of their buddies, in contrast to the effects of hospitalization, which necessitate a substantial temporal and spatial withdrawal with the accompanying loss of the informal social supports of their unit, impaired self-esteem and adaptation, and enduring symptomatology (29).

Amsterdam Experiment: The First Major Program

Between the two World Wars, in 1930, Querido established a community mental health program in the city of Amsterdam (16,22,63,76). He had been appointed city psychiatrist and, because of the economic depression, was instructed to cut the increasing costs for the care of the mentally ill. The most effective means of reducing the numbers in the mental hospitals, he observed, was not by discharging existing patients but by preventing the admission of new ones. Accordingly, he made it compulsory for all new patients to first be screened by a psychiatrist, which was accomplished by establishing a 24-hr service so that every patient could be promptly investigated in his own home. For administrative purposes the city of almost one million people was divided into sectors, each having a psychiatrist and two or more social workers. Sector psychiatrists saw patients in their own homes, and if hospitalization were absolutely necessary the sector psychiatrist continued to visit the patient in the hospital although treatment was conducted by hospital staff. The psychiatric service was supported by additional resources such as a sheltered workshop, foster homes, and an elaborate employment-finding system. About 40% of all adult psychiatric patients referred to the mental health service were never hospitalized. Ling (63) evaluated the effectiveness of the program by contrasting Amsterdam and London in 1941 on several indices. The suicide rate was 60% higher in London; there were 25% more patients in mental institutions; and the rate of hospital admission was three times greater than in Amsterdam. In 1963 Cath (16) visited Querido's successors and found the program still to be impressive, with more than one-third of the patients 65 years of age or older. Because of the effectiveness of this program for the elderly, with centralized responsibility and continuity of care in a large city, Cath expressed surprise that the model had not been copied in other countries.

Mapperley Hospital: Application of New Concepts

Perhaps the most gifted and thoughtful of the British psychiatrists who contributed to the community mental health movement and care of the aged was Duncan MacMillan (66–72,79). Immediately following World War II, at Mapperley Hospital in Nottingham, he pioneered some of the most innovative procedures of the time. Strong criticism was then being leveled at the mental hospital because it was believed that the institution itself had a noxious effect on residents, contributing considerably to their functional impairment. One type of response to this criticism was to alter the internal milieu of the institution by developing a therapeutic community, improving the communication between patients and staff, and giving patients more responsibility in their treatment (47,73). MacMillan (66), prior to the wide use of drug therapy, attempted to change the institutional atmosphere by opening up the previously locked hospital, which he started in 1945 and completed in 1952.

The geriatric part of his program was begun in 1948 with the advent of the National Health Service (68). Because of the difficulty in getting the elderly to come in for outpatient interviewing, he began a home care program conducted jointly by the psychiatrist and social worker. During the 10-year period from 1949 to 1959, 1,544 persons were seen in their homes. The geriatric day hospital was opened in 1955.

MacMillan was especially concerned about maintaining integration in the family. He believed that families went through a process of rejection when the burden of caring for the old person became too great or the separation lasted too long. Help given prior to the rejection, however, could forestall its development. He was one of the first to use "holiday relief" in which the aged person would go into the hospital on a scheduled basis to give his family free time. He also minimized rejection by the technique of time-limited hospitalization, explaining to the patient and family that hospitalization would last for a specified time period, usually 4 weeks. Under these conditions both maintained their expectation of return to the community. If further stay was required a formal letter to that effect was sent to the relative.

MacMillan (69) was particularly interested in the use of day care. He perceived it as a service for isolated people to whom it provided a regular routine, human relationships in a group setting, and essential nutritional needs, thereby arresting otherwise inevitable deterioration. He regarded its second major function as the relief of strain on the family, making it less likely that the family would find caring for the patient intolerable, leading to rejecting behavior. He also stressed day care for its primary prevention possibilities (67). In his experience, if one person of an isolated couple died, the other was likely to develop a senile reaction within a few months. Day care was often found to forestall this outcome. MacMillan (67) realized that there was not just one type of day care that was required in providing comprehensive services for the aged. He suggested a range of services, including community voluntary clubs, after-care centers, and day hospitals which would furnish "long-day" care, providing up to 7 days' care, if necessary, and keeping the patient until six o'clock or later until the relative was home. MacMillan was very aggressive in seeking out difficult problems. During one 3-year period he studied persons with a syndrome he called "senile social deterioration" (72). This was manifested by an extreme lack of hygiene and social deterioration, hostility, and withdrawal, and was often associated with alcoholism and a precipitous loss, e.g., death of a spouse.

He does not give figures, but claims day care was the most effective setting in treating this condition.

Most of the referrals to MacMillan's program were from general practitioners (68). Although the number of beds remained constant, the number of individuals admitted during the year rose from 178 in 1951 to 348 in 1958. For both periods, however, there were only 50 or fewer persons remaining in the hospital 4 months after the end of each 12-month period. In 1949, 201 elderly patients were seen for the first time in his program (68). Of these, slightly over 26% had senile dementia, with about half of all patients diagnosed as organic psychosis. Of all the aged, 45% were managed by care in the community, 16% were treated in the day care center, and only 37% were hospitalized.

Continuity of care was ensured by having the consultant who made the initial home visit also in charge of the inpatient beds. MacMillan was especially ingenious in achieving administrative arrangements which facilitated the effective coordination of mental health, social, and medical services. MacMillan himself was Medical Officer of Mental Health for the city, supervising all aspects of mental health activity including being superintendent of the mental hospital; he was, in addition, appointed policy advisor to the Medical Officer of Health, who was responsible for all community health care. The day center was administered by the local health authority with the psychiatric services provided by the Mapperley staff. He operated an assessment unit that was run jointly by three departments: Geriatric, Psychogeriatric, and the Local Welfare Authority Service (79). In this unit the Welfare Office functioned simultaneously as the hospital social worker. MacMillan had the law specially changed to permit the same staff to work with the patient whether in the hospital or on community care through administrative arrangements called "double appointments" (66); it was used for all levels of staff and served to make the professionals concerned with needs of the patient rather than their particular organization.

Chichester and Salisbury: A Controlled Study

Another early British program which demonstrated the capacity to manage elderly psychiatric patients on extramural treatment was the Worthing Experiment at Graylingwell Hospital (14,15,77,78). Started in 1957 because of overcrowded hospitals, the program added five basic ingredients to the original psychiatric hospital functions: extended outpatient services, home evaluation and treatment, establishment of a day hospital, close collaboration with the general practitioners, and immediate appointments for all urgent cases. About 30% of the new patients were 65 or over, but fewer than one-third were admitted to the hospital, a reduction of 43% compared to the year prior to the service (14). During 1957 there were 1,293 new patients of all ages evaluated, of whom 174 were diagnosed as having some condition of altered brain function, with 48 explicit diagnoses of senile dementia.

In 1958 that rare oddity—a controlled study of the community psychiatric service—was undertaken by Grad and Sainsbury (34–38,96–98). The experimental service centered on the Graylingwell program, which was now reorganized into the Chichester District, a catchment area of approximately 90,000 adults. The Salisbury District, with a similar population, located 60 miles away, but with a traditional hospital-based program, was used as the control group. A psychiatric register was established in each area for the year 1960 so that standardized information was obtained and referral rates were calculated that were specific for age, sex, marital status, social class, and household size.

The results were striking. It was found, for example, that the community program in Chichester had a much higher rate of severe mental disorder but a much lower rate of hospitalization. In 1960, 52% of the psychiatric referrals in Salisbury were hospitalized compared to only 14% in Chichester (36). Among referred persons aged 65 and over, 76% were hospitalized in Salisbury and 42% in Chichester. Although there was a significantly higher rate in Chichester for organic psychoses in the aged, including confusional states and presenile dementia, the hospitalization rate for those with this diagnosis was only 47% in Chichester, but 89% in Salisbury (35). The elderly apparently benefited most from the community service. There was a significantly higher total referral rate in Chichester, but the difference was especially marked for the very old (38); of those aged 75 or more, the referral rate per 100,000 was 1,125 in Chichester and only 624 in Salisbury. The community program was especially likely to recruit seriously mentally disordered persons who had previously been neglected. Socially, this included vulnerable groups such as widowed females, urban dwellers, single persons, and the poor. Clinically, a significantly greater number of persons with more psychoses but with shorter duration of illness were seen in Chichester.

Grad de Alarcón et al. (38) explained these results by the availability of psychiatrists and a range of services, the absence of waiting lists, and the general knowledge on the part of the general practitioners and families that they were welcome to telephone whenever they wanted advice. It was concluded that because there was less pressure to admit patients there was a greater willingness to refer them. These points must be kept in mind when considering that expanded services in this country had a substantially different consequence on the type of population served.

DEVELOPMENTS IN THE UNITED STATES

In contrast to the European experience, the development of community mental health in the United States after World War II has been associated with neglect of the aged. There has been an enormous expansion of interest in mental health and resources available, with the number of patient care episodes in 1973 being three times those reported in 1955 and twice the number in 1963 (84). Despite the increase for the population as a whole, treatment of the aged has consistently declined (51). Between 1946 and 1972, for example, the number of first admissions exhibited a dramatically opposite pattern to that of the prewar era, showing an increase in rate of almost 100% for the youngest age group, and a decrease of 71% for those 65 and over. Comparing just the years 1966 and 1971, there was an increase in patient care episodes for the whole population of 37% but a decrease of 22% for the aged. Even the general hospital psychiatric units showed a decrease of 45% in services to the aged during this period. Community mental health centers have shown a consistent decline in services for older persons (3,84,92).

Using an unduplicated count from the Monroe County Psychiatric Case Register, Babigian (3) found that during the period between 1963 and 1973 there was a progressive decrease in all kinds of services for the aged. A community mental health center was established in 1968, but it seemed only to accelerate the decline in services. Although the State of New York started restricting the admission of aged to the state mental hospitals in 1968, the register showed that instead of other resources taking up the slack the decline was characteristic of all services. Similar findings were obtained in a study of several catchment area programs in eastern New York State and in New York City (80). The aged were less likely than younger persons to receive inpatient treatment in state or general hospitals or to receive noninpatient admissions. Furthermore, of those aged 65 or older, more were admitted as inpatients than noninpatients, the reverse of the pattern for younger persons. The general discriminatory neglect of older people was shown by the United States Commission on Civil Rights in a study of the comparative percentage by age of the total population in areas covered by the services included and the proportion of new patients (108). Those aged 65 and over constituted 9.9% of the service population but only 4.1% of the new patients.

There are, of course, individual American programs which have focused on the aged (45). An early program was established at Montefiore Hospital in New York (86). Montefiore had a tradition of providing home care for the physically ill elderly and was receptive to a mental health program using the same principle. Basically, there was an age- and service-integrated catchment program with inpatient/outpatient, day and night care. All geriatric patients were evaluated in their own homes by the psychiatrist and social worker. In addition to the psychiatric services, the program developed a relationship with a community center down the street in which other old people from the neighborhood were included in a variety of social activities. The administrative device was an arrangement similar to MacMillan's technique, in which a social worker was jointly hired by the community center and the community mental health center. Through this overlap, the needs of the old persons, appropriate to either setting, could be accommodated with minimal dislocation.

From the evidence we have, the European and American community mental health programs have several characteristics in common. They have increased service utilization and broadened the base of the population served to include more disadvantaged persons in their programs (3,104), although this may be due to the effect of catchment itself as Klerman (59) pointed out. Tischler et al. (104) compared two catchment area programs, only one of which had a community mental health center, and found that the pattern of patient characteristics was the same in both. The European and American community mental health programs have also shown major differences in emphasis. The Chichester program, for example, compared to its control group, treated patients who were older and sicker (38). In the United States the community mental health centers serve not only younger patients, but also those with less severe illness (84,92). The general increase in accessibility of general mental health services does not automatically facilitate the treatment needs of categorical populations at risk (3).

Another perspective on contemporary mental health services for the aged is provided by Frankfather (27) who described the care of the elderly brain-damaged by observing their interaction in a number of settings in which they are likely to be screened, including senior centers, geriatric outreach programs, family counseling agencies, sheltered workshops, public welfare agencies, nursing homes, and neighborhood health centers. He found that all are alike in screening out these elderly. The psychiatrist at the general hospital, on the one hand, in labeling the elderly person as having organic brain damage, does not thereafter feel obligated to admit the person to a "treatment" ward. The intake worker at the Community Mental Health Center, on the other hand, when labeling the mental impairment as transient, can refer the older person to a local counseling agency or to a general hospital for treatment of an accompanying physical problem. However the elderly person is labeled, very few practitioners perceive the condition as tractable. According to Frankfather (27), the brain-damaged elderly are rarely accepted as desirable patients, clients, or residents because their liabilities to service organizations usually outweigh their assets.

With the failure of the state mental hospitals and the community mental health centers to deal with the major mental disorders of old age, there has been the emergence of a new custodialism and the accumulation of masses of elderly patients in nursing homes (91). This custodialism was fostered by the mass discharge of patients, largely chronic schizophrenics, from the state hospitals. Since many of these chronically institutionalized schizophrenic patients had already attained a chronological age of 65, their discharge from the state hospitals was fostered by certain stereotypes about the aged, mainly that they really had no mental illness but were in the hospital just because they were growing old (51).

CURRENT STATUS OF COMMUNITY TREATMENT

Although comprehensive community mental health programs for the elderly continue to be in operation in Europe (30), in the United States there is a proliferation of what could be called variant or partial community mental health programs. These have in common the emphasis on minimizing dislocation by preventing institutionalization and maintaining the person in his natural community; they differ from the original programs in their incomplete integration of psychiatric, medical, and social services, and in their concentration on broader segments of the population, including younger persons and those with less serious mental problems. When programs for the elderly were developed, they lacked a base in a psychiatric service, depended on just one service component, and lacked a geographically defined catchment area.

Although rare, it is possible to find programs that bridge or emanate from an inpatient psychiatric service and contain an array of community services. Some of these programs have the flavor of MacMillan's earliest efforts at Mapperley Hospital. Yet in the recent Glasscote et al. (30) review of 10 innovative programs, all the institution-based programs that used a mental hospital as a base were in other countries. The institution-based programs in the United States that were singled out emanated from sectarian long-term care facilities: Douglas Gardens, Miami Jewish Home and Hospital, and the Ebenezer Society in Minneapolis.

Protective Services

The absence of community mental health programs for the elderly, as well as the inattention by social service agencies to the needs of the impaired elderly, led to the National Council on Aging calling together in 1948 a group of social workers to develop "protective service" programs. Protective services for other age groups have been prevalent in social services, referring usually to children where a public or private agency may have to assume guardianship responsibility *in loco parentis*. Translated to the elderly, protective services refers to those situations in which the mental and physical status of the elderly person requires continuing supervision and assistance by a social agency because the older person is too impaired to do so himself and lacks significant others to assure protection. Examples of such services are health care, housekeeping help, nutritional assistance, and legal aid. The attention to this target population by social workers, predominantly from voluntary sectarian family service agencies, reflected the absence of a public policy toward the mentally impaired elderly. By default, because there was no community mental health initiative, the voluntary social service sector responded to the needs of the elderly who were unable to care for themselves.

The target group for protective service programs was estimated by Blenkner et al. (6) to be 7 to 10% of the elderly population. Although twice that estimate circumscribes the percentage of elderly with mental impairment as observed in community surveys in New York (7) and San Francisco (65), a lesser percentage apparently are mentally incompetent and lack interpersonal resources that can assure protection. Obviously this target group is not composed entirely of elderly with senile dementia nor are all community residents who have senile dementia included within the target group because those with adequate protection are excluded.

The most notable studies of comprehensive protective services have been undertaken by Blenkner and her colleagues (6,7,82). Their results were quite unexpected. In her first controlled study of a program of social work and public health nursing service for elderly applicants to the Community Service Society of New York, it was found that the greater the intensity of service the higher the death rate (7). Among the group provided maximal service, 24% died compared to only 6% receiving minimal service. Blenkner subsequently designed a social experiment to assess the use of professionally trained social workers in providing protective services (6). The design for the experiment was rigorous, given the nature of field studies. The Benjamin Rose Institute's Research Project randomly assigned protective service cases either to an experimental ($N = 76$) or a control ($N = 88$) group, as the cases were referred to the Project. If assigned to the control group, the client was served by one of 13 participating referral agencies. Clients in the experimental group were seen by one of the four highly trained caseworkers hired for the project. All 164 participants were interviewed by the research staff within 5 days after registration and before contact was made by the project staff. Clients were interviewed again 3 and 6 months later with short interviews, and after 1 year with a longer follow-up interview. Lastly, follow-up contact was made over a 5-year period to gather survival statistics.

Assessments made of service provided to clients showed that more service was provided to the experimental group than to the control group, although the types of services were similar. To evaluate effectiveness of the experimental services, three aspects were measured: competence, environmental protection, effect on others. Both groups showed deterioration in physical and mental competence, and at the end of the year the death rate for the experimental group was 25% and only 18% for the control group. Both groups show an upward trend on protection, but the experimental clients received more protection, particularly on the variable of concrete assistance, which was reflected in the data on supportive services. The difference in the amount of concrete assistance, however, was a function of rates of institutionalism: 34% among experimental clients and 20% in the controls. On effect, the trend was positive in both groups, the experimental group showing a nonsignificant but greater increase in contentment and nonsignificant but greater decrease in symptoms of emotional disturbance. On effect on others, both groups showed a diminution in collateral stress.

Follow-up data favored the control sample. By the end of 5 years, more of the experimental clients were institutionalized than the controls: 61% versus 47%, the same 14% difference that was found at the end of 1 year. Survival rates similarly were 37% for the experimental clients at the end of 4 years but 48% for the control clients. Correcting for age, sex, race, and geographic structure of the two groups did not appreciably alter the difference in survival rates. The authors concluded that the effect of more skilled social workers was an "overdosing" of clients that led to more concrete assistance, including institutionalization, and that institutionalization was responsible for the higher death rate.

A somewhat similar controlled study of the effectiveness of social work was undertaken by Goldberg (31) in England. Clients were selected, however, so that few persons with organic brain dysfunction were included. Outcome for the treated and control groups within a 10.5-month follow-up was similar in the areas of environmental change, changes in subjective attitudes, and changes in the social work assessor's judgment about the extent and nature of practical needs; the degree and type of problems experienced; and the client's contentment. Although more persons in the experimental group reported contact with the social worker, and although hospitalization and psychiatric referrals were used more frequently, there were distinct advantages to the experimental group in activity and affect state. Death rates were similar. Although Goldberg's results are decidedly different from those reported by Blenkner et al., it must be realized that in the English study the clients were healthier. It is also likely that the lack of available custodial institutional resources worked in favor of Goldberg's group. Her workers also had the greater degree of control over the delivery of services, providing empirical evidence for the benefits of continuity of care. In the Blenkner program, the social workers functioned less as coordinators of services under their control than as links between the client and services that were largely controlled by others. These workers were more likely to have serious reservations regarding the availability and usefulness of community services for the mentally impaired, and therefore were more likely to play it safe and recommend institutional care.

A community program that is more comprehensive than those of Blenkner or Goldberg was developed during the last few years and is described by Glasscote et al. (30) in their book on creative programs. The Council for Jewish Elderly (CJE), an agency of the Jewish Federation of Metropolitan Chicago, was developed with the intent of enabling older people to remain in the community. In contrast to previous emphasis on three distinct and unrelated long-term care facilities, a single community plan was developed with the purpose of providing a highly diversified service inventory, systems of proper evaluation of need and availability of needed services, the development of highly individualized service plans, rapid and effective delivery of services, and effective monitoring and follow-up on service plans (112). The services include a variety of home-delivered and day care services and a set of living facilities, including a group living apartment for 12 elderly persons (109) and a temporary holiday relief residence for 11 individuals. The personnel include social workers, nurses, outreach workers, and a psychiatrist who is employed for evaluation, consultation with the staff, and developing service plans. The services provided by the CJE are not unique in themselves. What is unusual is that the broad spectrum of services are delivered under the direction of a single agency (105,106). The entire program was mobilized as a unit, since the operation of any component depended on the whole. The possibility for this implementation was credited to the usefulness of a defined geographic catchment area, which in 1970 consisted of a total population of 61,000 with 22% aged 60 and over, and with an approximate elderly Jewish population of 7,000.

Basic to the system was making access easier for the elderly themselves rather than waiting for their adult children or relatives to seek service. Accordingly, intake was not restricted to a single location but was made accessible through a number of entry points, e.g., the outreach worker, the Area Service Center, and the Transportation Program (112). Area Service Center facilities serve as open "Drop-In Centers" or "Coffee Houses," providing a visible, unstructured operation the elderly can use on their own terms. Additional central concepts of the CJE program include responsiveness of staff workers who are close to the elderly and the community, giving the older person an individualized plan with continuity of care, protecting him or her from being overwhelmed by the availability of services, and, finally, giving the older person an opportunity to reduce or eliminate services (112).

Showing some features of a community mental health program, the CJE seems successful in caring for persons with dementia. Of the 33 clients served in day care, for example, 25 (76%) had notable mental impairment (severe in 10 persons). The day care seemed especially effective because more of the severely impaired were likely to be living alone (102). The part-time psychiatrist in the program was often able to become involved early, so that more serious emotional problems could be prevented and psychiatric hospitalization recommended early enough to permit the patient's return to the community services (25).

Single-Component Programs

Successful community treatment necessitates sufficient comprehensiveness so that one or more services can be mobilized on behalf of the elderly impaired individual (56). Any single component may be useful for select individuals but cannot suffice for a group of impaired elderly. A few single-component programs, however, do merit discussion.

An active intervention program among elderly living in age-segregated housing was reported by Sherwood et al. (101), who investigated the effects of a low-income public housing facility for the physically impaired elderly. Through the use of supportive services these elderly were helped to remain in their public housing apartments. To what extent the residents of this housing program were organically impaired is unknown. A study by Fisch et al. (26), however, does shed light on a sample of persons aged 65 and over who had demonstrable brain damage but were living in low-cost public housing. Each person was subjected to a standard, objective method of assessing brain damage, the Kahn-Goldfarb Mental Status Questionnaire (54), and a psychiatric examination. Two groups were compared: (a) 47% who had no evidence of organic mental dysfunction on either procedure, and (6) 17% who were regarded as definitely brain-damaged because they were positive on both procedures. Both groups had lived in the project for over 3 years, some for as long as 10 to 15 years, and both were physically healthy. The brain-damaged were more likely to live alone and have poorer social relationships, e.g., receive fewer telephone calls or have no person to call in emergencies. The principal support of the brain-damaged cases was from the housing assistants who maintained tenant relations and were in charge of each apartment. They were not aware that the old people had mental impairment but did know them as more complaining tenants. Each of the four most impaired persons showed a premorbid tendency to a strong, self-reliant personality, which seemed to be important in their present adaptation. This study is an excellent illustration of how persons with severe dementia, living alone and with little social contact, can be adequately maintained in the community by the minimal support provided by public housing and administrative supervision.

A sensible program, theoretically is foster family care, which, like day care, has a long tradition in other countries. Weinberg (111), relating his own successful experiences in placing elderly state mental hospital patients in foster families during the 1940s, noted that in 1885 the Board of Health of the State of Massachusetts enacted a law authorizing the placing of "insane persons of the chronic quiet class . . . into suitable families." Recently Sherman and Newman (99) interviewed caretakers of 100 adult foster family homes in New York City and reported that residents appeared well-integrated into their surrogate families and that caretakers reported a great deal of satisfaction. Of this alternative, Brody (9) noted that many foster homes function as the poorest kind of "mom and pop" boarding homes. Thus although foster family care has great potential for the mentally impaired elderly, it has not been used to great advantage.

Another example of a partial community mental health program is day care. This type of service played a major role in the comprehensive programs of Carse and MacMillan. However, despite their favorable reports, it has been surprisingly little copied in the United States (18), and then largely as an isolated unit. Controlled studies with younger patients (83) demonstrate that separate day care service can serve at least to prevent hospitalization (39), and it can result in better social adjustment and less likelihood of readmission (46).

For the demented aged, the British are continuing to describe day hospital programs in a more integrated structure (30). Baker and Byrne (4), for example, developed a day hospital program in Gloucestershire in which it was estimated there were 3,000 severely, and another 3,000 mildly, demented persons. It was decided to establish a psychiatric service to deal with the severe problems, including the dementias, and to develop extensive day hospital services. They reported that "almost without exception" patients responded better to day care than to inpatient care, particularly those with more severe dementia, who became disoriented on 24-hr care. In the day hospital the dementia patients showed less incontinence, less nighttime restlessness, and less excessive sedation. Of 100 consecutive new patients seen on home visits, 36% were treated in the day hospital, 18% were admitted to the hospital, and the remaining 46% were treated at home. The day hospital nurses do considerable home visiting for evaluation and continued care of discharged patients, as well as for treatment of new patients. On the basis of this experience, the authors claim that not more than 5% of all admissions to the service become long-stay patients, although there is some question whether all the severely demented are included in these figures. A different perspective is provided by the 5-year review of a geriatric psychiatric day hospital by Greene and Timbury (40). They observed that during this period the mean age of the patients increased from 72.8 to 77.7 years, and the percentage with organic disorders rose from 46% to 90%. Forty percent of the organic disease patients were living alone, and these were admitted with milder impairment than those living with families. Most of the organic disease patients remained in day care for less than 6 months and 75% were discharged to a long-stay ward. Greene and Timbury concluded that their day hospital provided short-term support, maintaining patients in the community until beds became available in long-stay institutions.

Weissert (113) studied 10 selected programs of geriatric day care in the United States and found two distinct models, one oriented to rehabilitation for the physically handicapped who would otherwise by institutionalized, and the other with a mixture of clientele including psychotic persons. Weissert noted that the kind of day care provided in a given setting depended on the contexts and purposes of the program, which ranged from filling a gap in service for a specific population to developing a service because funding was available. Many others (8,24,64,90) have also advocated a fairly rigid distinction between the medical and psychiatric aspects of day care. Although there are consistent reports that day care may be a cost-effective method of preventing hospitalization and further deterioration as well as aiding the family (61,75,89,93), there is some question concerning its limitation as a separate service. Goldstein and his colleagues (32,33) complained that by itself day care was not very successful in dealing with persons with moderately severe organic brain syndrome. They suggested that other services which should be linked to day care include a foster-home program and the services of parttime homemakers. They also found that patients become so attached to the program that none were discharged during the year despite improvement. They concluded that the patients should be gradually integrated into more social programs, such as Golden Age clubs or day centers.

Home evaluation and home care for the mentally impaired elderly is a *sine qua non* for community treatment and has been a cornerstone of the European community health services. Brown (13) found that hospitalization could be avoided with a home care program for younger patients. Paralleling the European experience is the finding by Pasamanick et al. (85) who used an alternative treatment design: providing home treatment to schizophrenics with at least as good results as hospital care but at considerably less cost. Appreciation for the value of home care, the major meaning of "alternatives to institutional care," has led to considerable development of home-delivered services. To what extent these services, provided usually without the benefit of a comprehensive system, have been helpful to the mentally impaired elderly is difficult to assess. An illustration of what could be accomplished is provided by Nielsen et al. (82) in one of the few systematic evaluations of home-delivered services. Participants 60 years of age and older who were discharged from a rehabilitation hospital did not require intensive nursing care after discharge and had dwellings in the community. The intervention was a home aide service developed for the project and based in a social agency. Outcome was assessed by measure of contentment, institutionalization, and survival before and 1 year after the demonstration project. The service group was more content than the control group, hospitalization was lessened, and survivorship was higher. The service was particularly helpful in reducing institutionalization of women 75 years of age and older when another person was in the household to provide additional care as needed.

COMMUNITY MENTAL HEALTH THEORY

There are many definitions of community mental health, as well as considerable controversy about how such programs should be implemented and how their effectiveness should be evaluated (2,82). On the basis of the available evidence of the last 30 years, however, there appears to be a fairly clear-cut set of principles and characteristics of programs that have been effective in treating the aged with altered brain function.

Unlike the custodial approach and its negative expectations, one principle that emerges from a historical perspective is that treatment will make a difference. Recently Wershow (114), approaching the subject from the viewpoint of institutional care, argued that "therapeutic omnipotence" on behalf of the elderly with organic brain syndrome leads to unnecessary costs for society. He portrayed organic brain syndrome as a progressive disease leading to incontinence and a state of vegetation, and added that to speak of community treatment or vigorous therapeutic intervention for these elderly is to ignore the realities of organic brain syndrome. Cohen (17), however, responded by first differentiating between patients with organic brain syndrome and pseudodementia, and then between those with organic brain syndrome stemming from different causes, emphasizing the variability in "individual reserve capacities" and "unpredictability in the course or rate of change."

A key position set forth by those who have developed outstanding programs for the aged was that the mental disorders accompanying dementia are partly organic and partly reactive. MacMillan (69) spoke of "secondary emotional disabilities" and stated that the chief manifestations of senile dementia are not organic but a response to emotional needs. It is not memory impairment but restlessness, nocturnal wandering, and incontinence which lead to difficulty. For example, MacMillan (68) believed, as did Newman (81), that nonorganic incontinence is an emotional reaction, an expression of unhappiness or dissatisfaction. Supporting this position is the common observation that older persons with organic brain disease often show a greater functional disability than is warranted by their health status. This condition is termed "excess disability" (49,50,53) and has been found prominently in nursing home (57) and home for the aged (10,11) populations. Persons showing this behavior appear apathetic and uninterested in performing motor or mental activities within their capability. In populations that have been institutionalized for any length of time, the excess disability is so powerful that even the most intense therapeutic efforts may induce no more than a transient response (10,11,51). Excess disability is often induced by our caring techniques, particularly severe and long-term dislocation (1,106). Gruenberg (43,44) described a similar acquired condition, the "social breakdown syndrome," in which persons with an initial symptom are treated in such a way, as by institutionalization, that additional impairment is superimposed on that due to the intrinsic properties of the pathology.

The basic principles of community mental health in care of the aged can be discussed in terms of four programmatic or conceptual areas: timing, minimal intervention, commitment to a population and guarantee of services, and the benefit of the service provided.

Critical Nature of Timing

The community mental health programs for the aged have emphasized secondary and tertiary prevention. They thus were directed at mitigating the pathological condition and reducing the disabilities consequent to the disorder. To achieve secondary prevention, the most compelling requirement is early identification and prompt treatment (5,19,88,95,103). MacMillan (71) was particularly concerned about timing, stating that it was important to become involved before a crisis developed in the family followed by rejection of the patient. Brothwood (12) pointed out that once social supports collapse, as when an old person is admitted to an institution, they may be extremely difficult to restructure. Intervention as early as possible is thus of the utmost importance, particularly because procedures that could help if provided early may have no effect after a relatively short delay. Although the reports of the European programs have been concerned with treating new patients, it is indicated that early intervention facilitates management of the chronic course of the illness as well by maintaining relationships with home, friends, and neighborhood and emphasizing established adaptive resources as much as possible.

Minimal Intervention

After early intervention, the second most important characteristic of the geriatric community mental health program is the emphasis on minimal intervention (19,20,51), including minimal dislocation (5). Home evaluation and treatment are preferred, and as much as possible the patient should stay in his own community, neighborhood, family, and home, performing his regular activities. Where intervention necessitates dislocation, the process should be structured to minimize disruption, e.g., by giving a time limit to the intervention, integrating the informal support systems into the mental health services, and treatment that minimizes family separation. Minimal intervention not only refers to how we intrude into the lives of patients and their families but also to the level or intensity of involvement. If we intrude too vigorously, there is a danger that in our eagerness to meet perceived needs for security and survival the patient will be infantilized by our doing too much, and we will be diminishing the old person's residual adaptive ability. Too vigorous intervention apparently accounts for the negative results of what were apparently well-designed programs of community treatment. This type of negative effect induced by the excessive helpfulness of the service providers was called "over-dosing" by Blenkner and "over-fostering" by Lear et al. (62).

Service Commitment

It is necessary to have flexible service alternatives in addition to hospitalization. Home evaluation and home care on the one hand and day care on the other are especially effective in dealing with the elderly population. To achieve the greatest effectiveness, the services must be part of an integrated program in which there is guaranteed commitment and trust. In the British programs the confidence that the professionals could be called at any time, that help was available when needed, and that there was no pressure toward institutionalization apparently was essential to the success of the programs. Continuity of care was required so that the same personnel had the responsibility for, and could work with, the client in different settings and at different times. One of the most difficult problems is dealing with the multiple needs of the old person, which may require the professional services of a variety of disciplines and administrative bodies. In particular it is difficult to integrate the various social services—and these with the medical and psychiatric services. No matter how cooperative or well intentioned the various professionals and agencies are, the client is likely to suffer from the lack of service coordination.

All of the notable British programs worked on the principle of a defined geographic catchment area. By itself this does not, of course, guarantee an adequate program for the aged, but it does appear to be a necessary prerequisite. With a catchment area it is possible to plan for a known population and thus offer the appropriate commitment or guarantee of a range of services, including continuity of care. A circumscribed geographic program also permits the optimum use of available community resources and the development of special arrangements, e.g., informal working relationships with family physicians and other key persons. Catchment areas also have provided an important methodology for evaluation of community programs (3,38,104). Combining the known population characteristics with the community-wide reporting techniques of a Psychiatric Case Register make it possible to determine specific utilization rates. It is apparent that a catchment program by itself broadens the social characteristics of the service utilization (3,104). If there is an attitude of confidence and trust built up, as in the Chichester study, by being available to help and without pressure for institutionalization, there can be a significant increase in utilization of services by persons who are more vulnerable and have more severe illnesses but who may also have a better prognosis because of the shorter duration of illness (38).

Program Benefits

A commonly cited criterion of community mental health program effectiveness is the impact on the family. However, as shown by Blenkner et al. (6), the relief to the relatives and the interests of the client do not coincide. The most systematic study of the impact on family burden was undertaken in the Chichester-Salisbury controlled study (34,38,98). These authors studied 119 elderly patients in the two areas and found that the families of over three-fourths said they were facing some burden, which was said to be severe in 40%. The burdens included nursing needs, demands for excess attention, the development of mental and physical ailments in family members, restriction on employment possibilities, and social and leisure limitations. They followed the group for 2 years; 44% of the patients had died and nearly one-third still had problems, with 12% severe. Although organic psychosis tended to be rated as a severe burden, and there were thus more difficult patients in the Chichester community health program, the amount of relief for families of the old persons who survived was approximately 80% and was the same in both communities at the follow-up. Interestingly, for young persons and less severely burdensome patients, the traditional program had a much greater effect on easing the impact on the family. Family burden is obviously a very complicated outcome variable and cannot be regarded as simply good or bad without considering the total context.

The selection of evaluative criteria can radically alter our perception of a program. Blenkner's experiments, as Weber (110) pointed out, could also have been counted as successful if she had focused on treatment effort such as duration of service and frequency of interviews or contacts while avoiding the damaging criteria of institutionalization and death. Examples abound where presumably benign benefit considerations are limited to relatively trivial criteria of effectiveness (52). Regarding care in extended care facilities, Kohen and Paul (60) noted that in Illinois the regulatory procedures avoid dealing with substantive psychological and health impact of these facilities by overwhelmingly concentrating on physical plant and physical aspects of care. In a similar vein, Weber (110) described the work of Katz and his associates who, when studying the effects of a public health nursing program, were so concerned with physical needs and protection that the clients showed the negative effects of reduced social interaction and minimal functioning. The combination of harmful and helpful aspects of a program is also related to the distinction which Kahn and Zarit (55) raised between basic and limited goals. A basic goal, for example, for an elderly person with early dementia may be to slow the intellectual deterioration as much as possible. If placed in an institution, however, the limited goal might be to follow the rules. However, achievement of this limited goal may contradict the basic goal, leading to a compliant, apathetic, deteriorated person. In contrast, the rebellious or aggressive person may actually be more effective in maintaining his intellectual function (106).

One of the earliest and still major criterion of program success is keeping persons out of institutions. The British programs, with their before and after data or controlled study information, clearly show that hospitalization is greatly reduced. There was originally a great emphasis on keeping people out of mental hospitals because of the overcrowding and economic costs, and because the state hospital itself, rather than its ideology, was blamed for the ills of the mental health system. Finding "alternatives to hospitalization" for the aged became one of the clichés of the time. The conceptual basis, however, that it was the dislocation and custodial orientation that caused the harmful effects, was often lost. With a confusion of cliché and theory, there has been widespread contamination of means and ends in the treatment of the mentally impaired elderly. The difficulties encountered following the recent rapid mass relocation of elderly schizophrenics from state mental hospitals "back to the community" have been cited as evidence of the failure of the community approach, but the management of these patients represents the antithesis of the basic community mental health ideology. Rather than being treated early in their illness, the change in management occurred after long years of being removed from their families, jobs, and neighborhood, and suffering the invalidism of chronic custodial care. Transferring these patients, if anything, removed the support of the familiar hospital environment which, at that stage of their lives and illnesses, may have been far more supportive than the boarding homes, foster care homes, and nursing homes to which they were relocated. It has been considered a triumph when old people were sent to other kinds of institutions, e.g., nursing homes or homes for the aged. Controlled studies have shown, however, that nursing homes, for example, are even more custodial and have a more damaging effect than state mental hospitals on elderly persons (23), and that relocation to even the best of long-term care facilities, the sectarian home for the aged, is associated with lessening of cognitive capacity (106). Indeed, Tobin and Lieberman (106) found that before a person actually entered the home for the aged but was still on the waiting list, a negative effect was produced by the experience of abandonment that precedes admission. They found that, even when controlling for degree of physical illness, double dislocation (e.g., going first to a general hospital and then to a long-term care institution) was associated not only with extreme mental deterioration but also with physical deterioration and death.

It is also a tragic irony that the policy of eliminating or reducing admissions of elderly persons to state mental hospitals in this country has resulted in a massive decrease in the provision of any psychiatric care at all (51). It was based on the remarkably false notion that the aged had previously been hospitalized incorrectly because they had not been suffering from psychiatric illness. This belief was maintained because the old people's psychoses and delusions typically occurred in a context of severe physical illness which was regarded as the primary disorder or because of the stereotype that dementia is just a manifestation of normal aging. So, instead of responding to the problem of the manifestly poor care that had been given to the elderly for so many years in the state hospitals by improving the quality of care, the response has been to stop treating them. Thus avoidance of hospitalization, which was originally a means for minimizing custodialism and dislocation, has now been converted into an end in itself even though it has become the cause of increased custodialism, major dislocation, and less treatment of any kind.

It is certainly preferable to maintain people at home rather than in an institution, but the management of individuals should rest on clinical substance rather than mechanical adherence to slogans. Institutional care by itself can be either custodial or therapeutic (21,87). An institution, for example, that is used for brief, time-limited crisis periods or for holiday relief and is part of a comprehensive system of continuity of care may be very therapeutic.

THE FUTURE: A PROPOSAL

Although there are a few controlled studies, there have been sufficient research and clinical data to indicate some direction for future activity. We seem to have learned little from our past experiences, however. The early European programs had remarkable characteristics and extreme effects, and the one controlled study clearly showed the advantage of a comprehensive type of community health program based on home care, but such programs are continuing today only in Europe (30). On the negative side, we have learned the deadly effect of providing services excessively attentive to physical needs (6,110), yet new service programs with similar characteristics are being developed. Although our past experience has shown that it is custodialism, not institutionalization per se, that has such negative effects, we continue to treat the elderly in custodial fashion (52). It has been found that even age segregation in special services for old people may have deleterious custodial effects (48), but many people insist that age segregation is necessary. It is noteworthy that the great European programs for the aged occurred as part of an age-integrated total program, although each adopted special administrative and service components for the elderly.

Not only do we have difficulty learning from others, we cannot draw on the lessons of our own research. In a maneuver that has been called the "last paragraph" phenomenon, Kahn (52) noted that many authors whose studies yield poor results will nevertheless write in a last paragraph which asserts that despite these results it is necessary to continue the same procedure. In part, this is because of the emphasis on quality of procedures used rather than outcome (28,100). It also arises because of the impact of social and political forces on professional judgment (59). It is, finally, an occupational failing of many professionals. In a long review of memory and verbal learning, Tulving and Madigan (107) concluded that whenever results conflict with theory "the last thing the typical experimenter does is to question the theory."

Comparable to the reaction against custodialism that set in after World War II, the time is again ripe for innovation. We are faced with the continued inadequate but expensive mental health services provided to the elderly with brain dysfunction, a situation that is more troublesome because of the increasing numbers of elderly persons, particularly those 75 years of age and older. Such old persons with altered brain function are especially difficult to manage because they require, in addition to mental health services, physical health and social services. Without this integration, even the most superior of programs may, at best, achieve a level of custodial care.

What is needed is the development of care for the mentally impaired aged that is more closely modeled on the European approach to community treatment. Using the principles that we outlined, we strongly urge that at least one demonstration controlled study be established in two or more comparable communities, e.g., cities of similar size and characteristics. Only through such an experiment can we fully learn the possibilities and limitations of the community approach in this country.

REFERENCES

1. Aldrich, C. K., and Mendkoff, E. (1963): *J. Am. Geriatr. Soc.,* 11:185–194.
2. Arnhoff, F. N. (1975): *Science,* 188:1277–1281.
3. Babigian, H. M. (1977): *Arch. Gen. Psychiatry,* 34:385–394.
4. Baker, A. A., and Byrne, R. J. F. (1977): *Br. J. Psychiatry,* 130:123–126.
5. Blain, D. (1975): *Hosp. Commun. Psychiatry,* 26:605–609.
6. Blenkner, M., Bloom, M., Wasser, E., and Nielson, M. (1971): *Soc. Casework,* 52:483–499.
7. Blenkner, M., Jahn, J., and Wasser, E. (1964): *Serving the Aging: An Experiment in Social Work and Public Health Nursing.* Community Service Society, New York.
8. Brocklehurst, J. E. (1973): In: *Textbook of Geriatric Medicine and Gerontology,* edited by J. E. Brocklehurst, pp. 673–691. Churchill Livingstone, Edinburgh.
9. Brody, E. (1977): *Gerontologist,* 17:520–522.
10. Brody, E. M., Kleban, M. M., Lawton, M. P., and Moss, M. (1974): *J. Gerontol.,* 29:79–84.
11. Brody, E. M., Kleban, M. M., Lawton, M. P., and Silverman, H. A. (1971): *Gerontologist,* 11:124–132.
12. Brothwood, J. (1971): In: *Recent Developments in Psychogeriatrics,* edited by D. W. Kay and A. Walk, pp. 99–112. Headley Brothers, Ashford, Kent, England.
13. Brown, B. S. (1962): *Arch. Gen. Psychiatry,* 7:98–107.
14. Carse, J. (1959): *The Worthing Experiment. A Report on the First Two Years of the Worthing and District Mental Health Service, Together With an Account of the First Year of the Chichester and District Mental Health Service.* Graylingwell Hospital Management Committee, England.
15. Carse, J., Panton, N., and Watt, A. (1958): *Lancet,* 1:39–41.
16. Cath, S. H. (1963): *J. Am. Geriatr. Soc.,* 11:679–698.
17. Cohen, G. D. (1978): *Gerontologist,* 18:313–314.

18. Cumming, J., and Cumming, E. (1975): In: *Modern Perspectives in the Psychiatry of Old Age*, edited by J. G. Howells, pp. 486–509. Brunner/Mazel, New York.
19. Daniels, R. S. (1966): *Commun. Ment. Health J.*, 2:47–54.
20. Daniels, R. S., and Kahn, R. L. (1968): *Geriatrics*, 23:121–125.
21. Davis, A. E., Dinitz, S., and Pasamanick, B. (1974): *Schizophrenics in the New Custodial Community: Five Years After the Experiment*. Ohio State University Press, Columbus.
22. Editorial Note (1954): *Br. Med. J.*, 2:1043.
23. Epstein, L. J., and Simon, A. (1968): *Am. J. Psychiatry*, 124:944–961.
24. Farndale, J. (1961): *Day Hospital Movement in Great Britain*. Pergamon Press, Oxford.
25. Finkel, S. (1978): *Personal communication*.
26. Fisch, M., Goldfarb, A. I., Shahinian, S. P., and Turner, H. (1968): *Arch. Gen. Psychiatry*, 18:739–745.
27. Frankfather, D. (1977): *The Aged in the Community: Managing Senility and Deviance*. Praeger, New York.
28. Freeman, H. E., and Sherwood, C. C. (1966): *J. Soc. Issues*, 21:11–28.
29. Glass, A. J. (1961): In: *Current Psychiatric Therapies*, edited by J. H. Masserman, pp. 159–167. Grune & Stratton, New York.
30. Glasscote, R. M., Gudeman, J. E., and Miles, D. G. (1977): *Creative Mental Health Services for the Elderly*. American Psychiatric Association, Washington, D.C.
31. Goldberg, E. M. (1970): *Helping the Aged: A Field Experiment in Social Work*. George Allen and Unwin, London.
32. Goldstein, S. (1971): *J. Am. Geriatr. Soc.*, 19:693–699.
33. Goldstein, S., Sevriuk, J., and Grauer, H. (1968): *Can. Med. Assoc. J.*, 98:955–959.
34. Grad, J., and Sainsbury, P. (1963): *Lancet*, 1:544–547.
35. Grad, J., and Sainsbury, P. (1966): *Milbank Mem. Fund Q.*, 44:246–278.
36. Grad, J., and Sainsbury, P. (1968): *Br. J. Psychiatry*, 114:265–278.
37. Grad de Alarcón, J. (1971): In: *Recent Developments in Psychogeriatrics*, edited by D. W. Kay and A. Walk, pp. 75–86. Headley Brothers, Ashford, Kent, England.
38. Grad de Alarcón, J., Sainsbury, P., and Costain, W. R. (1975): *Psychol. Med.*, 5:32–54.
39. Greenblatt, M., Moore, R. F., and Albert, R. S. (1963): *The Prevention of Hospitalization*. Grune & Stratton, New York.
40. Greene, J. G., and Timbury, G. C. (1979): *Age Ageing*, 8:49–53.
41. Grob, G. N. (1966): *The State and the Mentally Ill*. University of North Carolina Press, Chapel Hill.
42. Group for the Advancement of Psychiatry (1960): *Report No. 47, Preventive Psychiatry in the Armed Forces*. New York.
43. Gruenberg, E. M. (1967): *Am. J. Psychiatry*, 123:481–489.
44. Gruenberg, E. M. (1969): *Lancet*, 1:721–724.
45. Gurian, B. S., and Scherl, D. J. (1972): *J. Geriatr. Psychiatry*, 5:77–86.
46. Herz, M. I., Endicott, J., and Spitzer, R. L. (1971): *Am. J. Psychiatry*, 127:1371–1382.
47. Jones, M. (1953): *The Therapeutic Community*. Basic Books, New York.
48. Kahana, E., and Kahana, B. (1970): *Arch. Gen. Psychiatry*, 23:20–29.
49. Kahn, R. L. (1965): In: *Proceedings of the New York Institute On the Mentally Impaired Aged*. Philadelphia Geriatric Center, Philadelphia.
50. Kahn, R. L. (1971): In: *Clinical Geriatrics*, edited by I. Rossman, pp. 107–113. Lippincott, Philadelphia.
51. Kahn, R. L. (1975): *Gerontologist*, 15:24–31.
52. Kahn, R. L. (1977): In: *Geropsychology: A Model of Training and Clinical Services*, edited by C. D. Gentry, pp. 9–19. Ballinger, Cambridge, Mass.
53. Kahn, R. L., and Goldfarb, A. I. (1962): In: *Program Abstracts, Fifteenth Annual Meeting of the Gerontological Society*, p. 19. Washington, D.C.
54. Kahn, R. L., Goldfarb, A. I., Pollack, M., and Peck, A. (1960): *Am. J. Psychiatry*, 111:326–328.
55. Kahn, R. L., and Zarit, S. H. (1974): In: *Evaluation of Behavioral Programs, Fifth Banff Conference on Behavioral Modification*, edited by P. O. Davidson, F. W. Clark, and L. A. Hammerlynck, pp. 223–251. Research Press, Champaign, Ill.
56. Kamerman, S. B. (1976): *Gerontologist*, 16:529–537.
57. Kelman, H. R. (1962): *Public Health Rep.*, 77:356–366.

58. Klerman, G. L. (1961): In: *Mental Patients in Transition,* edited by M. Greenblatt. Charles C. Thomas, Springfield, Ill.
59. Klerman, G. (1974): *Am. J. Psychiatry,* 131:783–787.
60. Kohen, W., and Paul, G. L. (1976): *Schizophrenia Bull,* 4:579–594.
61. Kostick, A. (1972): *Gerontologist,* 12:134–138.
62. Lear, T. E., Corrigan, G., Bhattacharyya, A., Elliott, J., Gordon, J., and Pitt-Aitkens, T. (1969): *Lancet,* 2:1349–1353.
63. Ling, T. M. (1954): *Lancet,* 1:1127–1128.
64. Lorenze, E. J., Hamill, C. M., and Oliver, R. C. (1974): *J. Am. Geriatr. Soc.,* 22:316–320.
65. Lowenthal, M., Berkman, P., et al. (1967): *Aging and Mental Disorder in San Francisco.* Jossey-Bass, San Francisco.
66. MacMillan, D. (1958): In: *An Approach to the Prevention of Disability from Chronic Psychosis: The Open Mental Hospital Within the Community,* pp. 29–39. Milbank Memorial Fund, New York.
67. MacMillan, D. (1960): *Lancet,* 2:1429–1441.
68. MacMillan, D. (1962): *Canada's Mental Health,* Suppl. 29. Mental Health Division, Department of National Health and Welfare, Ottawa, Ontario.
69. MacMillan, D. (1963): *Lancet,* 1:567–571.
70. MacMillan, D. (1963): In: *Trends in the Mental Health Services,* edited by H. Freeman and J. Farndale, pp. 303–317. Pergamon Press, London.
71. MacMillan, D. (1967): *Br. J. Psychiatry,* 113:175–181.
72. MacMillan, D., and Shaw, P. (1966): *Br. Med. J.,* 2:1032–1037.
73. Main, T. (1946): *Bull. Menninger Clin.,* 10:66–70.
74. Malzberg, B. (1967): *Mental Disease in New York State 1910–1960: A Study of Incidence.* Research Foundation for Mental Hygiene, Albany, N.Y.
75. McComb, S. G., and David, J. D. P. (1961): *Gerontol. Clin.,* 3:146–151.
76. Millar, W. M., and Henderson, J. G. (1956): *Int. J. Soc. Psychiatry,* 2:141–150.
77. Morrissey, J. D. (1966): *Milbank Mem. Fund Q.,* 44:28–36.
78. Morrissey, J. D., and Sainsbury, P. (1959): *Proc. R. Soc. Med.,* 52:1061–1063.
79. Morton, E. V. B., Barker, M. E., and MacMillan, D. (1968): *Gerontol. Clin.,* 10:65–73.
80. National Institute of Mental Health (1976): *Services to the Mentally Disabled of Selected Catchment Areas in Eastern New York State and New York City.* DHEW Publication No. (ADM)76–372. Government Printing Office, Washington, D.C.
81. Newman, J. L. (1962): *Br. Med. J.,* 1:1824–1827.
82. Nielsen, M., Blenkner, M., Bloom, M., Downs, T., and Beggs, H. (1972): *Am. J. Public Health,* 62:1094–1101.
83. Ozarin, L. (1976): *Am. J. Psychiatry,* 133:69–72.
84. Ozarin, L. D., Redick, R. W., and Taube, C. A. (1976): *Hosp. Commun. Psychiatry,* 27:515–519.
85. Pasamanick, B., Scarpitti, F. R., and Dinitz, S. (1967): *Schizophrenics in the Community.* Appleton-Century-Crofts, New York.
86. Perlin, S., and Kahn, R. L. (1967): In: *Psychiatric Research Report 22.* American Psychiatric Association, Washington, D.C.
87. Polak, P., and Jones, M. (1973): *Commun. Ment. Health J.,* 9:123–132.
88. Querido, A. (1962): *Ment. Hyg.,* 46:626–654.
89. Rathbone-McCuan, E. (1976): *Gerontologist,* 16:517–521.
90. Rathbone-McCuan, E., and Elliott, M. W. (1976–77): *Soc. Work Health Care,* 2:153–170.
91. Redick, R. W. (1974): *Statistical Note 107.* Biometry Branch, Rockville, Md.
92. Redlich, F., and Kellert, S. R. (1978): *Am. J. Psychiatry,* 135:22–28.
93. Robertson, W. M. F., and Pitt, B. (1965): *Br. J. Psychiatry,* 111:635–640.
94. Rosenkrantz, B. G., and Vinovskis, M. A. (1978): In: *Aging and the Elderly: Humanistic Perspectives in Gerontology,* edited by S. F. Spicker, K. M. Woodward, and D. D. Van Tassel. Humanities Press, Atlantic Highlands, N.J.
95. Ross, H. E., and Dedward, H. B. (1976): *Soc. Psychiatry,* 11:121–126.
96. Sainsbury, P. (1975): In: *Handbook of Evaluation Research,* edited by M. Guttentag and E. L. Struening, pp. 125–159. Sage, Beverly Hills, Calif.
97. Sainsbury, P., and Grad, J. (1966): *Milbank Mem. Fund Q.,* 44:231–277.
98. Sainsbury, P., and Grad de Alarcón, J. (1970): *J. Geriatr. Psychiatry,* 4:23–41.

99. Sherman, S. R., and Newman, E. S. (1977): *Gerontologist,* 17:513–519.
100. Sherwood, S. (1972): In: *Research Planning and Action for the Elderly: The Power and Potential of Social Sciences,* edited by D. P. Kent, R. Kastenbaum, and S. Sherwood, pp. 70–96. Behavior Publications, New York.
101. Sherwood, S., Greer, D. S., Morris, J. N., and Sherwood, C. C. (1973): *The Highland Heights Experiment: A Final Report.* Government Printing Office, Washington, D.C.
102. Silverstein, D. (1978): *Personal communication.*
103. Stotsky, B. A. (1972): *Am. J. Psychiatry,* 129:117–126.
104. Tischler, G. L., Henisz, J., Myers, J. K., and Garrison, V. (1972): *Arch. Gen. Psychiatry,* 27:389–392.
105. Tobin, S. S., Davidson, S. M., and Sack, A. (1976): *Effective Social Services for Older Americans.* Institute of Gerontology, Ann Arbor, Mich.
106. Tobin, S., and Lieberman, M. (1976): *The Last Home for the Aged.* Jossey-Bass, San Francisco.
107. Tulving, E., and Madigan, S. A. (1970): *Ann. Rev. Psychol.,* 21:437–484.
108. United States Commission on Civil Rights (1977): *The Age Discrimination Study.* Washington, D.C.
109. Wax, J. (1976): *New York Times Magazine,* Nov. 22, p. 38.
110. Weber, R. E. (1977): In: *Evaluative Research on Social Programs for the Elderly,* pp. 50–80. DHEW Publication No. (OHD)77–20120. Government Printing Office, Washington, D.C.
111. Weinberg, J. (1977): In: *Creative Mental Health Services for the Elderly,* edited by R. Glasscote, J. E. Gudeman, and D. Miles, pp. XV–XIX. American Psychiatric Association, Washington, D.C.
112. Weismehl, R., and Silverstein, D. (1975): *J. Jewish Communal Serv.,* 51:260–266.
113. Weissert, W. G. (1976): *Gerontologist,* 16:420–427.
114. Wershow, H. J. (1977): *Gerontologist,* 17:297–302.
115. Zusman, J. (1966): *Milbank Mem. Fund Q.,* 44:363–394.

Clinical Aspects of Alzheimer's Disease and Senile Dementia, (Aging, Vol. 15), edited by Nancy E. Miller and Gene D. Cohen. Raven Press, New York 1981.

Natural Support Systems, Minority Groups, and the Late Life Dementias: Implications for Service Delivery, Research, and Policy

Ramón Valle

School of Social Work, San Diego State University, San Diego, California 92115

A FOCUS ON MINORITY AGED

There is a need to focus attention on the presence and impact of the later life dementias among minority elderly. A premise of this analysis is that caregivers in the 1980s and succeeding years can expect to see more minority elderly than ever before (51,71,81,92,95,100). This may come about not because of a new-found affinity for services but rather from the sheer presence of greater real numbers of such elderly in the social environment. Preliminary data, however sketchy, indicate that life expectancy is increasing for members of these groups, although the general estimate of 67 years for non-Whites still falls behind that of 72 years for Whites (See appendix Table 5). Also internal to their respective minority subgroups, the ratio of elderly to other age cohorts is increasing. For example, among the two largest minorities, Hispanics and Blacks, the percentage of elderly is beginning to approximate that of the elderly in the general White population (See Table 2). Given these trends, there is every likelihood that many more minority aged demented persons will likewise begin to surface.

Unfortunately there is an overall lack of preparation for this circumstance within the aging research and caregiving establishment. Not only is there a dearth of generalizable information about minority elderly as a whole, but a literature specifically on minorities suffering chronic brain disorders is nonexistent. A computer search of available information for this chapter revealed several thousand annotated citations on dementias and related impairments. Minorities, however, received no clear-cut mention. As a consequence, the issues discussed herein must of necessity be pieced together from various sources with resultant gaps in critical information.

Researchers and clinicians need to be aware that this circumstance is a direct outcome of methodological problems over and above inattention to minority group concerns. First, there has been a global pooling of data about minorities. This is evidenced in life expectancy information. For example, although Whites and Blacks are differentiated, Hispanics are aggregated with Whites, and all other minorities of color are indiscriminately counted together (88,93,101; see

TABLE 1. *Selected minority populations: Rank order by size*

Ethnic group[a]	Population	Percent
Black	22,580,289	11.11
Mexican-American[b]	5,023,000	2.47
American Indian	792,730	0.0039
Japanese	591,290	0.0029
Chinese	435,062	0.0021
Filipino	343,060	0.0017
Hawaiian	100,000	0.0004
Korean	66,000	0.0003
Samoan	35,000	0.0002
Total	203,211,926	100.00

[a] Data for other ethnic minority groups to be discussed in the narrative either were not available or incomplete.

[b] Updated estimates place the Mexican-American population at 9 million and other Latinos/Hispanics at 3 million, or 12 million Latinos as a corrected estimate. Data from ref. 8, based on 1970 Census.

also Table 5). This difficulty in the data base is also apparent in statistical analyses that fail to differentiate among poverty and ethnocultural factors. Often, "surname" is used as the critical identifier, such that Hispanics and several Asian American subgroups have been inappropriately counted together [some Asian Americans such as Filipinos and Guamanians have Spanish surnames (68,72)]. In short, the factor of intergroup heterogeneity has been mishandled.

Minorities have also been consistently undercounted. This phenomenon has been attested to by the Bureau of the Census' own admission as well as by

TABLE 2. *Selected minority elderly populations: Rank order by percentage of elderly*

Ethnic group	Percentage of population age 65 plus
Mexican-American[a]	8.44
Japanese	8.02
Black	7.03
Filipino	6.31
Chinese	6.22
American Indian	5.74
Hawaiian	4.00
Korean	3.30
Total population	9.89

[a] An HRC Report, *Theories of Gerontology* (1976), places the percentage of Spanish heritage at 4.1%, which would drop this group below the American Indian group. The author leans to the higher percentage because of the undercounts, which are acknowledged in the HRC Report.

Data from refs. 8 and 68, based on 1970 Census.

ethnic minority demographers and researchers. Estimates of undercounting vary from an admitted 7% undercount of Blacks to 38% of Latinos of Mexican heritage (91,92,94,95,97). What is important here is that such variance can have considerable impact on the recognized scope of problems such as the later life dementias—which may be underestimated in terms of the actual numbers within specific minority cohorts.

Not only have many groups been mislabeled and miscounted, but there are some ethnic minority subgroups on whom no information has been gathered or, if gathered, not reported. For example, urban and non-reservation-dwelling Indians are omitted in some key population counts (96). Likewise, it required a special effort by the Asian American research community to ferret out key information not only of special importance to specific regions of the country but also to the United States Asian community as a whole (69,70,72). A case in point is the Korean population. The 1970 Census enumerated approximately 66,000 persons representing 0.0003% of the nation's population (see Table 1). In the Southern California area, however, where a large proportion of the Korean community resides, this Asian subgroup and the needs of the elderly are very visible. This circumstance holds for many of the other smaller but very active minority populations. In this instance intragroup heterogeneity has been ignored.

The significant implications of these considerations for gerontologists, researchers, and human service providers are (a) the later life dementias cannot be considered nonexistent among minority groups just because we have no data, (b) where a database exists, it must be treated with caution because, until corrected, it may be less reliable than it appears, and (c) professionals interfacing with specific minority groups have to maintain a national rather than just a regional focus. The minorities they are working with are most likely represented elsewhere in the United States and its territories.

Despite these information handicaps, a number of key issues related to minorities and later life dementias can be discussed. First, chronic brain disorders are known to minorities, particularly as they affect the elderly and their families in the community. Second, what is known about minority lower income and lower class status must be sorted out from ethnocultural factors, as each area has a bearing on health-related coping patterns as well as the possible manifestation of the later life dementias. Third, a close examination of ethnocultural factors in terms of natural support system dynamics can serve as a vehicle for developing culturally syntonic interventive strategies for joint use by both the formal support network and the community. In point of fact, this chapter seeks to explore the role of a wide range of natural supports, i.e., family, self-help groups, and other community-based indigenous helpers as possible bridging mechanisms, bringing professional resources to bear on dementia-related needs.

It should be noted that by "minority elderly" we are referring specifically to members of the four populations of color residing in the United States and its territories, i.e., Asian Americans, Blacks, Latino/Hispanics, and Native Americans. Admittedly, in aging circles, the designation of "minority" often lacks specificity. For example, widows, rural aged, and physically handicapped elderly are often given the "minority" label. Sometimes all of the aged are so classified as a subgroup within the larger society. What distinguishes the term as used here, however, is the fact that the Asian Americans, Blacks, Latinos/ Hispanics, and Native Americans form ethnosystems, i.e., groups with organized modes of communication, social relations, values, and beliefs (80). Moreover, because of certain distinguishing characteristics such as skin color and/or physical features, members of these four populations have been singled out in the society and have been the object of discriminatory practices. In brief, they have been placed in what Butler and others term circumstances of multiple jeopardy (19,45,49,50).

PRELIMINARY NOTIONS ON MINORITIES AND THE LATER LIFE DEMENTIAS

Since the database is silent regarding the incidence of the later life dementias among minority groups, this chapter makes several assumptions about potential commonalities between minority and majority group elderly. First, until clarified by further research, chronic brain disorders among minorities are assumed to occur in at least the same proportion as within the general elderly population, i.e., 5 to 6% of the aged (28). Second, once present, organic brain syndromes, whether of the Alzheimers or multi-infarct type, would appear to have the same biophysical manifestations. Third, the increased sensory deprivations that accompany the aging process, and that may serve to exacerbate the behavioral effects of dementia, are likewise considered to be present among minority as among majority group elderly. Furthermore, minority elderly are seen as having the same high susceptibility to iatrogenic disorders resulting from inappropriately administered drugs (e.g., improper dosages, drug-drug interactions, negative side effects that are more pronounced with the very young and the very old, and dietary habits that may interact negatively with pharmacological interventions).

Given these possible commonalities, a number of questions relevant to potential differences between minority and majority culture elderly do emerge. For example, might not researchers need to explore whether the greater exposure of minority populations to high-risk, illness-producing occupations (such as field-hand and factory labor jobs, which tend to expose workers to greater amounts of toxic substances) has any differential manifestation in terms of dementia incidence and/or accompanying sensory deprivations. Might not investigators still need to evaluate the later life dementias in younger cohorts of some of the minority groups, say at ages 50 to 64, given the deleterious life conditions of these groups? At the other end of the age spectrum, might not researchers need to investigate the presence and significance of the actuarially identified "crossover effect" and its association with the late life dementias? (The crossover effect refers to the statistical finding wherein the survival potential for some

TABLE 3. Selected characteristics of minority elderly populations (65 and over)

Characteristics	Total elderly	White	Black	Spanish heritage	Spanish nationalities			Asian nationalities			Native American
					Mexican	Puerto Rican	Cuban	Japanese	Chinese	Filipino	
Number (in thousands)	20,050	18,360	1,586	382	189	34	35	47	27	21	44
Percent of total (all ages)	9.9	10.3	6.9	4.1	4.2	2.4	6.4	8.0	6.2	6.3	5.7
Median age of population	28	29	22	22	19	20	32	32	37	26	20
Age 75 and over as % of all elderly	38.1	38.6	33.4	32.4	32.5	32.7	33.8	41.2	30.0	20.8	35.2
Sex ratio (men per 100 women)	72	72	77	90	95	74	64	77	131	445	92
Percent living in											
Urban areas	73.0	72.6	76.6	86.3	86.3	98.0	98.5	84.8	97.0	77.9	42.7
Rural, non-farm	21.5	21.7	19.5	11.7	12.0	1.8	—	11.7	2.5	18.6	50.2
Rural, farm	5.5	5.7	3.9	3.5	1.7	0.2	—	3.5	0.5	3.5	7.1
Percent poor	27.3	25.3	49.3	32.2	36.7	29.1	24.3	20.0	28.9	25.3	50.8
Percent in labor market											
Men	24.8	24.9	23.5	24.8	24.1	22.6	32.6	29.3	24.8	32.1	17.2
Women	10.0	9.8	13.2	7.9	7.4	8.5	5.5	12.0	12.0	11.4	8.5
Percent completed high school											
Men	26.0	25.8	8.9	15.8	6.4	14.6	38.0	27.3	21.3	17.3	11.0
Women	29.8	30.6	11.5	15.5	7.4	9.2	21.5	25.4	15.5	16.6	14.9

From ref. 85, based on 1970 Census data.

TABLE 4. *Life tables: Expectation of life at single years of age by color and sex*

	White			All other		
Age	Both sexes	Male	Female	Both sexes	Male	Female
65	15.6	13.4	17.6	15.1	13.4	16.8
66	14.9	12.8	16.8	14.6	12.9	16.2
67	14.3	12.2	16.1	14.0	12.4	15.5
68	13.7	11.7	15.3	13.4	11.9	14.9
69	13.0	11.2	14.6	12.9	11.4	14.3
70	12.4	10.6	13.9	12.4	11.0	13.6
71[a]	11.9	10.1	13.2	12.0	10.6	13.6
72	11.3	9.6	12.6	11.7	10.3	12.9
73	10.7	9.2	11.9	11.4	10.0	12.6
74	10.2	8.7	11.3	11.1	9.7	12.3
75	9.7	8.3	10.7	10.8	9.5	12.0
76	9.2	7.9	10.1	10.5	9.2	11.6
77	8.7	7.5	9.6	10.2	9.0	11.2
78	8.3	7.1	9.1	9.9	8.7	10.8
79	7.8	6.8	8.6	9.6	8.5	10.5

[a] Start of "crossover in life expectancy."
Data from ref. 94.

minority cohorts—Blacks and others of color—appears to improve after age 70) (see Table 4). Could it be that the minority elderly of this age cohort survive with less proportionate senile dementias among their number, or are the dementias just played out in slower motion within these groups?

Although minority elderly may share with majority culture elderly similar heightened sensitivities to pharmacological agents, questions can be asked as to whether the chemistry of some medications might not indeed affect some minority elderly populations differently. For example, could research show either greater alleviation, or more serious exacerbation of the minority elderly's condition as compared with the reaction of the same biochemical agents with non-minority/White elderly? Moreover, since a number of the minority populations are still close to the natural medicines within their respective cultures, it would be important to determine if and how these substances facilitate or complicate the overall recuperative capabilities of the elderly subjects utilizing them. Another topic requiring study is whether or not the differential immune susceptibilities of certain minorities create any differences in the progression of chronic brain disorders. It would also be important to examine closely the dietary habits of a number of the minority groups to determine whether there are correlations between diet and presence and type of dementia. For example, might some minority groups be more prone to cerebroarteriosclerotic-related dementias which may be partly related to dietary factors? Might some others be less susceptible for the same reasons?

Obviously all of these preliminary notions about minorities and the dementias are highly speculative. Exactly how *ethnicity* enters the biophysiological picture remains as yet uncertain in either research or clinical terms and falls outside the scope of this chapter and its avowed purpose to discuss progressive chronic brain disorders in the context of the natural supports and ethnosystem dynamics of minority elderly.

Nevertheless, there are a number of outside-the-culture factors that do have immediate bearing on understanding the minority situation. The first relates to the minority elderly socioeconomic picture, given that an underclass status might affect health-related coping behaviors as well as access to formal caregiving systems (19,26,55,84,104). The second set of factors relates to what is known about the differential life expectancy, mortality, and morbidity rates among minorities as these might relate to the manifestation of chronic brain disorders. A careful distinction must be maintained through this phase of the analysis. Culture and poverty cannot be taken to be synonymous (87). For example, poor Blacks, Latinos/Hispanics, and Asian Americans do not share the same linguistic systems. In fact, even single ethnic minority cohorts do not always share identical languages. This becomes clear in working with Asian Americans. Within the Chinese community different dialects, such as Mandarin and Cantonese, can be found operating side by side (25,97). The same holds for the Asian American Pilipino group, wherein various dialects such as Tagalog and Ilucano (to name but two) can be found (72). Approximately 25% of American Indians are seen as more fluent in their native tribal language than in English (1). With regard to nutritional patterns, it is clear that different nationality groups, however poor, express different nutritional patterns. Poor Blacks, poor Latinos of Mexican heritage, and poor Chinese have quite different culinary traditions and expectations. The issues are complex and bear further examination.

SOCIOECONOMIC DIFFERENTIALS

In reviewing socioeconomic information, it is evident that minority elderly consistently occupy the lowest rungs of the economic ladder, placing them in a situation of multiple jeopardy (see Table 3).

The specific socioeconomic issues at hand with significance to minorities and the later life dementias are twofold. First, there are discernible longer inpatient hospitalization stays by lower income minorities. These lower socioeconomic elderly tend to have twice the number of inpatient days per hospitalization than White and upper income patients (26,104). Second, even though the hospitalization data do not contain specificity extending to the dementias, inferences may be drawn. For example, according to Weg, organic brain syndromes and depressive states account for approximately 42.2 and 18.3%, respectively, of state and county inpatient admissions of elderly over age 65 (105). There is a strong possibility, therefore, that minority cohorts, with more poverty in their ranks, will see their elderly—once classified as dements regardless of type— spending significantly more time as inpatients per treatment episode than their

TABLE 5. *Selected measures of health status by race and income*

Measure	White	Nonwhite[d]
Number of bed disability days per person, 1975[a]		
All incomes	6.2	8.8
Less than $5,000	10.9	13.5
$5,000–$10,000	7.2	8.8
Greater than $10,000	4.9	4.8
Number of bed disability days per person over 65, 1975[a]		
All incomes	11.7	24.6
Less than $5,000	13.8	29.6
$5,000–$10,000	10.2	19.5
Greater than $10,000	9.9	—
Average years of life expectancy at birth, 1974[b]		
All incomes	72.7	67.0
Age-adjusted deaths[c] per 1,000 persons, 1974[b]	6.4	9.0

[a] National Center for Health Statistics, unpublished data from the Health Interview Survey, 1975.

[b] National Center for Health Statistics, Advance Report, Final Mortality Statistics, 1974. *Monthly Vital Statistics Report,* 24:11:4–6 (Suppl.)

[c] If death rates for recent years are not age-adjusted, they are slightly higher for whites than for nonwhites. This reflects recent improvements in health status plus sufficient nonwhite deaths in the past to bias their average age downward, resulting in fewer deaths today.

[d] Nonwhite category excludes Latinos/Hispanics who have been grouped with whites in most morbidity/mortality/life expectancy data.

From ref. 93.

higher-income peers. If this pattern holds, minority group elderly will be severed, for longer periods, from their natural social supports, thus complicating clinical treatment and possibly interfering with the patient's recuperative abilities.

It should be noted that the lower occupational status for minority elderly goes hand in hand with their socioeconomic standing. Most minority elderly have had work careers in occupations that do not readily interface with the human service systems, mental health services in particular, where the later life dementias are often identified and treated. Moreover, the employment histories of minority elderly include occupations that often lack comprehensive insurance coverage which could facilitate linkages to formal health services at earlier points in their working lives. The occupational careers of minorities set patterns that tend toward catastrophic, advanced-stage-of-the-illness use of institutional caregiving facilities.

LIFE EXPECTANCY AND MORBIDITY FACTORS

Minority group life expectancy and specific morbidity factors also play a role vis-a-vis the manifestation and possible course of the later life dementias among the aged from these populations. With regard to life expectancy, however incomplete the data, there is an indication of increasing survival for the minorities, and specifically their elderly (8,15,42,66,97). Even American Indians, whose life expectancy still lags behind that of other minorities, appear to have made some gains from a 44-year-life expectancy, cited in reports relative to pre-1970 data, to an approximate 64-year life expectancy estimate in later documents (2,8,96,102). As seen here, this circumstance will have several effects. First, as noted earlier, the 1980s and subsequent years will see a growing number of minority demented persons given a larger pool of minority elderly. Second, this new and larger group of elderly will contain many more persons for whom an episodic relationship with the human services will be the norm. As a consequence, regardless of the need for earlier professional service intervention, these elderly demented persons will be showing up in the more advanced stages of their chronic brain disorders. In the interim, the already burdened minority group natural supports will find themselves even further strained to provide assistance without clear indication as to how to access services.

Gains in life expectancy promise additional potential complications for minority populations. Early in their lives minority group individuals are likely to have suffered from a number of diseases that no longer ravage Anglo-White populations (2,3,65). Solomon indicates that non-Whites are more vulnerable to such conditions as diabetes, hypertension, lung and heart disease (81). Blacks, for example, are three times as likely to die of hypertension (81). American Indians are ten times as likely to do so (3). From the standpoint of the later life dementias, the residual effects of these disorders may well compound the difficulties faced by the minority survivors who contract chronic brain disorders.

It is important to note than despite the higher vulnerability of minorities to many diseases, they continue to underutilize formal caregiving resources (26, 104). In discussing the issue, Solomon notes that such disparity can be traced to several factors. First, physicians are present in limited number in non-White areas and for non-White populations. Second, care is often received from hospital outpatient departments, emergency rooms, and clinics. This care, although perhaps adequate for the presenting condition, tends over the long run to be fragmented and episodic. Finally, even where non-Whites receive private physician care, this care may lack continuity (81). Generally, despite improving survival rates, the health care patterns and antecedent circumstances of minorities will make it particularly difficult for the elderly from these populations to coordinate their inpatient and outpatient care utilizing the formal service structures.

CLINICAL INTERFACE AND MINORITY RESPONSE DIFFERENTIALS: ISSUES AND CONSIDERATIONS

Since data available are so meager, it is difficult to draw firm conclusions regarding the late life dementias. Nevertheless, a schema of the typical course of intervention and support for demented elderly can be drawn. Figure 1 shows this course in a somewhat idealized and abbreviated format. The timeline between stages of progressive brain disorder can be hypothesized as extending over a

Independent living		Institutional living	
Stage I	*Stage II*	*Stage III*	*Stage IV*
Independent in community living with reliance only or primarily on natural networks and endogenous support systems	Independent community living with reliance on some mix of formal outpatient service and reliance on endogenous supports	Institutional semi-independent living with some elements of independent living (e.g., conservator relationship relation in foster home)	Institutionalized living, dependent care
Formal service delivery systems as auxiliary		Natural endogenous systems as auxiliary	

FIG. 1 The dementia continuum.

period as brief as 3 to 5 years or possibly as long as 15 to 20 years, depending on the severity of the disorder and speed of deterioration.

In general, the affected individual can be seen as hypothetically moving through various stages from independent community living (stage I), to institutionalized dependent care (stage IV), and back again. Some patients might experience occasional institutionalized, dependent care, as a result of acute confusional episodes that stem from a variety of circumstances, such as dietary deficiencies, the onset of sudden physical illness, emotional stress, and/or iatrogenic effects of medication. Proper intervention may return these individuals to stage I or II more independent type living formats. Figure 1 takes into account the fact that patients in an advanced stage of chronic brain dysfunction—e.g., of the Alzheimer's type—would be less tractable to independent living arrangements, regardless of the assistance to be obtained from their support systems (17,37,103).

The pattern outlined, however, may not obtain with regard to minority elderly. For the reasons listed earlier, the minority elder experiencing any of the later life dementia may for the most part remain in stage I despite manifesting stage II, III, or even IV disease behaviors. In addition, it is here that cultural propensities enter into the picture over and above already delineated underclass status dynamics. This is reflected in the consistent reports of the often expressed value of "caring for one's own" evidenced among minorities (48). It should be noted that the reasons given by the analysts for this expressed attitude are not always uniform. In some instances, linguistic communicational factors are listed as the rationale (33). In others, long-standing different-from-the-mainstream cultural helpgiving and helptaking values are cited (89,90). In still others, the lack of readiness among providers and their facilities to accommodate culturally diverse users are indicated as key factors in making services less accessible to elderly minorities (63).

From the writer's perspective, those professions interfacing with minority elderly populations, and specifically minority demented persons, are missing a good opportunity to enhance understanding of minority group cultural dynamics. This is evidenced in the directives to professionals emanating from the President's Commission on Mental Health (74). As a consequence, instead of the pattern in Fig. 1, this observer would suggest that for minority elderly dements, the alternate high human and dollar cost format outlined in Fig. 2 prevails.

Within the pattern seen in Fig. 2, the bulk of caregiving costs, both human and economic, for the elderly demented person will revert to the community and the affected individual's natural supports—in most instances the family but also friends, neighbors, and other endogenous helpers. This view is corroborated by a recent Comptroller General's study conducted in Cleveland, Ohio (32). The inquiry, although not focused per se on the chronic brain disorders, concludes that the natural supports, principally the family, do carry the major portion of the caregiving costs for the impaired elder. In this context, the immense effort necessitated to care for elderly dements may place added mental health stresses on minority kin and other natural supports over and above those accruing to other types of impairments. These stresses may come to a head, particularly in the more acute and/or advanced stages of the dementias, where institutionalization for the elder is clearly indicated. Uncertainties stemming from caring-for-one's-own value conflicts together with the lack of working knowledge about formal services will inevitably surface. Then, when the minority elder is finally encountered by the formal service system, providers will most likely be faced with less tractable states of dementia together with higher and longer term inpatient maintenance costs. By this time, also, the opportunity for some of the anticipatory/preventive type interventions, as suggested in Fig. 1, will have been lost (40,75). This includes the chance to use the patient's natural supports to postpone the precipitous deployment of stage IV institution-dependent care strategies (34).

Given these possibilities, it is not just an exhortation but rather a necessity that agencies and their staffs develop a natural network capability that will include not only a preliminary understanding of minority group endogenous support systems but also the relatively pragmatic ways to tie to these natural supports.

MINORITY ELDERLY NATURAL SUPPORTS

Admittedly, the literature on minority group elderly natural network stratagems and behaviors is largely impressionistic and often lacks empirical validation. Moreover, even in situations where the information is empirically based, the studies are quite localized in nature and therefore are not readily applicable to the total group studied and/or the minorities as a whole. Despite this, there is sufficient information from which to make inferences regarding those natural network cultural variables which may be playing a key role among minorities

	Stage I. Independent living	Stage II. Independent living outpatient intervention	Stage III. Semi-institutionalized living	Stage IV. Institutionalized living
Costs to minority elderly	• Low costs to *individual* re: self esteem (e.g., "*orgullo*" (sense of pride) "*giri*" Latino/Hispanic *(Japanese, not to burden others).* • All or most cost accrues to support systems natural networks (significant others).	• Cost to the minority elder individual's self-esteem may begin to appear. • Natural supports may not be included in the outpatient intervention. Natural network exclusion costs may begin to appear.	• These personal costs may increase. • These costs to natural systems may also increase.	• High costs to individual re: self-esteem, own posture, attitudes "orgullo," "giri" cost may be extremely high. • Cost to support systems may also be high in that networks are not invited to participate.
Systemic human service costs	• Apparent low cost formal service noninvolvement *but a* hidden problem may be present in that a hidden balloon-type cost may emerge at point of crisis.	• Apparent lower dollar cost in that minority elderly are not as evident in large numbers in out-patient intervention systems. • Preventive interventions may not be made available/accessible to the minority elderly. • Overall interventive inefficiencies will begin to appear in that support system resources may not be mobilized into the treatment plan.	• Continued apparent lower dollar cost re: minority elderly. • Semi-independent living services may appear as not available or accessible to minority elders. • Interventive inefficiencies increase. The dementia may be considerably exacerbated.	• Possibly high and sudden long-term maintenance costs. • Possibly higher interventive costs with less return in that the disease entity has reached a less tractable/reversible state because earlier preventive interventions were not available or accessible.
Overall	• Culturally holistic intervention is present in terms of natural network, endogenous support systems interventions. • Formal service systems are not in interventive picture.	• Physical/psychological stresses become more pronounced. Acute episodes occur, exacerbating underlying progressive chronic state. • Need begins to outstrip the support system capabilities. Some cultural supports are present but culturally holistic interventions from formal systems are missing.		• Culturally holistic formal system interventions are not present. Patients' recuperative-regenerative capabilities are diminished. • Natural networks, endogenous supports are not in interventive picture.

FIG. 2. Present intervention paradigm dollar and human costs: Minority elderly perspectives.

(6,11,14,22,27,40,59,61,62,77,82,83,98,101,102). In addition, available information can provide clues for bringing caregivers and their personnel together with natural helpers for the best interests of the minority aged demented person (10,12,16,18,20,23,30,31,54,73,75,77–79).

Within the literature, the general notion of natural supports can be refined into three distinct operational formats or levels to include: (a) aggregate (group) networks, (b) linkperson networks, and (c) kinship networks (60,102). Often without realizing it, clinicians and researchers may already be encountering the aggregate (group) type of natural network in the form of their ongoing interactions with various kinds of self-help groups such as ethnic benevolent associations, church-related social clubs, as well as in terms of their relationships with neighborhood or community service groups. For example, among Hispanics one can find many kinds of formal and informal cultural mutual aid organizations to include mutualistic lending societies that have long standing presence in the community and that help the elderly (102).

In the Black community one can also readily locate any number of both formally and informally chartered groups, many of which are church related and were formed years earlier for mutual assistance and that continue the same functions as their members proceed through the life cycle into their senior years. American Indian tribal councils can be seen concerning themselves with the needs of their seniors (2,3). Asian Americans have many similar aggregate or group type of natural networks (70,71). For example, both the Japanese and the Korean church ministry can be found actively meeting the human welfare needs of the populations they serve, including their seniors. Within the Pilipino community one can usually locate a wide variety of social organizations, a number of which focus primarily on the needs and concerns of their senior members (72). There are also Guamanian, Samoan, and Chinese self-help formal and informal associations wherever these populations reside (25, 46,47). These can be located whenever clinicians and researchers proceed to closely examine the infrastructure of the community of their minority patients, clients, and/or study respondents.

Linkperson natural networks are perhaps more difficult to see immediately. This is because they are composed of individuals with ties of friendship based on reciprocity and exchange behaviors rather than group membership (40,58). The bonds between the linked individuals tend to be kinlike, but lack the inherent formalities of familial relationships (61,62). In some instances, linkperson networks may be territorially fixed, for example, the informal helping systems located in inner city settings among the single room occupant elderly (37,38). In others, these natural networks may exceed the geographic boundaries of specific communities such as the Hispanic *consejeras* (community counselors) identified by Kent in Colorado and the *servidores* (natural helpers) identified in San Diego along with the Chinese *Yau Sum* (Cantonese for a "person of good heart" service broker). The Japanese also have the *Shinsetsu sva hito* ("kind person" service broker) (25,48,52,53,98).

The third form of natural supports are those networks composed of kin, extending through several degrees of such relationship. It should be noted that kinship networks can include individuals officially and/or unofficially adopted into the nuclear or extended family. Familial supports are the most common type of natural helping network ascribed to many minority populations, and their potential helping functions are variously described in the literature (44, 45,56,77,78). It is also important to note that researchers and clinicians caution against stereotyping the helping role of familial networks, particularly in the complex area of the later life dementias, which generate so many volatile feelings among family members.

Agencies and professionals interfacing with minority populations, especially with minority demented persons, need to recognize that in the three types of natural networks they have potentially very helpful supportive caregiving resources at hand. These endogenous systems constitute those key "significant others" already in contact with minority elderly (78).

These networks can provide an excellent point of entry to the study of the dementias in their natural crosscultural context. From a clinical perspective, natural network behaviors can be directly linked to current aging theory, which suggests that a continuity of earlier incorporated values persists over time (5, 9,57). These elderly generally seek to continue their preadmission life-styles (13). This dynamic is seen as even more powerfully at work among minorities.

Collectively, the three types of natural networks outlined provide clinicians with the following adjunct capabilities: (a) ongoing, already in place and culturally syntonic supportive assistance (38,99,101), (b) bilingual/bicultural communication linkages to the affected minority elderly populations (86), and (c) a variety of auxiliary service-delivery capabilities such as information and referral, community outreach homecare assistance, and natural counseling and advocacy support (6,38,75,77). From a still broader perspective, these endogenous systems embody a number of properties vital to future planning and decision making around service delivery for minority elderly demented persons that can be summarized as follows (101):

• Natural endogenous systems are operating parallel to and supportive of, existing human service systems. The natural helpers see their assistance as making program resources accessible to their linked members (61,62).

• These systems are in varying degrees of contact with many mental health and related human service programs at the line staff level. This contact is being actively maintained even if it is one-way only and even if it might be unknown to, or go unrecognized by, the higher administrative levels of agencies and service programs. A limitation, though, is that this contact may not be at the level to encompass a complete knowledge of the full potential of the human services on the part of the natural networks (86).

• These networks assist the elderly to maintain their residence in the community as long as feasible. This is particularly important to minority elderly, as

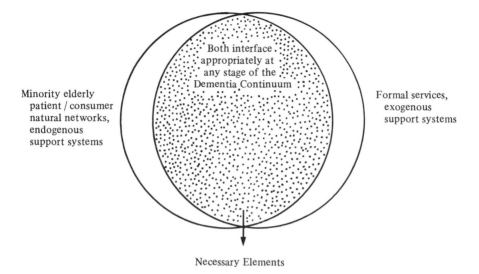

Minority elderly
patient / consumer
natural networks,
endogenous
support systems

Both interface
appropriately at
any stage of the
Dementia Continuum

Formal services,
exogenous
support systems

Necessary Elements

• *The Natural Networks/Endogenous Support Systems* are informed about the availability and accessibility of services

• The Networks are accepted as partners in the intervention

• The Networks are used to their maximum within each of the four stages of the dementia continuum including data collection and reporting activities

• *The Formal Services* maintain cross-cultural interventive and communicative capabilities either internally and/or through use of community brokers and resources

• The patient's cultural help-accepting values and outlooks are allowed to remain as intact as possible

• Reciprocity in use of Natural Networks and the interface relationships between the formal services and the natural networks is maintained over time

FIG. 3. A culturally holistic clinical interface approach.

well as to elderly in general, who prize their independence and who wish to stay in their home communities as long as possible (34,101).

• The three general types of networks are often tailored to, though not exclusively confined to, the needs of specific geographic locales and their minority populations (37,38).

Figure 3 summarizes those processes that facilitate the development of a natural network/formal caregiving joint system of interaction. The development of working ties between formal services and natural supports would not only assist the human services to incorporate cultural values into their interventive approaches, but it would also permit agencies to overcome the previously discussed "episodic type" relationship with minority elderly populations (23,24).

BARRIERS

This is by no means intended to indicate that a service panacea is at hand (4,35,39). Some elderly may in fact be isolated from their natural supports. In a New York study, 8% of the elderly sample did not have informal supports available to them (78). This finding may be duplicated elsewhere.

Recognition must also be given to the fact that a number of unanswered questions remain regarding any immediate attempt to implement a natural network technology for use with dementia-affected minority aged. The inherent gaps and limitations in the knowledge base regarding minorities and their natural supports cannot be overlooked (74). This barrier, although not insurmountable, requires careful research attention so that reliable information can be made available and rendered usable about natural supports by either the minorities themselves or program planners and providers despite the interest on both sides to be of immediate service to elderly minority demented persons.

An associated difficulty is the lack of clarity regarding cost-effectiveness of natural supports, particularly when utilized to bypass inpatient confinement (31). What is unclear in this equation is the displacement of such costs to other sectors of the caregiving system, for example, to outpatient community-based caregivers as well as to the patients themselves and/or to the patient's significant others. One area where natural networks may lower costs, for example, is in terms of "misinstitutionalization" in those cases where the minority older person may be inappropriately wrenched from natural supports and placed in circumstances where specific cultural helpgiving approaches are unavailable. The Cleveland Study and others provide hints in this direction (31,32,67). Unfortunately, though, the data are incomplete as to the actual savings involved.

There are barriers also at the direct clinical level (63). All too often, the intake process and/or diagnostic assessment does not pick up information necessary to map adequately the resource potential of the patients' significant others. In many instances, such persons may be summarily identified only as part of the client's problem, or simply left out of the assessment entirely. An unintended contributor to this negative manner of viewing natural networks may well be the multiplicity of professions who regularly interact with elderly demented persons (34). Each may not only have different areas of responsibility for the patient, but different understandings of the utility of others working with the patient's significant others. The positives of natural networks can easily get lost in this interplay. Caregivers are also hampered with regard to the professional development of their personnel. They cannot readily turn to gerontological training programs for assistance in learning to work with natural supports. Clinicians may therefore have difficulty getting their bearings on how to sustain relationships with minority endogenous systems. As a consequence, natural networks may come to be viewed as competitive rather than complementary.

There are also barriers at the policy level. Despite the strong endorsement of natural supports of the President's Commission on Mental Health, the report itself recognizes that the idea of incorporating social supports into the human services has not yet taken widespread hold at either service planning or service delivery levels (74). The community health and mental health movements, along with the current increase in home care approaches, and the standing use of community aides within programs for the elderly to some extent may be reversing prevailing attitudes. For the most part, these approaches lack clear-cut inclusion in long-range human service planning. Moreover, there is generally a lack of coverage within national and/or local agency reimbursement criteria for the wide variety of potential natural network services (7,36,41).

CONVERGING ISSUES AND CONCERNS

As discussed above there will be a probable rise in the visibility of later life dementias among Asian American, Black, Latino/Hispanic, and Native American populations during the coming decade. At the same time, both the formal caregivers and minorities lack the (protocols) for mutual interaction (64). It can be anticipated that human services agencies will be hard pressed to develop cross-cultural interventive strategies. For their part, minorities will be taxed to the limits of their self-help strengths. This situation can be remedied.

The Database

First, a concerted effort could be undertaken to create a viable database on the later life dementias and minority elderly for use in human service program development. This information would reflect the cultural heterogeneity of the four generic minorities of color, i.e., Asian Americans, Blacks, Latino/Hispanics, and Native Americans. Efforts to create the database should recognize that current informational problems are a consequence of a variety of factors, external to actual presence of minority demented persons in the social environment. These include (a) the previously cited methodological problems, along with generally poor quality of information gathering and record-keeping procedures within existing caregiving systems vis-a-vis minority elderly populations; (b) the lower level of interaction between caregivers and minorities; (c) the, until now, lesser real number of minority group persons in the age cohort under consideration (individuals age 65 plus) because of the lower life expectancy of these groups; and (d) the possible confusion arising as a result of the mixture of socioeconomic/multiple jeopardy variables with sociocultural dynamics. In addition, because of past experiences with various forms of discrimination, minority elderly and their social supports may be more oriented to keeping dementia-related information to themselves until the point of extreme need. The development of a statistically sound and ethnically relevant database will materially aid in the allocation of caregiving resources in a cultural context.

Clinical Interface Research

In a similar manner, an effort could be launched to generate a knowledge base for use by clinicians interfacing with minority populations and their significant others. This knowledge base would reflect not only the functioning of natural supports among minority elderly; it would also include identification of the actual strengths as well as the limitations of these endogenous systems, including their potential to serve as culturally attuned surrogate natural supports for isolated minority elderly. Through this research, the different help-giving and help-accepting expectations between minority elderly and professionals could be documented (29).

LOOKING AT THE COMING DECADE AND BEYOND

In the short run, and despite pending budget squeezes, national and local agencies serving demented populations could take steps that could change the quality of the database on minority elderly—almost overnight. Caregivers could look toward retrieving whatever unpublished and uncirculated information is present on minorities in their own files and databanks. Agencies could also undertake to build their own minority elderly databanks through relatively simple additions to existing intake assessment, patient diagnostic and biostatistical reporting forms (21). Moreover, despite the clearly recognized need for more research, caregivers could begin to reach out and establish working relationships with minority group natural networks within their local service environments. Finally, those federal agencies with major responsibility for services to the elderly could collectively develop training strategies for upgrading the professional community in natural network technology. However scattered, there are sufficient clues in the literature to guide badly needed, coordinated, training ventures.

All of this is not to underrate basic biophysiological, pharmacological, and sociopsychological research on the later life dementias among minority elderly populations. The above recommendations are likewise not intended to ignore the fact that the socioeconomic status of minorities will continue to interact negatively on their elderly over and above the normal aging process. Such concerns will remain outstanding for some time to come, no matter what other shorter run research, policy planning, and service delivery steps are undertaken. In this context, it may well be that future research will demonstrate no real biophysiological-biomedical differentials between minority and majority group aged with progressive chronic brain disorders—especially if the conditions leading to the socioeconomic/underclass status are controlled (8). However, the clinical arena, where coping customs and cultural values intersect, may prove to be the critical dimension in making services not only available but also accessible to minority demented persons and their endogenous helping networks.

ACKNOWLEDGMENT

The tables are provided through the courtesy of Human Resources Corporation, San Francisco, California, as contained in: *Issues Concerning the Minority Elderly: Report (1978)*. Submitted to Federal Council on Aging/Contract HEW 105–77–3004, 1978.

REFERENCES

1. American Indian Policy Commission (1976): Task Force on Alcohol and Drug Abuse, *Report on Alcohol and Drug Abuse: Final Report.* Government Printing Office, Washington, D.C.
2. American Indian Policy Review Commission (1976): Task Force on Indian Health, *Report on Indian Health: Final Report,* Government Printing Office, Washington, D.C.
3. American Indian Policy Review Commission (1977): *Final Report Vol. I.* Government Printing Office, Washington, D.C.
4. Arnoff, F. N. (1975): Social consequences of policy toward mental illness. *Science,* 188:1277–1281.
5. Back, K. W. (1976): Personal characteristics and social behavior: Theory and method. In: Binstock, R. H. and Shanas, E. (eds.). *Handbook of Aging and the Social Sciences.* Van Nostrand, Reinhold, New York.
6. Barg, S., and Hirsh, C. (1974): Neighborhood service support networks: Alternatives for the maintenance of active community residents by low income minority group aged of the inner city. *Paper presented at 27th Annual Gerontological Society Meeting, Portland, Oregon, October.*
7. Beattie, W. (1973): Designing systems of care planning: Issues and perspectives. In: Pfeiffer, E., (ed.) *Alternatives to Institutional Care for Older Americans: Practice and Planning A Conference Report.* Center for the Study of Aging and Human Development, Duke University, Durham, North Carolina.
8. Bell, D., Kasschau, P., and Zellman, G. (1976): Delivering services to elderly members of minority groups: A critical review of the literature. Rand Corporation, Santa Monica, Calif.
9. Bengston, V. F., and Cutler, N. E. (1976): Generations and intergenerational relations: Perspectives on age groups and social change. In: Binstock, R. and Shanas, E. *Handbook of Aging and Social Sciences.* Van Nostrand, Reinhold, New York.
10. Bild, B., and Havighurst, R. (1976): Senior citizens in great cities: The case of Chicago. *Gerontologist,* 16 (Part 2):4–88.
11. Blau, Z. S. (1978): Aging and social class and ethnicity. In: *The Leon and Josephine Winkelman Lecture Series.* School of Social Work, University of Michigan, Ann Arbor.
12. Bowles, E. (1976): Older persons as providers of services: Three federal programs. *Social Policy,* 7:81–88.
13. Brody, E. (1981): The formal support network: Congregate treatment setting for residents with senescent brain dysfunction. In: *Clinical Aspects of Alzheimer's Disease,* Miller, N. and Cohen, G. T. (eds.). Raven Press, New York.
14. Brotman, H. B. (1975): The black aged as good neighbors: An experiment in volunteer service. *Gerontologist,* 15:554–559.
15. Brotman, H. B. (1977): Life expectancy: A comparison of national levels in 1900 and 1974 and variations in state levels. *Gerontologist,* 17:11–22.
16. Buchanan, B., and Choca, P. R. (1979): Mutuality of expectations and cultural etiquette: Some considerations and a proposal. In: Martin, P. (ed.) *La Frontera Perspectiva: Providing Mental Health Services to Mexican Americans,* pp. 35–41. La Frontera Center, Tucson, Ariz.
17. Burnside, I. M. (1979): Alzheimer's disease: An overview, *J. Gerontol. Nurs.,* 5:14–20.
18. Burrul-Fornam, G. (1979): The definitional process among Mexican Americans and its effects on the utilization of mental health services. In: Martin, P. (ed.) *La Frontera Perspectiva:*

Providing Mental Health Services to Mexican Americans, pp. 3–10. La Frontera Center, Tucson, Ariz.

19. Butler, R. (1975): *Why Survive: Being Old in America.* Harper & Row, New York.
20. Cantor, M., and Mayer, M. (1975): Health and the inner city elderly. *Gerontologist,* 16:17–24.
21. Cantor, M., and Mayer, M. (1975): Factors in differential utilization of services by urban elderly. *J. Gerontol. Soc. Work,* 1:47–63.
22. Carp, F., and Kataoka, E. (1976): Health care problems of the elderly in San Francisco's Chinatown. *Gerontologist,* 16:30–38.
23. Chavez, N. (1975): Mexican Americans' expectations of treatment, role of self and therapist: Effect on utilization of mental health services. Ph.D. dissertation, University of Denver.
24. Chavez, N. (1975): Mexican Americans' expectations of treatment, role of self and therapist: Effects on utilization of mental health services. In: Martin, P., *La Frontera Perspectiva: Providing Mental Health Services to Mexican Americans,* pp. 11–33. La Frontera Center, Tucson, Ariz.
25. Chen, N. (1978): *The Elder Chinese,* Campanile Press, San Diego, Calif.
26. Christmas, J. J. (1977): How our health system fails minorities. *Civil Rights Dig.,* 10:3–11.
27. Clark, M., and Kiefer, C. W. (1969): Social change and intergenerational relations in Japanese American and Mexican American females (mimeo). *Paper presented at the Annual Meeting of the American Sociological Convention,* September.
28. Cohen, G. (1979): *Senile Dementia Alzheimer's Disease Fact Sheet.* Center for Studies of the Mental Health of the Aging, National Institute of Mental Health, Rockville, Md.
29. Cohen, C. I., and Sokolovsky, J. (1979): The clinical use of network analysis for the psychiatric and aged populations, *Commun. Ment. Health J.,* 15:203–213.
30. Collins, A. M., and Panacost, D. L. (1976): *Natural Helping Networks: A Strategy for Prevention.* National Association of Social Workers, New York.
31. Comptroller General (1977): *Home Health—The Need for a National Policy to Better Provide for the Elderly.* Government Accounting Office, Washington, D.C.
32. Comptroller General (1977): *The Well Being of Older People in Cleveland, Ohio.* Government Accounting Office, Washington, D.C.
33. Cuellar, I. (1980): Service delivery and mental health services for Chicano elders. In: Miranda, M. and Ruiz, R. (eds.) *Chicano Aging and Mental Health.* National Institute of Mental Health, Washington, D.C.
34. Doherty, N., Segal, J., and Hicks, B. (1978): Alternatives to institutionalization for the aged. In: *Aged Care and Service Review,* 1:1–16.
35. Doll, W. (1976): Family coping with the mentally ill: An unanticipated problem of deinstitutionalization. *Hosp. Commun. Psychiatr.,* 27:183–185.
36. Eisele, F., and Hoke, R. R. (1979): Health care policy and the elderly. Toward a system of long-term care. *J. Health, Polit. Policy Law,* 3:452–455.
37. Erikson, R., and Eckert, K. (1977): The elderly poor in downtown San Diego hotels. *Gerontologist,* 17:440–446.
38. Evans, R., and Northword, L. (1979): The utility of locally based social networks. *J. Minority Aging,* 3:199–211.
39. Faulkner, A., Heisel, M., and Simms, P. (1975): Life strengths and life stresses: Explorations in the measurement of the mental health of the Black aged. *Am. J. Orthopsychiatry,* 45:102–11.
40. Faulkner, A. (1975): The Black aged as good neighbors: An experiment in volunteer services. *Gerontologist,* 15:554–559.
41. Hammerman, J. (1974): Health Services: Their success and failure/reaching older adults. *Am. J. Public Health,* 64:253–256.
42. Hamlow, J. J. (1979): Minority aging populations: Mortality and morbidity issues. In: *Minority Aging Research: Old Issues, New Approaches,* E. P. Stanford (ed.). Campanile Press, San Diego, Calif.
43. Hernandez, J., Estrada, I., and Alvarez, D. (1971): Census data and the problem of conceptually defining the Mexican American population. *Soc. Sci. Q.,* 53:671–687.
44. Hill, C. A., and Spector, M. (1971): Natality and mortality of the American Indian compared with U.S. Whites and Nonwhites. *HSMHA Health Report,* 86:229–246.
45. Hill, R. B. (1972): A profile of Black Aged. In: *Minority Aged in America,* pp. 35–50. Institute of Gerontology, University of Michigan, Ann Arbor.

46. Ishikawa, W. (1978): *The Elder Guamanian.* Campanile Press, San Diego, Calif.
47. Ishikawa, W. (1978): *The Elder Samoan.* Campanile Press, San Diego, Calif.
48. Ishizuka, K. (1978): *The Elder Japanese.* Campanile Press, San Diego, Calif.
49. Jackson, J. J. (1967): Social gerontology and the Negroes: A review. *Gerontologist,* 7:168–178.
50. Jackson, J. J. (1970): Aged Negroes: Their cultural departures from statistical stereotypes and rural-urban differences. *Gerontologist,* 10:140–145.
51. Kelley, C. B. (1979): *U.S. Immigration: A policy analysis.* The Population Council, New York.
52. Kent, D. P. (1971): *Needs and Use of Services Among Negro and White Aged: Social and Economic Conditions of Negro and White Aged Residents of Urban Neighborhoods of Low Socioeconomic Status.* Pennsylvania Department of Public Welfare, Harrisburg.
53. Kent, J. A. (1971): Descriptive approach to a community. Western Interstate Commission on Higher Education (WICHE), Boulder, Col. *(A videotape lecture).*
54. Killilea, M. (1976): Mutual help organizations: Interpretation in the literature. In: Caplan G., and Killilea, M. (eds.) *Support Systems and Mutual Help Multidisciplinary Explorations.* Grune & Stratton, New York.
55. Lambing, M. (1972): Social class living patterns of retired Negroes. *Gerontologist,* 12:285–288.
56. Lebowitz, B. D. (1979): Old age and family functioning. *J. Gerontol. Social Work,* 1:111–118.
57. Levine, E. S., and Padilla, A. M. (1980): *Crossing Cultures in Therapy: Pluralistic Counseling for the Hispancis.* Brooks Cole Publishing Company, Monterey, Calif.
58. Lomnitz, T. A. (1976): *Networks and Marginality.* Academic Press, New York.
59. Lurie, E., Kalish, R. A., Wexler, R., and Ansak, M. L. (1976): On Lok Senior Day Health Center: A case study, *Gerontologist,* 16 (Part I):39–46.
60. Martinez, C. (1980): Informal support systems: A valuable resource for providing care to the non-instutionalized elderly. School of Urban and Regional Planning, University of Southern California, Los Angeles, Calif. *(Unpublished paper.)*
61. Mendoza, L. (1980): *The Servidor System: Policy Implications for the Elder Hispano.* Campanile Press, San Diego, Calif.
62. Mendoza, L. (1980): Los servidores natural helpers among Hispano Mexicano elderly. United States International University, San Diego. *(Unpublished dissertation.)*
63. Montiel, M. (1978): Chicanos in the United States: An overview of socio-historical context and emerging perspectives. In: Montiel, M. (ed.) *Hispanic Families.* National Coalition of Hispanic Mental Health and Human Service Organizations, Washington, D.C.
64. Moore, S. S. (1971): Situational factors affecting minority aging, *Gerontologist,* 11 (Part 2):88–93.
65. Mortality Differentials Among Nonwhite Groups (1974): *Metropolitan Life Insurance Company Statistical Bulletin,* July.
66. Olmo, W. (1979): The elderly in Puerto Rico. *Unpublished master's essay research project,* School of Social Work, San Diego State University.
67. Owan, T. C. (1978): Improving the productivity in the public sector through bilingual-bicultural staff. *Soc. Work Res. Abstr.,* 14:11–17.
68. Pacific Asian Elderly Research Project (1977): *Census and Baseline Data: A Detailed Report.* OHD-AOA, grant 90-A-980/02. Los Angeles, Calif.
69. Pacific Asian Elderly Research Project (PAERP) (1978): *Understanding the Pacific Asian Elderly: Working paper on Unmet Research Needs in the Pacific/Asian Elderly Community.* Los Angeles, Calif.
70. Pacific Asian Elderly Research Project (1978): *Critical Factors in Service Delivery,* Los Angeles, Calif. OHD-AOA grant 90-A-980/02.
71. Pacific Asian Elderly Research Project (1978): *Final Report,* Los Angeles, California, OHD-AOA-90-A-980/02.
72. Peterson, R. (1978): *The Elder Filipino.* Campanile Press, San Diego, Calif.
73. Phillipus, M. J. (1971): Successful and unsuccessful approaches to mental health services for an urban Hispano population. *Am. J. Publ. Health,* 61:820–830.
74. President's Commission on Mental Health (1978): Report to the President, Vol. I, *Executive Summary,* Vols. II and III, Government Printing Office, Washington, D.C.

75. Salber, E. (1979): The lay advisor as a community health resource. *J. Health Polit. Policy Law,* 3:409–478.
76. Seward, J., and Marnor, J. (1956): *Psychotherapy and Culture Conflict.* Ronald Press, New York.
77. Shanas, E. (1973): Family-kin networks and aging in cross cultural perspective. *J. Marriage Fam.,* 35:505–511.
78. Shanas, E. (1979): The family as a social support system in old age. *Gerontologist,* 19:169–174.
79. Smith, S. A. (1975): *Natural Systems and the Elderly: An Unrecognized Resource.* School of Social Work, Portland State University, Portland, Ore.
80. Solomon, B. (1974): Growing old in the ethno-system. In: Stanford, E. P. (ed.). *Minority Aging.* Center on Aging, San Diego State University, San Diego, Calif.
81. Solomon, B. (1978): Minority group issues and benefit programs for the elderly in policy issues concerning minority elderly. Final report, Human Resources Corporation (Groundwork paper 2, pp. 69). San Franciso, Calif.
82. Stack, C. B. (1974): *All Our Kin: Strategies for Survival in a Black Community.* Harper & Row, New York.
83. Steglich, W. C., Cartwright, W., and Crouch, B. (1978): *Study of Needs and Resources Among Aged Mexican Americans.* Texas Technological College, Lubbock, Texas.
84. Stretch, J. J. (1976): Are aged Blacks who manifest differences in community security also different in coping reaction. *Aging Hum. Dev.,* 7:2.
85. Stutsman, L. (1976): *Theories of Gerontology.* U.S. Human Resources Corporation, San Francisco, Calif.
86. Sussman, M. (1977): Family, bureacracy and the elderly individual: An organizational/linkage perspective. In: Shanas, E. and Sussman, M. (eds.) *Family Bureaucracy and the Elderly,* Duke University, Durham, North Carolina.
87. Swanson, W. C., and Harter, C. (1971): How Do Elderly Blacks Cope in New Orleans, *Aging and Human Development,* 2.
88. Terris, M. (1973): Desegrating health statistics. *Am. J. Publ. Health,* 63:477–480.
89. Torres-Gil, G. (1978): Age health and culture: An examination of health among Spanish-speaking elderly. In: Montiel, M. (ed.) *Hispanic Families,* pp. 83–113. National Coalition of Hispanic Mental Health and Human Services Organizations, (COSSMHO), Washington, D.C.
90. Torrey, E. F. (1972): The irrelevance of traditional mental health services for urban Mexican Americans. In: Levitt, M., and Rubenstein, B. (eds.) *On The Urban Scene.* Wayne State University Press, Detroit, Mich.
91. U.S. Bureau of the Census (1973): Current Population Reports Series P-23, No. 43. Government Printing Office, Washington, D.C.
92. U.S. Bureau of the Census (1974): *Current Population Reports, Population Characteristics: Persons of Spanish Origin in the United States,* March 1972 (Advance Report), Series P-20, No. 259. U.S. Government Printing Office, Washington, D.C.
93. U.S. Congress, Congressional Budget Office (1977): *Health Differentials Between White and Non-White Americans.* U.S. Government Printing Office, Washington, D.C.
94. U.S. Department of Health, Education, and Welfare (OS) 75-120 (1974): *Study of Selected Socio-Economic Characteristics of Ethnic Minorities Based on the 1970 Census: Vol. I, Americans of Spanish Origin.* Prepared by Urban Associates Incorporated for the Office of Special Concerns, Assistant Secretary for Planning and Evaluation.
95. U.S. Department of Health, Education and Welfare, Public Health Services Health Resource Administration (1974): *Life Tables: Vital Statistics of the United States, Vol. II.*
96. U.S. Department of Health, Education and Welfare (1977): American Indian population 55 years of age and older: Geographic distribution, 1970, *Statistical Reports on Older Americans,* U.S. Government Printing Office, Washington, D.C.
97. Valle, R. (1974): *Amistad-Compadrazzo* as an indigenous network compared with the Urban Mental Health Network. University of Southern California, Los Angeles *(unpublished dissertation.)*
98. Valle, R., and Mendoza, L. (1978): *The Elder Latino.* Campanile Press, San Diego.
99. Valle, R. (1978): The knowledge base for planning services to minority elderly. In: *Policy Issues Concerning Minority Elderly: Final Report.* Human Resources Corporation (Groundwork Paper 1, 106 pp.). San Francisco, California.

100. Valle, R. (1978): An innovation for tomorrow's elderly: Incorporating helping networks in the human services. In: *Future Aging/Impact of Jarvis-Gann, Part I,* Hearing before the Subcommittee on Human Services of the Select Committee on Aging, House of Representatives, Ninety-Fourth Congress, July 5, 1978, San Diego, California, Comm. Public. 95-108.
101. Valle, R., and Martinez, C. (1980): Natural networks of Latino aged of Mexican heritage: Implications for mental health. In: Miranda, N., and Ruiz, R. (eds.) *Chicano Aging and Mental Health,* National Institute of Mental Health, Washington, D.C. *(unpublished manuscript).*
102. Velez, C. (1980): *Una Union de Confianza* (A Union of Mutual Trust). The Cultural Meaning of Urban Mexican/Chicano Rotating Credit Associations, University of California at Los Angeles, Los Angeles, California *(unpublished manuscript).*
103. Verwoerdt, A. (1976): *Clinical Geropsychiatry,* Waverly Press, Baltimore.
104. Weaver, J. (1976): *National Health Policy and the Underserved: Ethnic Minorities, Women and the Elderly.* C. V. Mosby Company, St. Louis.
105. Weg, R. B. (1978): *The Aged: Who, Where, How Well,* Andrus Gerontological Center, Los Angeles, California.
106. Wu, F. (1975): Mandarin speaking aged Chinese in the Los Angeles area. *Gerontologist,* 15:271-275.

Clinical Aspects of Alzheimer's Disease and Senile Dementia, (Aging, Vol. 15), edited by Nancy E. Miller and Gene D. Cohen. Raven Press, New York 1981.

The Formal Support Network: Congregate Treatment Settings for Residents with Senescent Brain Dysfunction

Elaine M. Brody

Department of Human Services, Philadelphia Geriatric Center, Philadelphia, Pennsylvania 19141

In the absence of a generally accepted definition, it is suggested that long-term care refers to one or more services provided on a sustained basis to enable individuals whose functional capacities are chronically impaired to be maintained at their maximum levels of psychological, physical, and social well-being.[1] The recipients of services can reside anywhere along a continuum from their own homes to some type of institutional facility. Characterization of care as "long-term" flows from the chronicity of the disabilities of the population in need of it, which in turn dictates continuing rather than episodic or time-limited supports, services, and treatment. Any definition should view the family of the older person, where family exists, as the focus of planning rather than simply as a care-giving resource for the impaired elderly individual. The family focus has been emphasized by professionals, supported by the research literature, and recently was enunciated by the Secretary of the U.S. Department of Health, Education and Welfare (25). However, it has not been put into operation in social policy (9).

To implement that definition and its goals, an adequate formal support system of congregate treatment settings for residents with senescent brain dysfunctions should be coherent and comprehensive. It should include thorough multidisciplinary assessment; a spectrum of facilities providing options for a population whose needs are diverse despite the fact that they share a common diagnosis; criteria for matching the individual to the most appropriate setting; monitoring over time and reformulation of treatment goals; and linkages among facilities and services to facilitate orderly movement along the continuum of care as changing needs dictate. It also implies that the social and physical environments of the congregate settings are truly "supportive," that they provide the treatment

---

[1] This definition is a composite of those suggested by Brody (12), HRA's Division of Long-Term Care (HRA) (51), and the Technical Consultant Panel on the Long-Term Health Care Data Set of the United States National Committee on Vital and Health Statistics (124).

indicated, and that the care is available and accessible to those who need it.

What does exist at present is an incomplete network of facilities and services that does not constitute a system fulfilling those conditions. Nor does the existing partial network address itself specifically to those with a diagnosis of senescent brain dysfunction in the sense that they are sorted out by clear diagnosis and effective screening from those whose needs for care result from physical ailments, developmental disabilities, or functional mental problems. On the contrary, the vast majority of programs and facilities serve people with all of those diagnoses despite the efforts of some to screen for particular groups. Efforts at segregation are frustrated not only because mental and physical ailments in the aged are highly correlated, but because an aged population with one primary diagnosis is likely to develop others as it continues to age. As a result, an unresolved issue in institutions for older people is the "mix"—that is, whether residents with varying degrees of brain dysfunction should share living quarters with those who are cognitively intact. A parallel issue in congregate housing for the elderly is the management or discharge of those whose mental and/or physical capacities change over time after they first became tenants. It is unlikely, then, that individuals with a particular diagnosis can ever be served by either separate institutions or a separate system in which those institutions are embedded.

The categories of formal community care, institutional care, and the informal network of family and friends are not discrete. Some facilities (e.g., high-rise apartment buildings and smaller congregate arrangements) offer services and have many elements of the institution "restructured and made palatable with a new acceptable facade" (126). Some services (e.g., day care and respite care) are a "mix" of institution and community. Some institutions have created new forms of living arrangements and reached out to deliver services to clients living in their own homes in the community. Some community dwellers receive a combination of various types of services. Contrary to popular belief, the informal family support system does not cease its supportive activities abruptly upon the older person's entry into an institution; it continues them to varying extents depending on factors such as previous relationships and the degree to which such in-reach is tolerated or encouraged by the institution.

This chapter reviews what now exists by way of a formal support system of congregate treatment settings, the nature of the facilities, the characteristics of the residents, how decisions are made for admissions, the effects of institutionalization, and existing programs of treatment. It also suggests areas for future investigation. First, it is necessary to make explicit the goals and philosophy that are the context of these remarks.

Facilities that are institutional in nature and in which so many older people with brain dysfunction reside are an important, appropriate, and necessary component of any long-term care system. The current climate favoring "deinstitutionalization" and alternatives places community care and institutions in a false position of competition. As the review of the health, functional, and social characteristics of institutionalized older people indicates, there will always be a residual proportion of the elderly for whom institutional care is a necessity.

Community care services should be expanded enormously to serve those who live in the community and need but do not have them, as well as the 10 to 18% of institutional residents who could live in a community if those services were available. [See Lawton (77) for review of estimates of inappropriate institutionalization.] However, no matter how many services and facilities are developed that are inaccurately called "alternatives" and inaccurately viewed as less expensive in dollars,[2] the number of institutionalized older adults will increase in the future. The very rapid increase of the very old will increase the number and proportion of those who are most vulnerable to senile dementia and to institutionalization. It is projected that during the last quarter of this century people under 65 will increase by 21%, those between 65 and 75 by 23%, and those 75 and over by 60%. During the 6 years between 1970 and 1976 alone, the total 65-plus population increased by 14.8%, but those 85 and over increased by 39.6% (115).

Even if offset by full development of community care services and facilities, the institutional beds freed would be filled not only with the larger number of those who will need them but with those who now need but cannot obtain them. Broad social trends also are influential. Women's changing life styles, specifically the rapid increase in their labor force participation,[3] will make them less available to give the 80 to 90% of all home health services they provide at present. It is impossible to forecast the future impact on family service provision of the high rates of divorce and remarriage, with the multiple and complex filial loyalties resulting.

In any case, response to conditions of abuse or poor care in institutions should not take the form of mindless slogans such as "de-institutionalization." That approach would perpetuate the horrors initiated during the 1960s by the dumping of patients from state psychiatric hospitals without appropriate services and facilities in place. There has been a wave of reaction and thoughtful reviews of studies and experiences concerning those programs. Without exception they point to the dangers to the old people and their families of mounting such programs indiscriminately on the basis of misguided social reform rather than the needs of the people themselves (4,34,36). The conditions of impaired older

---

[2] The recent General Accounting Office survey in Cleveland showed that the cost of home care for extremely disabled older people (and for some who are moderately disabled) is greater than the cost of institutional care when the value of family services was included in the calculations (74). The social cost to families was not calculated, but other studies [e.g., Grad and Sainsbury (48)] identify negative stress on families.

[3] In August 1978, 50.2% of all women 16 years of age and older in the United States were in the working force. This represented a steady increase from 31.8% in 1947, 37.8 in 1960, and 43.4% in 1970 (119). Particularly significant is the increase in the proportion of middle-aged women who work, as they are the traditional and principal caregivers to dependent older people. Between 1940 and 1978, the proportion of working married women between the ages of 45 and 54 rose from 11% to almost 54%. Rates for single, separated, widowed, and divorced women are even higher, so that about 57% of all women in that age group are now working.

people in poor quality institutions are matched by the conditions of many older people in what is often euphemistically called the "community."

The goals should be to have a complete spectrum of high quality community services and congregate facilities, to identify those for whom each arrangement is appropriate, and to determine the nature of the services and environments that foster maximal well-being for each individual.

At present, the lack of clear definitions for long-term care facilities reflects a lack of clarity as well as a lack of commitment to that goal. Titles such as nursing home, personal care home, geriatric center, home for the aged, chronic disease facility, and others may reflect individual institutional goals and history, a philosophy of care, the characteristics of the residents, the nature of the sponsoring organization and its service emphasis, or the perceptions of third-party payors as to the appropriate functions to which they key reimbursement. There are also regional variations not only in nomenclature but in the number of levels of care identified, with wide disparities in reimbursement.

This picture is due in part to the rapid growth of facilities and their mixed ancestry, e.g., voluntary sectarian homes for the aged, the almshouse, the county home, the convalescent home, the psychiatric hospital, and the acute general hospital. By borrowing from such institutions, long-stay facilities now are a patchwork of borrowed identities. They have failed to develop a consistent value system or "personality" determined by the nature and needs of the populations to be served (15). An acute care model has been imposed inappropriately on chronic care.

The net effect is that older people with chronic organic brain syndrome (COBS) reside in a bewildering array of long-stay facilities that frustrates efforts at assembling coherent data. The U.S. Senate Subcommittee on Long-Term Care stated: "Nursing home statistics are as controversial as the nursing home industry itself. There has been an absence of universally accepted data" (125).

Differences in definitions and nomenclature also prevent precise cross-national comparisons of the proportions and characteristics of older people in long-term care institutions. Available information indicates that the United States, France, and the Federal Republic of Germany each have about 5% of their older people in institutions; in Yugosalvia there are more than 4%, in Canada 9%, and in Poland 1% (considered inadequate) (59). In Great Britain in 1971, 5% of all older people did not live in private households; slightly more than a third of that 5% were in local authority or voluntary association homes for the elderly, slightly less than a third in nonpsychiatric hospitals, a sixth in psychiatric hospitals, and the remainder in hotels or private residential establishments (56). About 4.2% of older people in Great Britain, then, can be said to be institutionalized. In Holland 10% of the elderly are in institutions (104). In Switzerland 7% of older people are in old age and nursing homes, in Israel 4%—and it is considered that the demand is not met in either country. In Sweden about 9% of those 65 and over and 12% of those 70 and over are in long-stay facilities of various types. In Norway (in 1970) 4.5% of those 70 and over were in "somatic" nursing homes alone, and policy plans were to increase that figure to 7% (95).

GROWTH OF LONG-TERM CARE FACILITIES
IN THE UNITED STATES

It is clear that there has been an enormous growth in the number of elderly in institutions, although, again, data are not precise because of different definitions and lack of data collection during earlier decades. In 1939 the Bureau of the Census estimated 25,000 nursing home beds in the United States in about 1,200 homes; by 1954 there were about 450,000 beds and by 1970 almost a million. The 1973–1974 survey of the National Center for Health Statistics reported 1,075,800 residents (almost 1.2 million beds) in 15,033 nursing homes (123). The most recent data available, from the 1977 National Nursing Home Survey, show an increase to 18,300 nursing homes containing a total of 1,287,400 residents (1,383,600 beds) of whom 1,097,900 were 65 or over (120,121). The vast majority of residents in all facilities are elderly (95.5% of those in voluntary homes, 86% of those in proprietaries, and 87% of those in government facilities). Between the 1973–1974 and the 1977 surveys, the institutionalized proportion of the total elderly populations remained the same despite the 20% increase in their total number.

Factors giving impetus to the growth of institutional facilities (which occurred primarily after World War II) were: (a) the increasing number of older people, especially those reaching the advanced old age at which vulnerability to institutionalization is greater; (b) federal programs making funds available to purchase long-term care (Old Age, Survivors, and Disability Insurance; Kerr-Mills; Medicare and Medicaid) and federal grants and loans enabling sponsors to construct, equip, and rehabilitate facilities [Hill-Burton Act, Small Business Act and Small Business Investment Act (1958), National Housing Act (1959)]; and (c) large-scale programs to discharge elderly mental patients from state hospitals to the community, spurred by the Mental Health and Retardation Acts of 1963 and 1965. [For detailed description of these developments see Brody (12) and Kramer et al. (73).][4]

The latter development was the catalyst for redistribution of beds among facilities with various types of auspices. In 1960 the bulk of the institutionalized elderly (92%) were distributed in roughly equal proportions among psychiatric hospitals (28.9%), nursing homes (28.1%), and domiciliary homes (35%) (mainly homes for the aged). Of those in domiciliary homes and nursing homes together (63.1%), one-fourth were in nonprofit facilities, three-fifths in proprietary facilities, and about 15% in county or city facilities.

---

[4] Pollak's (97) careful analysis indicates that between 1960 and 1970 the nursing home/home for the aged population increased by 105% (408,000 people), the absolute use of mental hospitals by the elderly declined by 36%, and the use of all institutions by the elderly increased by 58%. The percentage of all institutionalized older people in mental hospitals fell from 29% to 12%, and the percentage in nursing homes rose from 63% to 82%. He attributes the 105% increase in the nursing home population to the following factors: increased elderly population (29% of the increase); changing age composition of elderly (14%); substitution of nursing home for mental hospital care (25%); and advances in medical care that permit survival with greater impairments, changes in age structure *within* the 5-year brackets usually used to describe age-structure change, and changing social/cultural patterns.

Subsequently, there was a sharp drop in the number of people of all ages in psychiatric hospitals and a corresponding rise in the nursing home population. Between 1965 and 1975 the total population of all ages in state and county mental hospitals decreased by 60% (from 475,202 to 191,391 persons), and those 65 and over by 61.4% (from 140,330 to 54,195) (117). By the time of the 1973–1974 National Nursing Home Survey, 73.3% of the nursing homes were proprietary and contained almost 70% of the beds; 26.7% were either government operated (about 6% of the homes and 10.5% of the beds) or voluntary (about 20% of the homes and the beds) (123). In 1977, 74.3% of the facilities were proprietaries and contained 67.8% of the beds, whereas 21% and 11% of the beds were under voluntary and governmental auspices, respectively[5] (121). That is, during the past few years, the proportion of the proprietary facilities remained about the same (a growth of only 1%) and the proportion of beds they contained dropped slightly (about 3%) (121).

Overall, the massive increase in beds has occurred largely in the profit-making sector, and the proportion of beds under governmental auspices has decreased. Although the absolute number of voluntaries and their number of beds has increased, the proportion of beds and facilities they represent dropped sharply but seems to have leveled off during the past few years. This pattern of auspices is unique in the United States.[6] Elsewhere there is a conspicuous absence of a profit-oriented institutional system (65).

CHRONIC OBS AND INSTITUTIONS

Attempts to estimate the number of institutionalized older people with senile dementia suffer from variations in diagnosis, lack of standardized techniques for data collection, and observer and sampling biases (55). Although there is no assurance that the people so diagnosed do not actually have other conditions with similar symptoms, it appears that senile dementia afflicts about 60% of those in nursing and old age homes, or 660,000 people. The National Survey found 34% with what it called "advanced senility" and 27% with "less serious" senility. In 1975 an additional 16,008 people 65 or over with diagnoses of "organic brain syndrome associated with cerebral arteriosclerosis and senile and presenile brain disease" resided in psychiatric facilities[7] (116). Thus the indications are that there is a minimum of about 675,000 older people with senile dementia in "official" institutions.

---

[5] Data from the 1976 Survey of Institutionalized Persons are somewhat different, identifying 18,261 nursing homes and homes for aged of which 4.8% are under government auspice (but not federal), 61.4% are proprietary, and 33.8% nonprofit (115). The survey estimated 1,027,850 institutionalized people 65 or over at that time, a number that undoubtedly is higher now.

[6] For example, 90% of the facilities in the United Kingdom are public, 54% of the facilities in Israel are voluntary (serving 80% of the institutionalized aged) (64), and in the Federal Republic of Germany 61% of facilities are governmental, 20% public, and 19% proprietary (59).

[7] Such diagnoses were second only to schizophrenia in the mental hospitals, accounting for 17.2% of all the residents (15% of the males and 19.9% of the females).

Complicating the picture in the United States is the existence of facilities called boarding homes, hotels, foster homes, or places by other names that contain many older people with mental and physical disabilities similar to those of the residents in facilities formally designated as institutions. Those individuals are not included in the customary 5% estimate of institutionalized old people, and no exact information exists about their number or characteristics. A recent hearing of the U.S. House Committee on Aging estimated that there are about 500,000 older people (about 2% of the total elderly population) in adult care homes (112). A few scattered studies indicate that this may be an underestimate.

An Allegheny County report on boarding homes indicated that a minimum of 3% of the aged in that area resided in such facilities. The residents had a median age of 73, with one-third 80 or over; most were impaired, with about half showing symptoms, e.g., confusion and memory loss (99). A Philadelphia conference estimated that there are more than 1,000 boarding homes (without licensure or controls) containing as many as 10,000 people, many of whom were of questionable competency and should have been in nursing facilities (8). A study in New York State found that as many as 15 individuals often resided in places called foster homes, raising question as to how many people reside in facilities that are actually boarding homes bearing different labels (13,105).

It is suggested, therefore, that the current 5% figure used in the United States as the proportion of institutionalized older people is an understatement. Boarding homes and other facilities may be called by other names, not licensed as nursing homes, and lack even minimal services. Nonetheless, the impaired residents are in the main elderly and are institutionalized.

If, as seems likely, half of the 2 to 3% of the older people or about 225,000 individuals in such unofficial institutions suffer from senile dementia, as many as 900,000 older people with that diagnosis may reside in offical and unofficial institutions together. Added to those are an unknown number in quasi-institutions such as age-segregated apartment buildings with services. Acute general hospitals also merit attention as they frequently are sites for care of this group. Older people are hospitalized three times as often as younger patients, their average length of stay is twice as long, and they utilize one-third of the general hospital bed days. Hospitals and long-stay facilities are major sources of referrals to each other.

CHARACTERISTICS OF THE RESIDENTS

Available data about the characteristics of institutionalized older people are not specific to the subgroup of those with COBS. It is not known, therefore, whether they are a representative group demographically, in social or health characteristics, or in functional capacities. The following summaries pertain to all institutionalized older adults.

Age

Those in nursing and old age homes are in advanced old age. The median age of those 65 or over is 82, or almost a decade older than that of the total elderly population. Eighty-three percent of them are over 75, with 43% being 85 or over (123). The chances of admission to an institution increase with advancing age: in 1970, 1% of the 65–69 group, 2% of those 70–74, 4.3% of those 75–79, 9% of those 80–84, and 16.5% of those 85 or over were in institutions (97). Older people in psychiatric facilities are somewhat younger than those in nursing homes; 56% are 65–74 and 44% are 75 or over (116).

Sex

More than 70% of institutional residents are women, with the discrepancy between the sexes widening with advancing age (62% of those between 65 and 74, but 75% of those 85 or over are women) (122). One factor contributing to this imbalance is the longer life span of women, which in turn makes them more vulnerable to the social, physical, and mental disabilities associated with advanced old age; another is the fact that men tend to marry women younger than themselves. The discrepancy is not as great among mental hospital patients, with 59% being female (116).

Race

Ninety-two percent of residents are white (120). Minority groups (Blacks, Spanish Americans, and Asian Americans) are underrepresented in long-stay facilities. For example, Blacks constitute 6.6% of those in skilled nursing facilities (SNFs) (118), although they constitute about 11% of the total population and about 8% of the elderly. In addition to minorities having shorter life spans, other contributing factors may be economic factors, culture, and discriminatory practices.

Economic Status

Institutionalized people have a significantly lower economic status than the general population of older people owing to a constellation of factors: (a) They are primarily elderly women whose economic status is lower than that of elderly men. (b) Resources may have been depleted by long periods of retirement, inflationary trends, long illnesses prior to institutionalization, and the cost of institutional care itself. (c) People with ample resources can create one-bed nursing homes in their own homes. Medicaid and Medicare pay more than half the nursing home bill, but inadequate reimbursement levels have resulted in two systems of care which are very different in quality: one for the poor, and one for those whose resources are sufficient to purchase care (2,44,72).

Health

Mental impairment of one kind or another is the most common diagnosis of the institutionalized elderly. In addition to the mental hospital population, about 60% of those in nursing homes have COBS and 17% have either functional disorders or retardation. The proportion of the institutionalized with senile dementia rises with advancing age; 62% of those 75–84 have that diagnosis, as do 70% of those 85 or over (123). These conditions coexist and are highly interrelated with physical impairments (61) of which the most frequent are circulatory disorders such as heart disease (37%), stroke and associated disorders (25%), arthritis (33%), other skeletal disorders (42%), and digestive disorders such as diabetes (29%) (122).

The salient fact about these multiple health problems—of which most institutionalized old people have three or four—is that they are *chronic* and result in *functional disability*. Disability impairs the capacity of these individuals to care for themselves in normal living situations and leads to dependence on others for ongoing services. The universal emphasis of geriatricians and gerontologists has therefore been on *function* as the key to treatment plans for the impaired older adult.

The most common functional disabilities in nursing homes are in ambulation and personal self-care. Estimates of those who can walk without assistive devices range from 80% (49) to 60% (45) to 22% (122). Estimates vary also as to the amount of help required with activities of daily living. The Long-Term Care Facility Improvement Study (118) of SNFs and the 1977 National Nursing Home Survey (120) were in rough agreement about the proportion needing help with bathing (93% and 86%), dressing (72% and 68%), and eating (50% and 32%) as well as the proportion of those who are incontinent (between 45% and 55%). The two studies disagree in estimates of the proportions of those in need of help in toileting (68% and 42%, respectively). The Survey of Institutionalized Persons (SIP) (115) estimates that 14.4% are bedfast, whereas the National Center for Health Statistics report 5%. The latter survey reported that a startling 35% of residents are confined to their rooms. Bedsores afflicted almost 10% of the residents of the Long-Term Care Improvement Study (118); over half of the patients had difficulty in their awareness of their situation in respect to time, place, and self-identification; and one out of every seven was not aware of the environment or was comatose.

REASONS FOR ADMISSION TO LONG-TERM CARE FACILITIES

Poor health is identified by surveys as the primary reason for admission in the vast majority of cases. For example, the SIP (115) cites medical reasons for 79.3% of admissions and family inability to care for the person at home for 12.4%. According to the 1977 National Nursing Home Survey (120), poor physical health accounted for 76% of admissions, lack of social or economic resources and disruptive behavior for 12%, mental illness for 7%, and mental retardation for 5%. The explanation for the predominance of physical health conditions as the admitting diagnoses is probably because in many areas diagnosis of senile dementia is not considered sufficient to establish eligibility for nursing home care. Those completing the Medicaid certification of need therefore emphasize medical conditions.

Although institutional residents undeniably are in poor health, it is simplistic and inaccurate to explain admissions on that basis. For example, since disabled older people in the community outnumber their institutionalized peers in a ratio of about 2:1, other factors must be at work. For more than a decade, data have accumulated which demonstrate unequivocally that when older people are in advanced old age, are mentally and/or physically impaired, and are functionally disabled, the critical determinants of who is admitted to institutions and who remains in the community are the social supports available (primarily family).

The family status of the institutionalized is dramatically different from that of the total population of older people. The three surveys cited are in rough agreement that only about 14% of elderly institutional residents are married, compared with 56% of all older people. About 60% of the institutionalized are widowed, 6 to 7% are separated or divorced, and almost 20% had never been married (in contrast to 5.6% never-married in the general population). Further, whereas four out of five older people have at least one surviving adult child, almost half of the institutionalized elderly are childless and more of them have only one child rather than two or more (45,113). The size of the family is directly related to the proportion of elderly women living with relatives and inversely related to the proportion institutionalized. Thus childless women at any age have higher rates of institutionalization than their counterparts with children; those with the largest familes have about half the rate of institutionalization of childless women of the same age (108).

If disabled older people in institutions are compared only with their disabled peers in the community rather than with the total population of older people, the significance of family is further highlighted. In one study of a sample of severely or totally disabled older people living in the community and being served by a Home Health Agency, none lived alone: 46% lived with children, 20% with a spouse, and 34% with other relatives or friends. In contrast, those who were only moderately impaired and were in private SNFs had few family supports: 54.5% had never been married, 40.9% were widowed, 4 to 5% were divorced, and 68.2% of the total group were childless (24).

Beyond the sheer existence of family members are the characteristics of the family members themselves. People in advanced old age are likely to have children who themselves are approaching or already in the aging phase of life. The capacities of such children to provide care for disabled parents is qualified by their own age-related problems, e.g., the appearance of chronic disabilities, lowered energy levels, interpersonal losses, retirement, and lowered income. Thus that proportion of increased institutionalization which is attributed to the increase in the very old is due not only to the functional incapacities of advanced old age but to the social losses that are age-related. For example, in a study of applicants to a voluntary home, 40% of them had at least one adult child 60 years of age or over and the children's ages ranged as high as 74. In half the cases, application was precipitated by the death or severe illness of a spouse (25%) or adult child or child-in-law (25%) (18).

More subtle factors also are at work. There often is an accumulation or clustering of stresses. The applicant's personality (independent or more reliant on protection), the quality of family relationships, the capacity of individual and family to tolerate stress and their coping abilities, and socioeconomic factors play their roles (16,19). Geographic distance of children makes the older person more vulnerable to institutionalization (113). Behavior that is socially unacceptable or that brings the older person to the community's attention may precipitate admission to a psychiatric facility; at the other extreme, "social invisibility," or the capacity for sheer self-maintenance, may keep them out (89).

In short, there is no one "reason" for institutionalization; it is multiply determined. The accumulated evidence is definitive: admissions are due to varied social/health problems for which social/health solutions have been sought. The inventory of research studies that disproves the myth of abandonment by families and that documents their attempts to avoid insititutional admissions is so long and the findings so consistent that the issue should require no further discussion. [See Brody (12) for review.] Rather, professional and research efforts should be directed to ways of supporting and supplementing the care-giving efforts of families who are being subjected to increasing demands (whether the older person is in an institution or in the community). Ways should also be explored of substituting for family care when needed for the approximate 7 million older people without families, whose families are not close at hand, or whose relationships are impaired historically (10).

There are no studies that focus specifically on the reasons for the admissions of those with COBS as they may differ from the reasons other population groups are admitted. At the Philadelphia Geriatric Center (PGC) more than one-third of applications for long-term care note symptoms of confusion and disorientation as major reasons for requesting care (19). Years of experience with thousands of older people and their families lead to the conclusion that senile dementia is the most socially disruptive ailment of all (17). The anxiety, fear, panic, and sense of loss of control on the part of the elderly sufferer has its parallel in the anxiety, fear, panic, and inability to cope on the part of the family. The need for constant surveillance; the inappropriate, unpredictable, often embarrassing behavior; the fear of leaving the old person alone lest he wander away or leave the water tap or gas jet open; the nature of the care needed for those who are incontinent; the inability to communicate as formerly with the older person; the stimulation of fears of one's own aging in general and of "inheriting" the disease in particular all extract a heavy toll and place a particularly severe burden on family members.

In that context, although being married is a major factor enabling an older person to avoid institutionalization, brain impairment may play a more significant role than does physical impairment in the reluctant decision to institutionalize one's spouse. This hypothesis is supported by the fact that, at present, of the 36 residents at the PGC's long-term care facility who have spouses living in the community, 30 of them (83%) suffer from COBS. Of the remaining six, two are incapacitated from CVAs, two from brain tumors, one from brain damage due to a car accident, and one is blind and mentally retarded. It is striking that in each situation some form of impaired brain function is present. Parenthetically, the distress of the intact spouses of these residents is so great that a therapy group was established to help them.

A caveat is in order on the subject of the overall characteristics of institutionalized older people. Advanced old age, impairments in various spheres, and absent or diminished social supports do not make them a homogeneous group. They represent several generations, come from different socioeconomic–cultural–ethnic–educational backgrounds, and function at different levels. They may be institutionalized for different periods of time: for many years or temporarily for convalescent or terminal care. They vary widely in personality, life experience, and life style. Therefore the tendency to generalize about them should be resisted lest their similarities to each other obscure their differences and lest any shared diagnosis obscure the individuality of response, behavior, adaptation, and treatment needs.

DECISION-MAKING PROCESS

The demographic, health, and socioeconomic characteristics of the impaired aged and their families are not, of course, the only determinants of whether admission takes place or of the choice of the particular facility to which access is sought. Important roles are played by social policy, as reflected in the existence, availability, and accessibility of resources, and by the perception of the providers as to their missions. Resources are created or made to disappear by policy decisions and by the various streams of reimbursement for which the individual is eligible. Thus as noted above, the development of long-term care facilities followed the flow of the federal dollar in fostering construction, equipment, and reconstruction of facilities and in reimbursing for care. Similarly, policy decisions closed the doors of state psychiatric facilities, and funding availability opened the way for a mushrooming of nursing and boarding homes.

Diagnoses have been flexible in their adaptability to the admission criteria of any particular facility. In 1965 Camp (26) pointed out that the same elderly man who was "confused and depressed with somatic delusions" on the doorstep of a mental hospital might be "rather forgetful with some preoccupations about food" at the door of a home for the aged, or have a "gastrointestinal disorder with relatively intact sensorium" on the way to a nursing home. "Abdominal distress requiring diagnostic studies" might provide entrée to a general hospital.

Now, 14 years later, the perceptions of the older person and family or those of professionals as to needs and appropriate settings to meet them are still often subordinate to such considerations as the availability of any bed, particularly a Medicaid bed. The family may initiate placement in the crucible of an acute crisis preceded by long periods of severe strain. The Medicaid certification of need by the physician is often a pro forma paper review. Transfers from hospitals frequently are precipitated at the eleventh hour when the doctor enters the discharge note on the chart because hospital care is no longer needed or in response to pressure from the Utilization Review Committee. In the main, assessment and orderly planning do not occur. It is rare for the old person to receive careful preparation for transfer or admission, let alone be afforded the participation in the decision-making process which is a predictor of adjustment and well-being. *The great majority of older people with mental diagnoses enter nursing homes without any contact with any part of the mental health system* (41).

Although there is universal agreement about the critical need for thorough multidisciplinary evaluation and functional assessment as part of the decision-making process, it rarely occurs. Many systems of assessment have been developed, but none is universally used. In general, emphasis has been primarily on physical and mental function and diagnosis; neglected in this process is an assessment of: (a) instrumental behaviors; (b) needs for socialization, recreation, and creativity; (c) the availability of social supports; and (d) the physical environment. Lawton (78) proposed a classification that provides a theoretical framework for a rounded assessment system, and he is currently engaged in putting this concept into operation in the form of a multilevel assessment instrument.

Enthusiasm for even the most sophisticated assessment system should not obscure the fact that it is only part of the decision-making. Other considerations are the treatment potential of the individual and the preferences and attidues of the older person and family (16,19). The *process* of decision-making and the people who make the decision are as important as the professional assessment.

RELOCATION

No matter the nature of the decision-making process, every older person in an institution has been subjected to at least one relocation and in many instances several relocations. Various studies have noted an acceleration in mobility prior to institutionalization with several moves made in rapid succession (16,40,113). In one of them, applicants had moved five times more frequently in the course of the year preceding admission than the total 75 and over population: 80% had moved at least once; more than 25% had moved two or more times (16).

National data on movement into and out of facilities indicate that more than half of the residents (54%) are admitted from another health facility (32% from hospitals, 13% from another nursing home, and the remainder from other types of facilities) and 41% from residences in the community (12% of them had lived alone) (120). The SIP (115) identifies 28% as having lived with next of kin prior to admission.

The median length of stay in nursing homes nationally is about 1.6 years.

However, nearly a third of the residents have been in the facility for 1 to 3 years and nearly another third for 3 years or more (120). More than 20% of the residents have lived in the facilities for more than 5 years (115).

Statistics on discharge can be deceptive. Of the 973,100 persons of all ages counted as "discharged" from nursing homes during 1976, one-fourth were deceased. The number of persons 65 or over discharged alive was about 600,000 (120). Those discharged had more social supports (20% married compared to 13% of the residents, and 11% never married compared to 21% of the residents). Only about one-third of those discharged alive went to a private or semiprivate residence and the remainder to another health facility (44.7% to a hospital and 13.3% to another nursing home). Thus for two-thirds of the "discharges" the word "transfers" would be more accurate, and in many instances the transfer to other institutional facilities was because of deterioration of health and the need for more intensive care. This is supported by the fact that 20% of those discharged were bedfast compared with only 5% of the residents. Undoubtedly, many nursing homes are reluctant or do not have the capability to deal with the dying resident, who is therefore transferred to a hospital.

The minority of residents who return to private residences more often had been admitted for short-term or recuperative care (e.g., those with fractures). The NCHS study concluded that there are two groups of persons who use nursing homes: those admitted for relatively short periods of time for recuperative care and those admitted for relatively long periods of time because there is little chance of improvement in their chronic problems (120). Undoubtedly, those with senile dementia are in the latter group.

The overall picture is one of considerable movement of older people, who are circulated among institutions of various types. Once "boosted" into the institutional nonsystem, they move from hospital to nursing home, from nursing home to hospital, and from nursing home to nursing home. Frequently they move from one room or floor to another within the facilities as their changing needs dictate, to resolve roommate problems, or in response to reimbursement criteria.

EFFECTS OF LIVING IN AN INSTITUTION

There is an extensive literature on the negative effects of living in an institution. Many thorough reviews are available (6,47,80,82,84), but, again, almost none of the work on this subject is specific to those with senile dementia. Where that group is mentioned, its special vulnerability is highlighted.

The institutionalized compared poorly to the noninstitutionalized in cognitive, emotional, and social functions. A list of their characteristics includes poor adjustment, depression, unhappiness, intellectual ineffectiveness, negative self-image, apathy, feelings of insignificance and impotency, docility, submissiveness, withdrawal, and unresponsiveness (84). Those effects have been attributed to institutionally induced lack of privacy, restricted mobility, separation from family and society, routinization, depersonalization, desexualization, loss of self-determination, lack of productive or enjoyable activity, and the transfer of power and surrender of control over one's own life to staff.

There is general agreement that negative effects cannot be attributed simplistically to the fact of living in an institution. Much research remains to be done, but those who attempt to sort out contributing factors now recognize that differences between institutionalized older people and those who are not in institutions are often due to: (a) pre-existing population differences (which are related in part to the reasons for institutionalization); (b) the experiences of applying for admission, waiting for admission for varying periods of time, and actually making the transition to institutional living (relocation); and (c) the social and physical qualities of the particular institutional environment.

Selection biases such as more disability, pre-existing poor psycho/emotional status, and different socioeconomic backgrounds are thought not to be explanatory when accounting for the poor status of the institutionalized as compared with community dwellers (84). However, institutional residents have experienced more familial losses, which in turn contribute to the needs for admission. The role of those losses in producing negative psychological status requires additional exploration.

The stream of research on the relocation effect (i.e., excess morbidity and mortality as a result of environment change) is of special interest in view of the particular vulnerability of those with COBS and the multiple moves to which they often are subjected prior to their admission. Soon after the early studies documenting the existence of the relocation effect, additional research made it apparent that the negative impact of moving cannot be attributed globally to the change in environment per se. Relevant matters are the special vulnerability of subgroups of movers, the reasons for the move, its meaning to the mover, the ways in which moves are managed, and the quality of the environments from and to which the moves are made.

The most vulnerable were found to be the physically ill, the depressed, the confused and disoriented, and those who were moved involuntarily. The older person with senile dementia who is selectively at risk and is being institutionalized is often characterized by all those conditions. Disorganization during and immediately after a move increases mortality, although the stress of several successive changes in environment has not been calculated.

Improvements in movers have been noted for those who were physically well and those who chose to move. Other factors that reduce or avoid negative effects are the provision of opportunities for choice, careful individualized preparation through counseling and premove orientation to the receiving facility, and participation of the older person in the decision-making process. Again, it is those with senile dementia who are most often denied such techniques and processes because of negative attitudes; their capacities to participate are underestimated. Further, there has been little exploration of helping techniques that do not rely on intact cognition. Some work along those lines has been done clinically at the PGC and involves gradual admission and "acting out" rather than verbal interchanges [see case example in Brody (12)].

One explanation suggested for the negative effects of moving on the confused individual is that while "not sufficiently in contact to understand advance explanations of a move [he] is nevertheless sufficiently aware of environmental cues to become disturbed when the cues are no longer at hand" (1). The hypothesis advanced was that the demented individual cannot prepare for a change and lacks the adaptive capacity to cope with it. In the same vein, a theme reiterated in the literature on stress is that its negative impact is due to the existence of a stress which is perceived as such, coupled with an inability on the part of the individual to cope with it (30,53,98,103). It is suggested that because of the very nature of the ailment the individual with COBS has diminished capacity to cope with relocation stress and the accompanying feelings of helplessness and hopelessness. At the PGC it was observed that there is often a sharp increase in confusion on admission which recedes when appropriate concentrated services are given.

The role of the environment itself was highlighted by several studies. Lieberman's (84) study of the effects of entry into institutions attributed negative effects to institution-like environments—vastly different from previous more natural living styles—that overloaded the old person's adaptive capacities. In his report on the relocation of elderly mental patients, the strongest association with outcome status was the psychosocial milieu of the receiving environment. "Patients placed in cold, dehumanized, dependency-fostering environments show declines. The psychological characteristics of the relocation environments were considerably more influential on outcome than any combination of the characteristics of the discharged patients themselves" (86).

Marlowe's (90) study also assessed environmental dimensions. Two groups of highly comparable individuals experienced diametrically opposed outcomes: one group did very well and the other "fell apart." "The answer to this anomalous situation," she wrote, "is to be found in a consideration of the environments." The improvers went to environments that encouraged autonomy (the resident's control over his own life), fostered personalization (privacy and respect), offered less succoring (did not foster dependency by doing things for an individual that he could, with encouragement, do for himself), fostered community integration (access to the outside world), had a lower tolerance for deviance, encouraged social interaction and did not expect docility or passivity, and treated residents with warmth and positive attitudes. Under opposite conditions, the same type of people withdrew and deteriorated. Marlowe's (90) finding that the characteristics of the improver environments cross-cut different types of facility comments on the heterogeneity of institutional environments and their positive potential.

Institutional residents tend to try to continue their preadmission life styles (7), and adjustment is affected by the extent to which that continuation is permitted by the institution. For example, Kahana (57) found that congruence between individual needs and environmental opportunity, mainly for privacy and impulse expression, were important to adjustment. Those patients with personalities described as "vigorous, hostile-narcissistic" have been found to make better adjustments to institutional life (114). That finding is consonant with the results of a PGC study in which subjects with COBS who were described as "aggressive" improved the most in response to psychosocial treatment (69).

The overwhelming impression given by a review of the literature on the process of institutionalization and the experience of living in such facilities is that: (a) psychosocial care is not an ethical matter alone; lack of it contributes to decline and can even be lethal (87); and (b) in general, positive effects accrue when the institutional environment is modified in the direction of being less "total," i.e., when the institution itself is deinstitutionalized.

With respect to the relocation effect, there are other issues that deserve more attention than they have received. First, the phenomenon is usually discussed in terms of moves into or between institutions. However, ill effects can also occur when people are moved out of institutions (38,110,111). Further, about 17% (4 million people) of the total elderly population are admitted to an acute care hospital at least once in the course of a year, and 25% (a million individuals) of these are admitted at least twice. It is not known what proportion suffer from COBS or to what extent such relocations and inpatient experiences have a negative impact. Studies of such relocations and programs to ease such moves or to mitigate the effects of the hospital environments for those with COBS are virtually nonexistent.

Secondly, there has been little work and almost no attention to the negative effect of *not* moving when indicated. One study found negative effects of waiting on a list for admission (85), and in another study wait-listed applicants reported more problems than their peers who had been admitted (16). A more intact group of elderly under environmental stress who had expressed but not carried out a need to move experienced a precipitous drop in psychosocial adjustment (11). The latter study led to the hypothesis that an "immobilization effect" exists, i.e., negative effects of not changing one's environment when a move is needed and wished for, or of the environment changing while the older person remains in place, or of failure to modify the environment supportively when indicated. The net effect is a lack of congruence between the environment and the individual's capacity to function in it (14).

The issue of quality, then, pertains to community care as well as institutional care. Admittedly, the institutional setting by its very nature is more vulnerable to abuse (42), but the quality of care in the community directly affects the status of those who are subsequently institutionalized.

INSTITUTIONAL PROGRAMS OF TREATMENT

It is safe to say that by the time older people (including those with senile dementia) arrive at the institution, all are in need of psychosocial treatment intervention. The relationship between the degree of organic brain impairment and the level of individual functioning is not always absolute (31,101), and there is every reason to believe that many of those who are institutionalized with senile dementia are functioning below their maximum levels of well-being. They have experienced many of the assaults linked to senile dementia as correlates, precipitants, or contributing factors, e.g., physical illness and traumatic events (100). Many have already experienced and many will be living under adverse environmental conditions, e.g., restrictive institutions (27,71,75). Some have had life-long difficulties in adapting to stress which exacerbate the problems of adjusting to such a dramatic change in life style (62). All have diminished capacities to adjust and to replace the psychosocial supplies they have lost.

A variety of formal treatment approaches have been applied to institutionalized older people. Only the few that included or focused on those with COBS are reviewed here.

Among the best known treatments that have been tried are milieu approaches (e.g., the well known studies in Michigan, at Fergus Falls, in Minnesota and at the Philadelphia State Hospital) as well as group activity and occupational and social therapies. All reported favorable results. Almost all included people with a variety of diagnoses, and some specifically excluded the extremely confused individual. The target populations most often consisted primarily of functionally disturbed individuals whose median age was a decade younger than the median age of all institutionalized old people. The facilities in which much of the research took place generally offered relatively low levels of basic care. [For review of these studies, see Gottesman and Brody (47) and Bennett and Eisdorfer (6).]

Two substudies of the Michigan milieu series focused on the "senile" patient. Donahue et al. (37) reported that extremely confused "senile" patients responded to work and recreation therapy but were slow to do so and in need of constant stimulation for gains to be maintained. Ibsen's (54) report, which describes the use of similar modalities, found that close personal attention resulted in improved behavior, gains which were reversed when the attention was withdrawn.

In two studies in England, Cosin and his co-workers (32,33) applied domestic activity, social groups, occupational therapy, crafts, and other group activities with resultant improvements in conversation and general activity level. However, in the first study the treatment modalities were not sorted out. Although they subsequently were contrasted, neither study was well controlled and they were unsophisticated methodologically.

Another study limited to the institutionalized with moderate to severe COBS used a sheltered workshop program as the treatment element. The participants were able to sustain effective participation for at least 3 months (94).

An experiment on the effects of segregating/integrating the mentally impaired and intact on floors of an institution was inconclusive but did point up the effectiveness of stimulating staff and improving their attitudes (58). Experience at the PGC points to segregated areas within the facility for those who are extremely confused or whose behavior is severely disordered. The solicited opinions of staff and families overwhelmingly support this view.

REALITY ORIENTATION

The form of treatment called reality orientation (RO) (for descriptions see refs. 3,39,83,96) has achieved widespread interest approaching the proportions of a fad despite the fact that there have been no definitive studies of its effectiveness. Although generally understood to be used for the "senile," RO most often includes all individuals who exhibit confusion or disorientation regardless of age or of the etiology of the symptoms.

One report of RO treatment of 125 men ranging in age from the mid-forties to the nineties noted that 80% of them had "organic brain syndrome due to cerebral arteriosclerosis" (although there is no description of diagnostic criteria), 15% had had cerebrovascular accidents (CVAs), and 6% unspecified organic brain damage; 40% of the total also had "other forms of brain damage" (83). More traditional techniques were used simultaneously. The staff rated 32% of the patients as improved with respect to level of nursing required, and 68% remained the same. The conclusions drawn were that disorientation is not necessarily a permanent consequence of brain damage, that RO successfully prevented decline in those who had remained the same, and that as part of the total rehabilitation program RO can be rated highly successful. There was no way of evaluating the differential impact of RO and the other aspects of treatment.

Another report studied the effects on six patients of a 6-week program utilizing the classroom aspect of RO (5). All were diagnosed as having senile dementia, and their mean age was 81. There were no pre/post significant differences on informational scores or behavioral ratings. However, the investigator stated that personnel unanimously reported improvements that did not show up on the measures.

A controlled study of RO was conducted in a state hospital (50). Improvements were found in the treated group but not in the controls. However, the two groups of women were relatively young (mean age 66.6 years for experimentals and 71.1 for controls), had mixed diagnoses, and had been hospitalized for an average of 24.6 and 23 years, respectively. The investigators pointed out the possible role of the sheer extra attention on the improvers and emphasized the positive effect on staff morale.

Twelve experimental subjects in another RO study were compared with 13 controls (mean ages 84 and 83) in a large geriatric institution (28). The treated group improved on information, but not in behavioral, functioning. Although selected on the basis of being "moderately disoriented," there is no description of how the subjects were screened and no mention of random assignment to the two groups. The investigators were frank in stating that perhaps the program content was not as important as the structured contact between residents and staff.

RO teaches all staff to create a quiet, friendly atmosphere, to call residents by name and to repeat their own names, and to tell residents where they are being taken when going to various places, e.g., the bathroom or the doctor's office. This seems useful in that it trains staff to do what they should be doing anyway. However, the practice raises the question as to whether constant indiscriminate repetition can insult or infantilize those who do not require it. A careful study of RO found that the training had a positive effect on staff attitudes (107), an improvement that seems to be a common thread in many reports. That aspect of RO which prescribes a specific, consistent attitude for staff to adopt toward each resident is a debatable practice in the light of the variations within each human personality and the reasons for behaviors.

In view of the lack of evidence of RO's success, the phenomenon of its popularity as a treatment for senile dementia is puzzling. Perhaps it speaks to the hunger of care-givers for treatment methodology. Its appeal may be that in prescribing a relatively simple, easily learned technique it relieves the staff of the more difficult demand that individuals and their varied behaviors be understood; or, since it focuses specifically on the symptoms of confusion and disorientation, to the unsophisticated it appears to hold promise of reversal or "cure" of the actual impairment. One danger is that hailing RO as a panacea can close off experimentation and multiple avenues to treatment. In addition, the fact that it "rejects the idea that there are erudite and definite explanations for senility" (96) disregards the critical necessity for careful differential diagnosis and therefore for a variety of treatments appropriate to those diagnoses. Perhaps the lesson to be learned is that a structured program which conveys optimism to staff, compels staff–resident interaction, and fosters positive attitudes pays therapeutic dividends.

INDIVIDUALIZED TREATMENT

Little is known of the effects of interventions defined more specifically than milieu and group programs. A highly focused program called Individualized Treatment of the Mentally Impaired Aged[8] was designed at the PGC to examine the effects of individualized interdisciplinary treatment on institutionalized women with COBS (22). The target group differed from subjects of other studies in that all suffered from moderate to severe chronic brain syndrome, were in advanced old age (average age about 82), and were free from a history of early life functional psychosis. Diagnosis was established by neurological examination and the Kahn-Goldfarb Mental Status Questionnaire (mean scores of 3.3 correct answers). The 64 subjects were assigned randomly to experimental and control groups.

A key concept of the project was that of "excess disabilities," a term originated by Kahn and Goldfarb (60). An excess disability (ED) is the discrepancy which exists when the individual's functional capacity is greater than that warranted by the actual impairment, i.e., the gap between actual function and potential function. It was hypothesized that EDs could exist in all spheres of functioning (physical, social, psychological), and that they could be reduced or eliminated

[8] Research described was supported by grant MH15047, National Institute of Mental Health.

by appropriate therapeutic intervention. Basic features of the treatment program were individualization, an interdisciplinary approach, the setting of specific goals (realistic rather than global), assignment of definite tasks to team members in order to implement goals, careful monitoring to ensure implementation, and re-evaluation to determine whether goals had or had not been met. Each subject received detailed multidisciplinary pre- and post-treatment clinical assessment and ratings. Treatment for the experimental group focused on the specific EDs identified. Both groups continued to receive the usual institutional services.

At the end of the treatment year it was found that the EDs of experimental subjects had improved significantly compared to those of the controls (22), particularly in the categories of family relationships and activities. Improvement of family relationships points up the importance of attention to this aspect of life among the institutionalized. Improvements in the sphere of activities were attributed to individualization; i.e., in developing treatment there was heavy reliance on the individual's history, past interests, skills, and experiences. There was also some evidence of improvement in the treated subjects in caring for their clothing and personal effects. However, improvements in the main were limited to the specific EDs with no definitive evidence of spillover into other areas of function.

Both groups showed an overall decline in physical health status during the year despite meticulous medical care. Thus improved physical health status was not a prerequisite for improvement in other spheres of functioning. Significant death predictors indicated that those who died had at baseline greater incapacities in interpersonal responsiveness, bowel control, self-care, and psychological functioning. They also had been viewed by the physicians and psychiatrists prior to treatment as being in greater need of care and supervision than the survivors (21).

The main predictors of favorable response to treatment were personality traits of the subjects (68,69). Those who profited the most were those with characteristics described within the "aggression" factor, which accounted for 60% of the prediction of improvement in their EDs. Apparently these "fighters" were able to improve when the project structure offered help to retrieve functions; the treatment capitalized on the constructive aspect of the behavior of this traditionally hard-to-care-for group.

The personality studies of the project strongly supported the continuity of personality over time, even for women in advanced old age with moderate to severe COBS. Although there was diminished functioning on the 50 personality traits rated for their middle years and for the time of the study, they were essentially the same. An interesting finding was that the personality factor labeled "emotional investment in family and people" had risen in relative importance from the middle years to impaired old age. That the need for emotional closeness becomes more visible and more important may relate to the loss of other functions. In any case, it again attests to the centrality of family relationships and underlines the importance of treatment, taking note of the finding that improvement in such relationships is possible even at such a late hour in the family life cycle.

The project also provided evidence that families continue their involvement with their elderly relatives after institutionalization. Eighty percent of the "significant others" visited at least once weekly and reported discussing a wide range of subjects with the impaired old people. However, the more deeply impaired the resident, the shorter and less enjoyable were the visits (92). Research elsewhere indicated that there is continuity of the amount of family involvement with the older person before and after admission; the number of visits were not related to the amount of impairment, but enjoyment of those visits diminished significantly when the older person was mentally deteriorated (128).

After termination of the treatment in the PGC project, an additional study followed the same individuals longitudinally to determine long-range effects. Nine months after cessation of the experimental treatment the gains in EDs made by the experimental subjects had dissipated substantially (20). When reporting their findings, the investigators emphasized that such findings do not imply "failure" of that or any treatment program. No other treatment modality with this population has demonstrated maintenance of gains without sustained treatment input. The nature of chronicity dictates continuing treatment rather than an inappropriate orientation to "cure."

During the course of the longitudinal study, a new instrument was tested that was developed at the PGC to assess cognitive functioning (76). A previously developed instrument, the widely used Kahn-Goldfarb-Pollak Mental Status Questionnaire (MSQ) correlates significantly with psychiatric diagnosis of COBS (62) and is predictive of death in an institutional setting (43). However, many of the severely impaired are not able to respond to any of the items at all (79). The Extended Mental Status Questionnaire (EMSQ) was developed to discriminate among those severely impaired. It adds to the 10 questions of the Kahn-Goldfarb MSQ 16 new items which tap areas suspected to be less vulnerable to erosion: family relationships, orientation to the immediate institutional environment, and meaningful religious/cutlural past events (76). Although tested with a small, homogeneous population in the project, it differentiated well among the subjects. The group showed strong linear declines in cognitive functioning over a 4-year span. The total set of 26 questions was better able to identify decreases in functioning than either the 10 Kahn-Goldfarb questions alone or the new 16 items alone (91).

The longitudinal study also included behavioral observations of the elderly subjects over a 2-year period. Contrary to popular expectations, and despite the declines in physical health and cognitive functioning, only 37% of the group declined in terms of concrete behavioral functioning. A similar proportion remained stable in that respect, and the remainder actually improved. Baseline predictors of decline proved to have been more psychopathology, more serious medical conditions, and less comprehension of the immediate living environment (70).

CLINICAL REPORTS OF TREATMENTS

There are many descriptive reports of a host of other treatments such as remotivation, behavior modification, resocialization, sensory retraining, and self-image therapy. There is also a long inventory of activity therapies based on productive, creative, or diversional pursuits enjoyed by people of any age or health status, e.g., dance, arts, crafts, movement, music, work, writing. A recent report from England emphasizes the "support of the intellect of the person who is showing dementia." The program uses many techniques such as an interdisciplinary team, development of 24-hr individualized programs, memory cues, a prosthetic physical environment, communication therapy, and a variety of activities (52).

Although a search of the literature fails to reveal any programs that report failure, that statement is not to be interpreted as deprecating them. Clinical experience and descriptive reports are important resources and should not be ignored in the search for psychosocial treatment methodologies. It is likely that all of the programs did indeed achieve some success for some people. Experience at the PGC leads us to believe that any specific treatment element is successful to the extent that it taps the individual's past experiences, interests, skills, preferences, culture, and residual healthy areas of function. Since, like all people, those with COBS respond to different stimuli, this should be reflected by variety in programming. Further, the ever-changing characteristics of the institutionalized as new cohorts of older people are admitted indicate programming that is flexible in responding to those changing needs and interests.

Beyond the intrinsic importance of any particular treatment element, success may be attributed in part to the fact that all the programs inevitably involve the stimulation of increased relationships, contact, and interest on the part of staff. The positive effects on staff attitudes that result from active treatment efforts speak not only to the benefits that therefore accrue to the residents but to the value of such programs in adding interest and status to jobs that are in the main ill paid and unattractive in a field that has difficulty recruiting and retaining personnel.

Regarding families of the institutionalized, the clinical literature has described the interlocking of the well-being of family members in all generations with the well-being of the institutionalized older person (12,23,35,88,102,109). The focus on the older person therefore should not obscure the experiences of family members and their need for help during the stressful time preceding institutionalization, the emotional crises of decision-making, and the relocation of their relative. Their need for help continues with ongoing problems related to the institutionalized relative and ultimately in their bereavement.

In addition to ongoing social services addressed to these matters, there are at the PGC and some other facilities many special family groups designed to: (a) mitigate the negative psychosocial concomitants of institutionalizing an elderly family member with COBS; (b) involve them positively in institutional programs; and (c) give them information about the nature and management of that particular form of mental impairment. Much in demand is a booklet designed for families that was inspired by Weinberg's paper "What Do I Say to My Mother When I Have Nothing to Say" (127).

The absence of family also has program implications. Since many institutional residents do not have close family members or do not have them close at hand, special services are required to replace that serious lack.

DISCUSSION OF TREATMENT PROGRAMS

Review of treatment efforts, whether clinical or experimental, must conclude that no dramatic breakthroughs have been achieved. No form of psycho/social/behavioral treatment has demonstrated any cure or reversal of the organic damage that afflicts this population. Certainly, much research is required, and research strategies have been suggested regarding institutions in general and specific treatment interventions in particular (47,67,80,84). Kahn and Zaritt (63) point out a variety of research problems, including the confounding of different institutional populations.

At the same time it is apparent that much can be done to improve functioning and quality of life for this group and their families. Therapeutic nihilism is unjustified and probably flows from inappropriate and unrealistic expectations and goals. Cohen (29) states that pessimistic therapeutic attitudes err in attributing homogeneity, rather than wide variation, to the degree, manifestation, and course of COBS. In light of hard evidence that this group is responsive to such stresses as relocation and negative institutional environments, it is a peculiar assumption that it is impervious and unresponsive to positive treatment efforts. Can it be that only negative stimuli penetrate the barrier of that disease?

Pessimism regarding treatment potential also may rest on inappropriate goals such as "cure" or "improvement" measured with a yardstick calibrated to other populations. Small gains, maintenance of existing function, and retardation of decline are also legitimate goals, as are the introduction of interest, enjoyment, and some degree of psychic/emotional comfort. The criterion for success in treating a chronic illness should not be improvement that is maintained when treatment is withdrawn. A related error is the expectation of spillover from treatment of a targeted deficit. The apathetic, withdrawn, mentally impaired resident who is stimulated to some social participation or enjoyment of a recreational activity will not suddenly recover from incapacitating arthritis or resume personal self-care functions.

The weight of accumulated evidence makes a powerful argument for social, recreational, and work-oriented activities. The need is in marked contrast to evidence that most of the waking hours of nursing home residents are spent doing nothing at all, and that staff interacts with residents less than 9% of the time (46).

STATUS OF BASIC SERVICES

Experimental treatment programs do not substitute for, but must go hand-in-hand with, skilled interdisciplinary professional services in a favorable psycho-social and physical milieu that includes a prosthetic and attractive physical environment, positive optimistic respectful staff attitudes, support of social relationships, good basic care and services, and the utilization of teams whose members represent different perspectives. Those with senile dementia are not exempt from the concept of the whole person, which has been one of the major philosophical thrusts of this century.

Regarding the physical environment, some aspects of care are a matter of right. Privacy, respect, dignity, control over one's life to the fullest possible extent, and opportunity for choices are *rights* to be enforced for people of all ages, sick or well, institutionalized or in the community. Those rights are now too often denied the population with whom this volume is concerned.

Needed health services are often absent. Surveys that describe the health and functional characteristics of the population at any given moment do not reveal whether treatment can improve their functioning. However, there is no doubt but that gross undertreatment is widespread. Lawton juxtaposed data from a survey of institutional services with those from a survey of SNFs which counted those residents actually receiving certain services. He concluded that fewer than one-third of those needing physical therapy actually received it, and only 11% of those in need received occupational and speech therapy (77). Other measures of services are that 29% of SNF residents had not been seen by a physician during the previous 2 months, and only 10% of homes had a registered nurse in charge of all three shifts. The Long-Term Care Facility Improvement Study (118) reported that one-third of the recorded diagnoses (e.g., decubi, fractures, genitourinary and respiratory infections) may be directly linked to the quality of care. Chronic brain syndrome was on the list of underreported impairments. Only 6% of all facilities surveyed met all Life Safety Code requirements.

In the main, psychiatric services in nursing homes are conspicuous by their absence, a situation that was deplored by the report of the American Psychiatric Association (41). That report also spoke to the need for full-time trained social work and activity personnel.

The Long-Term Care Facility Improvement Study's indictment of the existing psychosocial environments and services was also severe. "In the greater number of facilities there was very little understanding of the importance of psychosocial services. The goal of enriching the daily environment . . . was frequently cited in the policies, but rarely implemented" (118). Fewer than half of the residents have psychosocial data recorded on their charts. The study stated that one-fourth of SNFs had full-time and another fourth part-time employees performing social work, and that 44% had activities coordinators and 28% activities consultants. However, those data are not informative about the actual extent of services, since the Social Security Act's Conditions of Participation (405.1130 Social Services) require only that a facility has "satisfactory arrangements for identifying the medically related social and emotional needs of the patient." Neither the social work "designee" nor the activities worker need be professionals; someone on staff in another capacity or a parttime consultant can fulfill the requirements. It is estimated that only a small minority of facilities, primarily those under voluntary auspices, have a full-time professional social worker (66).

Where there are activities staff, because of their limited number and inadequate skills, the greatest portion of program time is devoted to working with alert, mobile patients, rather than those who are room-bound or a "problem," a categorization that surely includes those with senile dementia (118). In short, those who need more get less.

All of these issues and others relate to one of the major planning and research tasks ahead: the exploration of new models of institutional care that would put the critical elements together in new ways. If this is to be done, it is necessary to put aside the fruitless territorial debate about the appropriateness of the medical versus the social model. The desirability of a social/health model as the goal has been underscored by three recent international conferences.[9] That model implies profound renovations in the physical environment, staff roles and attitudes, and the total institutional life style, as well as the testing of new experimental treatment programs. Institutions are living arrangements, and the role of the full-time professional patient should not be the only role an individual plays over the long years of residence, a role symbolized by the constant characterization of the resident as a patient.

In this, the institutional issue reflects the broader issue regarding long-term care that exists in most countries, i.e., the jurisdictional dispute between social and health authorities (65). The summary of one major conference stated: "Perhaps the single and most pervasive theme throughout the discussion was the deficiencies and dangers of applying a strictly medical model based on acute episodic care to long-term care" (93). Nevertheless, from a practical standpoint the medical model prevails in long-term care in institutions and in the community, with the physician made the gate-keeper whether he will or no. This direction is reinforced by federal regulations that leave no options.

SOCIAL CONTEXT OF INSTITUTIONAL CARE

Another set of issues concerning institutional care are broad social issues such as the share of the national dollar that should be allocated to it, the

---

[9] The Long-Term Care Data Conference in Tuscon, Arizona in May 1975; the Conference on Care of the Elderly, Meeting the Challenge of Dependency, co-sponsored by the U.S. Institute of Medicine of the National Academy of Medicine and the Royal Society of Medicine in Washington, D.C., May 1976; and the Institut de la Vie's Conference on Aging: A Challenge to Science and Society, April 1977, in Vichy, France.

nature of auspices that should be encouraged, regulation and quality control, and legislation. Although not within the scope of this chapter, these issues cannot be separated from treatment. Thus the number and types of personnel and the nature of treatment programs that are required or can be mounted are related to reimbursement and governmental regulations. Similarly, aspects of physical design are dictated by the Life Safety Code and other criteria set by the three levels of government.

In any event, a focus on specific treatments for elderly institutional residents with senile dementia is self-defeating unless viewed in the context of the macrocosm of the community as well as the microcosm of the particular facility. Attempts to "treat" must go forward on many levels. Just as the whole institution in every one of its aspects is part of treatment, so too is the system part of treatment. It is not necessary to await the fruits of badly needed research or of a major biomedical breakthrough to bring order to the chaotic long-term care nonsystem, to begin to modify institutional environments in the indicated directions, and to improve the quality of life within them. The broad system of long-term care should include community service to individuals and families to prevent or interrupt the downward spiral of decline, orderly decision-making, a range of facilities to meet varying needs, services to avert unnecessary relocation and to mitigate the effects when relocation is a practical necessity, and an institutional environment that supports psychosocial as well as physical functioning.

After looking at the long-term care scene at present, the conclusion is inescapable that in the main it is nontherapeutic, even antitherapeutic. To treat the group about which we are concerned, we must also treat professional and popular attitudes, and mount educational programs for all levels of staff and the general public. Any review of treatment methods therefore must take note of the general conditions under which this population now lives. Clinical and research efforts will have been in vain if we let persist the abuses that erupt periodically as scandals, make headlines and feature stories, are investigated, engender governmental commissions and reports, and are then forgotten.

Finally, the fact that this chapter dwelled on the deficiencies of care for the institutionalized older people in general and those with senile dementia in particular should not be interpreted as pessimism. Experience with that population indicates a responsiveness to high quality, thoughtful treatment and a capacity for improvement in well-being. As for the broader picture, the fact that this volume is being published is a signal that there is hope for these uniquely deprived human beings who cannot themselves articulate their needs.

REFERENCES

1. Aldrich, C. K. (1964): *Gerontologist,* 4:92–93.
2. Anderson, N. (1969): *Policy Issues Regarding Nursing Homes.* Institute for Interdisciplinary Studies, Minneapolis.
3. APA Hospital and Community Psychiatry Service (undated): *Reality Orientation.* APA, Washington, D.C.

4. Arnoff, F. N. (1975): *Science,* 188:1277–1281.
5. Barnes, J. (1974): *Gerontologist,* 14:138–142.
6. Bennett, R., and Eisdorfer, C. (1975): In: *Long-Term Care: A Handbook for Researchers, Planners and Providers,* edited by S. Sherwood, pp. 391–454. Spectrum, New York.
7. Bennett, R., and Nahemow, L. (1965): In: *Mental Impairment in the Aged,* edited by M. P. Lawton and F. G. Lawton. Philadelphia Geriatric Center, Philadelphia.
8. *Boarding Home Conference* (1973): YWCA, Philadelphia (mimeo).
9. Brody, E. M. (1978): *Ann. Am. Acad. Polit. Soc. Sci.,* pp. 13–27.
10. Brody, E. M. (1978): *Aged Parents and Aging Children.* Presented at National Conference on You and Your Aging Parents, Ethel Percy Andrus Gerontology Center, University of Southern California, Los Angeles.
11. Brody, E. M. (1978): *Gerontologist,* 18:121–128.
12. Brody, E. M. (1977): *Long-Term Care of Older People: A Practical Guide.* Human Sciences Press, New York.
13. Brody, E. M. (1977): *Gerontologist,* 17:520–522.
14. Brody, E. M. (1977): In: *Care of the Elderly: Meeting the Challenge of Dependency,* edited by A. N. Exton-Smith and J. G. Evans. Academic Press, London.
15. Brody, E. M. (1973): *Gerontologist,* 13:430–435.
16. Brody, E. M. (1969): *Gerontologist,* 9:187–196.
17. Brody, E. M. (1967): *Geriatr. Dig.,* 4:25–32.
18. Brody, E. M. (1966): *Gerontologist,* December:201–206.
19. Brody, E. M., and Gummer, B. (1967): *Gerontologist,* 7:234–243.
20. Brody, E. M., Kleban, M. H., Lawton, M. P., and Moss, M. (1974): *J. Gerontol.,* 29:79–84.
21. Brody, E. M., Kleban, M. H., Lawton, M. P., Levy, R., and Woldow, A. (1972): *J. Chronic Dis.,* 25:611–620.
22. Brody, E. M., Kleban, M. H., Lawton, M. P., and Silverman, H. (1971): *Gerontologist,* 11:124–133.
23. Brody, E. M., and Spark, G. (1966): *Family Process,* 5:76–90.
24. Brody, S. J., Poulshock, S. W., and Masciocchi, C. F. (1978): *Gerontologist,* 18:556–561.
25. Califano, J. A., Jr. (1978): *Ann. Am. Acad. Political Social Sci.,* pp. 96–107.
26. Camp, W. P. (1965): In: *Mental Impairment in the Aged,* edited by M. P. Lawton and F. G. Lawton, pp. 130–137. Philadelphia Geriatric Center, Philadelphia.
27. Chalfen, L. (1956): *J. Genet. Psychol.,* 88:261–276.
28. Citron, R. S., and Dixon, D. N. (1977): *Gerontologist,* 17:39–43.
29. Cohen, G. D. (1978): *Gerontologist,* 18:313–314.
30. Colligan, D. (1975): *New York Magazine,* July 14:28–32.
31. Corsellis, J. A. N. (1962): *Mental Illness and the Aging Brain.* Oxford University Press, London.
32. Cosin, L. Z. (1957): *Int. J. Social Psychiatry,* 3:195–202.
33. Cosin, L. Z., Mort, M., Post, F., Westropp, C., and Williams, M. (1958): *Int. J. Social Psychiatry,* 4:24–42.
34. Cramer, P. K. (1978): In: *Commentaries on Human Services Issues.* Health and Welfare Council, Philadelphia.
35. Dobrof, R., and Litwak, E. (1977): *Maintenance of Family Ties of Long-Term Care Patients: Theory and Guide to Practice,* U.S. Government Printing Office, Washington, D.C.
36. Doll, W. (1976): *Hosp. Community Psychiatry,* 27:No. 3.
37. Donahue, W., Hunter, W. W., and Coons, D. (1953): *Geriatrics,* 8:656–666.
38. Epstein, L., and Simon, A. (1968): *Am. J. Psychiatry,* 124:955–961.
39. Folsom, J. C. (1968): *J. Geriatr. Psychiatry,* 1:291–307.
40. Friedsam, H. J., and Dick, H. R. (1963): Decisions leading to institutionalization of the aged. Unpublished final Report, Social Security Administration Cooperative Research and Demonstration Grant Program, Project 037(C1) 20–031.
41. Glasscote, R. M. (1976): *Old Folks at Homes: A Field Study of Nursing and Board-and-Care Homes.* American Psychiatric Association and the National Association for Mental Health, Joint Information Service, Washington, D.C.
42. Goffman, E. (1962): *Asylums.* Aldine, Chicago.
43. Goldfarb, A. I. (1961): In: *Psychopathology of Aging,* edited by P. H. Hock and J. Zubin. Grune & Stratton, New York.
44. Gottesman, L. E. (1974): *Am. J. Public Health,* March:269–276.

45. Gottesman, L. E. (1971): *Report to Respondents.* Nursing Home Project, Philadelphia Geriatric Center, Philadelphia.
46. Gottesman, L. E., and Bourestom, N. C. (1974): *Gerontologist,* 14:501–506.
47. Gottesman, L. E., and Brody, E. M. (1975): In: *Long-Term Care: A Handbook for Researchers, Planners and Providers,* edited by S. Sherwood, pp. 455–510. Spectrum, New York.
48. Grad, J., and Sainsbury, P. (1966): *Milbank Mem. Fund Q.* 44:246–278.
49. Grintzig, L. (1970): *Selected Characteristics of Residents in Long-Term Care Institutions,* Long-Term Care Monograph No. 5 (mimeo). Research Division, Department of Health Care Administration, George Washington University, Washington, D.C.
50. Harris, C. S. and Ivory, P. B. C. B. (1976): *Gerontologist,* 16:496–503.
51. Health Resources Administration, Division of Long-Term Care (1977): In: *The Report of the Task Force,* HSA, Washington, D.C.
52. *Help Age International* (1978): Vegetables brought to life. No. 8, March-April.
53. Holmes, T. H., and Masuda, M. (1974): In: *Stressful Life Events: Their Nature and Effects,* edited by B. S. Dohrenwend and B. P. Dohrenwend. Wiley, New York.
54. Ibsen, E. (1963): *Besketigelses Terapeuten,* 24 (9).
55. Jarvik, L. F. (1976): *Aging and Mental Health: Research Needs* (mimeo). December.
56. Jefferys, M. (1977): In: *Care of the Elderly: Meeting the Challenge of Dependency,* edited by A. N. Exton-Smith and E. J. Grimley, pp. 5–20. Grune & Stratton, New York.
57. Kahana, E. (1971): Effects of matching institutional environments and needs of the aged. Presented at the Annual Meeting of the Gerontological Society, Houston.
58. Kahana, E., Kahana, B., and Jacobs, K. (1970): Functionally integrated therapy programs for the elderly. Presented at the Meeting of the Gerontological Society, Toronto.
59. Kahn, A. J., and Kamerman, S. B. (1976): *Social Services in Institutional Perspective,* U.S. Government Printing Office, Washington, D.C.
60. Kahn, R. L. (1965): In: *Proceedings of the York House Institute on the Mentally Impaired Aged,* edited by M. P. Lawton and F. G. Lawton. Philadelphia Geriatric Center, Philadelphia.
61. Kahn, R. L., Goldfarb, A. I., Pollack, M., and Gerber, I. E. (1960): *Am. J. Psychiatry,* 117:120–124.
62. Kahn, R. L., Pollack, M., and Goldfarb, A. J. (1961): In: *Psychopathology of Aging,* edited by P. H. Hoch and J. Zubin. Grune & Stratton, New York.
63. Kahn, R. L., and Zaritt, S. (1973): Evaluation of mental health programs for the aged. Presented at the 5th Banff International Conference on Behavior Modification.
64. Kamerman, S. B. (1976): *Gerontologist,* 16:529–537.
65. Kane, R. L., and Kane, R. A. (1976): *Long-Term Care in Six Countries: Implications for the United States.* Fogarty International Center, Proceedings No. 33. U.S. Government Printing Office, Washington, D.C.
66. Kaplan, J. (1975): *Gerontologist,* 15:280–281.
67. Katz, D., and Kahn, R. L. (1966): *The Social Psychology of Organization.* Wiley, New York.
68. Kleban, M. H., and Brody, E. M. (1972): *J. Gerontol,* 27:69–76.
69. Kleban, M. H., Brody, E. M., Lawton, M. P. (1971): *Gerontologist,* Part I:134–140.
70. Kleban, M. H., Lawton, M. P., Brody, E. M., and Moss, M. (1976): *J. Gerontol.,* 31:333–339.
71. Kleemeier, R. W. (1961): In: *Aging and Leisure: A Research Perspective into the Meaningful Use of Time,* edited by R. W. Kleemeier. Oxford University Press, New York.
72. Kosberg, J. I. (1973): *Gerontologist,* 13:299–304.
73. Kramer, M., Taube, C. A., and Redick, R. W. (1973): In: *The Psychology of Adult Development and Aging,* edited by C. Eisdorfer and M. P. Lawton, pp. 428–528. American Psychological Association, Washington, D.C.
74. Laurie, W. F. (1978): In: *Advances in Research,* Vol. 2, No. 2. Duke University, Center for the Study of Aging and Human Development, Durham, N.C.
75. Laverty, R. (1950): *J. Gerontol.,* 5:370–374.
76. Lawton, M. P. (1980): In preparation.
77. Lawton, M. P. (1978): *Health Social Work,* 3:109–134.
78. Lawton, M. P. (1972): In: *Research, Planning and Action for the Elderly,* edited by D. P. Kent, R. Kastenbaum, and S. Sherwood, pp. 122–143. Behavioral Publications, New York.
79. Lawton, M. P. (1971): *J. Am. Geriatr. Soc.,* 19:465–481.
80. Lawton, M. P. (1970): *Gerontologist,* 10:305–312.

81. Lawton, M. P., and Lawton, F. (eds.) (1965): *Mental Impairment in the Aged: Institute on the Mentally Impaired Aged.* Philadelphia Geriatric Center, Philadelphia.

82. Lawton, M. P., and Nahemow, L. (1973): In: *The Psychology of Adult Development and Aging,* edited by C. Eisdorfer and M. P. Lawton, pp. 619–674. American Psychological Association, Washington, D.C.

83. Letcher, P. B., Peterson, L. P., and Scarbrough, D. (1974): *Hosp. Commun. Psychiatry,* 25:801–803.

84. Lieberman, M. (1969): *J. Gerontol.,* 24:330–340.

85. Lieberman, M. A., Prock, V. N., and Tobin, S. S. (1968): *J. Gerontol.,* 3:343–353.

86. Lieberman, M. A., Tobin, S. S., and Slover, D. (1971): The effects of relocation on long-term geriatric patients. Final Report to Department of Mental Health, State of Illinois, Project No. 17-328 (mimeo).

87. Liebowitz, B. (1974): *Gerontologist,* 14:293–295.

88. Locker, R., and Rublin, A. (1974): *Gerontologist,* 14:295–299.

89. Lowenthal, M. F., Berkman, P., et al. (1967): *Aging and Mental Disorder in San Francisco: A Social Psychiatric Study.* Jossey-Bass, San Francisco.

90. Marlowe, R. A. (1973): Effects of environment on elderly state hospital relocatees. Presented at 44th Annual Meeting of the Pacific Sociological Association, Scottsdale, Arizona (mimeo).

91. Moss, M. S., Kleban, M. H., Brody, E. M., and Lawton, M. P. (1972): Longitudinal measurement of cognitive functioning in the mentally impaired aged. Presented at 25th Annual Meeting of the Gerontological Society, San Juan, Puerto Rico.

92. Moss, M., and Kurland, P. (1979): *J. Gerontol. Social Work,* 1:271–278.

93. Murnaghan, J. H. (1976): *Med. Care,* 14(Suppl.):1–25.

94. Nathanson, B. F., and Reingold, J. (1969): *Gerontologist,* 9:293–295.

95. Nusberg, C. (1978): Data supplied to the author, October.

96. Phillips, D. F. (1973): *Hospitals,* July 1.

97. Pollak, W. (1976): In: *Community Planning for an Aging Society,* edited by M. P. Lawton, R. J. Newcomer, and T. O. Byerts, pp. 106–127. Dowden, Hutchinson and Ross, Stroudsburg, Pa.

98. Rahe, R. H. (1974): In: *Stressful Life Events: Their Nature and Effects,* edited by B. S. Dohrenwend, and B. P. Dohrenwend, pp. 73–86. Wiley, New York.

99. Roberts, P. R. (1972): *Human Warehouses: A Boarding Home Study.* Congressional Record, April 11, pp. E3515–E3518.

100. Rosow, I. (1963): In: *Processes of Aging,* edited by R. H. Williams, C. Tibbitts, and W. Donahue. Atherton Press, New York.

101. Rothschild, D., and Sharp, M. L. (1941): *Dis. Nerv. Syst.,* 2:49–54.

102. Safford, F. (1980): *Developing a Training Program for Families of the Mentally Impaired Aged.* Isabella Geriatric Center, New York.

103. Selye, H. (1970): *J. Am. Geriatr. Soc.,* 18:669–680.

104. Shanas, E., and Maddox, G. L. (1976): In: *Handbook of Aging and the Social Sciences,* edited by G. L. Maddox and E. Shanas, pp. 592–614. Van Nostrand, Reinhold Company, New York.

105. Sherman, S. R., and Newman, E. S. (1977): *Gerontologist,* 17:513–520.

106. Silverstone, B. (1978): Testimony at public hearings held by the Health Care Financing Administration of the Department of Health, Education and Welfare, July 19, Washington, D.C.

107. Smith, B. J., and Barker, H. R. (1972): *Gerontologist,* 12:262–264.

108. Soldo, B. J., and Myers, G. C. (1976): The effects of life-time fertility on the living arrangements of older women. Presented at the Annual Meeting of the Gerontological Society, October, New York.

109. Spark, G., and Brody, E. M., (1970): *Family Process,* 9:195–210.

110. Stotsky, B. (1967): *J. Genet. Psychol.,* 3:113–117.

111. Stotsky, B. (1967): *Genet. Psychol. Monogr.,* 76:257–320.

112. *Supportive Services* (Care Reports, Inc.) (1977): June 24, pp. 1–2.

113. Townsend, P. (1965): In: *Social Structure and the Family: Generational Relations,* edited by E. Shanos and G. Streib, pp. 163–187. Prentice-Hall, Englewood Cliffs, N.J.

114. Turner, H., Tobin, S., and Lieberman, M. A. (1972): *J. Gerontol.,* 27:61–68.

115. U.S. Bureau of the Census (1978): *1976 Survey of Institutionalized Persons: A Study of Persons Receiving Long Term Care.* June. Washington, D.C.

116. U.S. Department of Health, Education and Welfare (1978): Na
March.

117. U.S. Department of Health, Education and Welfare (1968): Nat
Mental Health Statistical Note No. 146, March.

118. U.S. Department of Health, Education and Welfare (1975): Ir
provement Study, Introductory Report. U.S. Government Prir
D.C.

119. U.S. Department of Labor (1978): Bureau of Labor Statistics,

120. U.S. National Center for Health Statistics (1978): *Advance De
Home Residents and Discharges from the 1977 National Nursing*
U.S. Department of Health, Education and Welfare, PHS, No.

121. U.S. National Center for Health Statistics (1978): *Advance Di
Home Characteristics: Provisional Data from the 1977 National*
Department of Health, Education and Welfare, PHS, No. 35, Se

122. U.S. National Center for Health Statistics (1973): *National Heal:
Residents in Nursing Homes and Personal Care Homes,* U.S. Jur
No. 19, HSMHA.

123. U.S. National Center for Health Statistics (1975): *Preliminary Da
tional Nursing Home Survey.*

124. U.S. National Committee on Vital and Health Statistics (1978):
Minimum Data Set, Preliminary Report of the Technical Consu
Term Health Care Data Set, PHS, NCHS, September 8.

125. U.S. Senate Special Committee on Aging, Subcommittee on Long-T
Home Care in the United States: Failure in Public Policy, Introductory
Printing Office, Washington, D.C.

126. Waldman, A. (1965): In: *Selected Papers, Fifth Annual Conference
Aging.* U.S. Government Printing Office, Washington, D.C.

127. Weinberg, J. (1974): *Geriatrics,* 29(11):155–159.

128. York, J. L., and Calsyn, R. J. (1977): *Gerontologist,* 17:500–505.

*Clinical Aspects of Alzheimer's Disease and
Senile Dementia,* (Aging, Vol. 15), edited by
Nancy E. Miller and Gene D. Cohen.
Raven Press, New York 1981.

The Social Strategy of Disease Control:
The Case of Senile Dementia

Odin W. Anderson

Center for Health Administration Studies, University of Chicago, Chicago, Illinois 60637

Previous chapters in this volume have presented in great detail the psychological, neurological, and physiological characteristics of patients with senile dementia. Others have considered formal and informal medical and social supporting
services such as the role of and the effect on the family.

Perhaps it would be useful to place this problem in the framework of formulating and implementing public policy to cope with senile dementia, drawing on
the rather fragmentary data on costs, family structure, the helping services,
and the social and political system through which we deal with health and
welfare problems. The continuing tendency seems to be to present data on
disease characteristics, including need/demand for services, and possible costs
and then assume that the solutions are self-evident and that a rational society
will react accordingly. We know that this is not true but we nevertheless seem
to believe that society is completely plastic. Given competing interests, differential
perceptions, and scarce resources in relation to all our wants, we use either
the private market, where choices are made by buyers, or the political market,
where choices are made by voters, or a combination of both. More precisely,
people who are classified as suffering from senile dementia are a small minority
in relation to all voters and, even worse, are incapable of voting. They then
need friends in court and in the political market. Thus far, senile dementia
has not received the interest shown other more politically prestigious illnesses
such as kidney disease, heart disease, and cancer.

Rarely, then, are health and welfare problems analyzed carefully and data
related to the social, economic, and political crucible in which policy is formulated and programs implemented. Regarding particular diseases, common sense
would dictate that each disease require a strategy of control and management
more or less peculiar to that disease—ease of diagnosis, specificity of therapy,
curability, and preventability, or if it were not either curable or preventable,
possibilities for stabilization, incidence, and prevalence, age group and sex most
affected, and even parts of the body. Such data should be used to formulate
public policy and programs, taking into consideration resources in personnel

and facilities, costs, methods of finance, and special interests in the body politic that are supportive, or indifferent, or even hostile.

A certain tradition in the history of public health is embodied in an annual volume, *Control of Communicable Diseases in Man,* which in 1915 listed 38 communicable infectious diseases and by 1965 presented 148. It is a manual detailing incubation time, period of communicability, modes of transmission, and recommendations for control. The manual revealed more knowledge of the behavior of microbes than the behavior of humans and political systems (5).

Several years ago I made a study of the history of syphilis control in the United States since World War I (1). The spread of syphilis is a product of a certain type of human behavior that if stopped completely for 2 years would break the chain of infection. To suggest seriously total abstinence as a public policy would, of course, be ludicrous. Short of this drastic step, nevertheless, I despaired that we could wipe out syphilis because of our value of individual privacy which inhibits inquiring about sex partners. I concluded, not whimsically, that a certain incidence of syphilis was necessary for a certain degree of individual privacy and civil liberties. What are the characteristics of senile dementia and what does it imply for public policy and program formulation?

CHARACTERISTICS OF SENILE DEMENTIA BEARING ON SOCIAL STRATEGY

Let me select the salient characteristics of senile dementia that have a direct bearing on social strategy of control and management (2,3,4,6,8,11–13,22).

1. People with senile dementia present a ponderous behavior problem regarding self-care, perceptions of reality, age, independence, and size and weight. They need to be taken care of like small children, but to make matters worse they are bigger and heavier, and have had a history of self-reliance that lingers. It requires drastic adjustment on the part of healthy adults to handle other adults as incompetent individuals.

2. A characteristic of senile dementia is progressive deterioration. This characteristic places extreme strain on the helping professions and next of kin. In fact, a basically religious attitude of inevitability and its compassionate and stoic acceptance is required.

3. The great majority of those with this diagnosis are 65 years of age and over; most are 80 and over. The pressures on our still fragmenting nuclear family are intense. The nuclear family—father, mother, and children—are geared to an outside-of-the-home workaday world and not to the care and nurturance of old parents, grandparents, and increasingly, even great-grandparents who are sick and deteriorating. Indeed, the nuclear family finds it difficult to care for short, acute illnesses in the home, let alone long-term intractable ones.

Some descriptive statistics will help to quantify the problem for social strategy and public policy purposes. Indeed, given the current undeveloped level of social strategy thinking, I believe we have enough data to gain a perception of the overall problem and to suggest tentative social strategies as the body politic becomes increasingly aware of possible approaches. All data point in the same direction—grimness and exceedingly difficult answers.

The actual number of people suffering from senile dementia is not known with any degree of precision. In fact, there are differences of opinions among psychiatrists about definitions. For policy purposes this lack of precision should not cause concern unless Congress attempts to force the health field into precise definitions for particular program purposes, as in renal dialysis and black lung pensions. Even then we should be candid and not play with numbers.

I am quite satisfied, however, that we know with sufficient precision for social strategy purposes the proportion of people 65 years of age and over who need total surveillance daily. Certainly it can be assumed that senile dementia is a subgroup of this element of the population. This group is a hidden segment of a serious problem because they are a relatively small minority who are not reached adequately by the general provisions of Medicare and Medicaid and the social services.

Careful estimates from national household surveys reveal that 12 to 14% of the population 65 years of age and over can be left by themselves for only short periods of time. Shanas (12) estimates that among the older population who are not institutionalized, 10% of all older persons interviewed (8% of all men and 12% of all women) were "very sick." These include all conditions. Referring mainly to the American scene, although this survey was conducted over 20 years ago, I am assuming that a similar survey today would not yield significantly different figures for policy purposes. There have been no medical breakthroughs to affect the sick aged in this respect. Indeed, some of the high technology and chemotherapy may well have perpetuated more physically and psychologically dependent aged today than 20 years ago. This has been suggested by Gruenberg (6), who demonstrated in a Scandinavian sample that the greater increase in the life span has occurred in the sickest persons, probably because of the introduction of sulfa drugs.

Using 10% as the base figure for those interviewed in their homes, older persons in institutions should also be added. This latter group is usually estimated at 4 to 5% of the persons 65 years of age and over. Thus the total is approximately 14 to 15% of this age group. In another household survey in the United States conducted concurrently with comparable surveys in Great Britain and Denmark in 1962, Shanas estimates that 8% of the elderly population living at home are bedfast and housebound or both (13). If the institutional population in this age group is added, the total percentage then approaches 12 to 13. There need be no dispute over specious precision as to what percentage is exactly right. It will suffice to work with a range of 10 to 15%, given the fact that public policy has dealt inadequately if at all with only a small percentage even within this range.

As a compromise, we shall consider a figure of 13% who are bedfast and homebound, both at home and in institutions. In the last estimate of the Bureau of the Census (1975) 10.5% of the population or well over 22 million were 65 years of age and over. The middle-range estimate for 1990 (there are three projections—low, middle, and high) is that 11.8% of the population will be 65 years of age and over, or very close to 29 million. For the year 2000, the percentage seems to be stabilizing at 11.7% given current population trends, but the absolute number will increase to 30,600 million (16). The percentage and absolute number of people 65 years of age and over is significant enough, but even more important is that age groups 75 and 80 and over are increasing faster than younger age groups in the 65 and over category. It was estimated that in 1975 there were almost 4.5 million people 80 years of age and over, in 1990 there will be 6 million, and in the year 2000, 8 million.

Fortunately, and contrary to a stereotype that I believe is no longer held, only a minority of older people are sick or helpless, as is true of the younger elements of the population. A larger and more intractible minority of older people, however, are sick and helpless than younger persons. A crude indication of this is given in provisional data from the 1973–1974 Nursing Home Survey of the National Center for Health Statistics. It is estimated that among primary diagnoses for residents 65 years of age and over in nursing homes, 13.6% are diagnosed "senility, old age, and ill-defined conditions." This diagnosis is applied to 8.5% of the residents between 65 and 74 years of age, and 18.5% of those 85 years of age and over. Associated diagnoses of hardening of the arteries, stroke, and diseases of the nervous system, sense organs and mental disorders, inflates this percentage considerably. Insofar as senile dementia is a specific diagnosis, it obviously becomes lost in this diagnostic maze.

A detailed and recent survey of nursing homes released by the Bureau of the Census reveals that 23% of the patients 65 years of age and over in nursing homes in this country are unable to walk at all, over 11% cannot hear, and about 11% have severe speech handicaps. Of helpless older people living at home, and if we accept Shanas' estimate that 8% of them are bedfast or house-bound or both, we emerge with an absolute figure of 1,700,000 of such patients in that age group. Various estimates of the degree of mental incompetence among people 65 years of age and over is 5%, which rises to 20% among those 80 years of age and over. This means that almost 900,000 persons in this group are regarded as mentally incompetent. I do not pretend that these estimates, or other estimates I have reviewed, are precise, but they are probably adequate for policy formulation at present. It is safe to assume that, at any rate, no program will initially meet the problems optimally.

Current evidence suggests that the modern nuclear family is attempting to cope seriously with its helpless aged members, and that nursing homes and mental institutions are used as a last resort. The pressure on nursing homes resulting from specific legislation occurs concomitantly with changes in family structure and the increasing survival of dependent aged.

Starting with the entire population 65 years of age and over, the Bureau of the Census estimates that 15% of the males and 36% of the females constitute one-person households (16). This does not mean, of course, that they are isolated and not looked after by nearby relatives and friends, but it does mean that a drastic change in their living arrangements becomes necessary as they become dehabilitated (it will be remembered that 4 to 5% are in institutions). In addition, of those under 75 years of age and over, 23% are widowed; for females in the same age group the figure is 69% (19). As a result, a higher proportion of nursing home residents are widowed than those outside of the institutions. Because of greater longevity, the vast proportion of widowed are women.

These data are fragmentary, but even so, reveal that the care and management of long-term illness among the aged crosses medical and social helping services. They occupy a gray area between these professional helping services sectors. Our knowledge of the interrelationships between family structures and the professional helping services, and of the care of the helpless, is exceedingly primitive. Research on these interrelationships is urgently needed in order to fit services, family structure, and helplessness.

ESTIMATES OF COST AND USE OF SERVICES

Again it is difficult, if not impossible, to factor out the costs for health services and their use for senile dementia for reasons already described. A safe assumption, as stated, is that senile dementia patients comprise a subgroup of the 13% of the people 65 years of age and over. The last estimate of total expenditures for personal health services for those in this age group was in the neighborhood of $1,500 a year per person. This was for 1975, but since that time, health care expenditures have increased 30%, resulting in roughly $2,000 per person 65 years of age and over (7). People who have senile dementia probably incur costs considerably in excess of the average of $2,000 per year. For example, nursing homes alone cost about $7,000 a year per inpatient and a significant number of nursing home residents have senile dementia. Because of this, and difficulties with self care and accidents, an estimate of $4,000 per patient is not unrealistic. If I apply this estimate of $4,000 a year to the entire 13% of the aged over 65 who need total care, then $12 billion would be spent for personal health services, exclusive of social services for this group, and $44 billion would be spent for all the aged. Since the total expenditures for the aged is $44 billion and $12 billion is estimated as being spent for the very sick aged, then the very sick aged accounts for 27% of all expenditures. For simplicity then we can speculate that 10% of the total population accounts for 30% of the expenditures, but of this 10%, 13% account for 30% of the expenditures. I take no stock in elaborate model building; thus, my crude method is, I feel, good enough for the purpose.

So far, health legislation has not adopted this kind of estimating for problem amelioration. Medicare, for example, was designed primarily for relatively short-term acute and costly illness episodes. Long-term chronic illness like senile dementia, constitutes not an episode, but a way of life until death with a high and constant drain on health resources. It appears that of the total per capita expenditures for those 65 years of age cared for, 45% goes for general hospital care, 23% for nursing home care, and only 16% for physicians services, leaving another 16% for all other personal health services and goods. Indeed, it can be seen that institutional care accounts for almost 70% of all personal health services for the aged, an exceedingly expensive service component.

So far, the private profit and nonprofit sectors have formed the supply backbone of the American personal health services, with increasing financing for day-to-day services by the various levels of government. In the nursing home industry, the private sector has responded dramatically to changes in legislation regarding reimbursement. A recent survey of nursing homes revealed that 67% of the nursing home beds are privately owned whereas 33% are owned by various levels of government (21). The relative slowness of government to provide the supply is not peculiarly American. All developed countries with some form of national health insurance or national health service have difficulties financially and conceptually in expanding out-of-hospital services to include the increasing number of aged patients with long-term and intractable illness. The difference between the United States and other industrialized countries in Western Europe is that in Europe, government is expected to do almost everything; there is no entrepreneurial concept embedded in the private sector for health services. The governmental programs in Western Europe are ahead only in degree and in part because their populations begin to age earlier than that of the United States (7).

To state a truism, personal health services must have personnel of various types. The more the needs of the patients are care-oriented, particularly long-term care, the more difficult it seems it is to attract the proper type of person. In nursing homes today, for example, there are 45 employees per 100 beds. (General hospitals employ 300 personnel per 100 beds.) Of these 45 employees, 66% are nurses' aides, 13% are licensed practical nurses, and 10% are registered nurses. The remainder, 11%, are administrative, medical, or therapeutic personnel. The lower the skill grade of caring personnel the higher is the annual turnover, and therefore, the greater is the presence of the stranger and discontinuity in care. This characteristic is inherent in the type of service function.

There is a great deal of discussion about the expansion of home-care services, a largely undeveloped service area. Home care for the homebound aged from physician to housekeeping services has eminent logic, but so far there is little knowledge of the nature of the demand, methods of paying for the service, and the possible support services in the homes themselves.

WHAT ARE THE STRATEGIES?

The foregoing data and information do not suggest a social engineering type of solution to the care of the helpless aged of which the senile patients are a part. This problem strains the family, does not arouse enthusiasm among the helping services and the medical and nursing professions, and gets obscured in the political process. It is a problem that ramifies systemically so widely that there is hardly any handle to take hold of which will move it toward neat solutions.

I believe that although important, money itself is of less importance for problem amelioration than the sheer ability of the body politic to face senile dementia realistically and with compassion. I believe that the kind of care the helpless aged need is in essence not purchasable. It is the kind of care that can be expected only of relatives and close friends. It is the kind of personal concern that cannot be expected of strangers short of sisterhoods and brotherhoods and the like who are dedicated to service.

The service concept, directed to caring for others, has eroded during the last couple of generations. I do not mean to romanticize the extent and nature of service and duty of simpler days because families were larger, helping to assure that one of the children would take care of the aging and ailing parents, and then the aging parents obliged by not living as long as they do now. Further, amenity and psychological standards are higher today, straining the helping services financially and psychologically.

In the past, women were regarded as the chief reservoirs of service and duty, but with increased employment outside of the home and fulfillment regarded as residing in an occupation, strangers more and more need to be hired to care for the helpless. For example, in 1940, 36% of the female labor force was married. In 1976 this percentage had increased to 62%. In 1940, 17% of the married females were in the labor force, and in 1975 46% were in the labor force. This shift in women's situations must clearly have an impact on the ability of households to take care of homebound aged (19). I am not making a moral judgment here. All personal and social objectives demand tradeoffs. Institutionalization of the aged is a tradeoff in the range of values that a society tries to attain simultaneously. Concepts of individual self-fulfillment have ramifications.

The health professionals are asked to take more interest in the helpless aged exhorting that the problems they present are more challenging and interesting than appears on the surface. This may be true, but it will require a drastic change in attitude.

In 1972 an article appeared in the *New England Journal of Medicine* by Dr. William D. Poe calling for a new medical specialty called marantology. Marantology is derived from the Greek word *Marantos,* meaning withered, faded, turned, as leaves become withered in the autumn. The primary tenet of marantology would be that it would not accept any patient anybody else wanted. Who would make good marantologists according to Dr. Poe?

> Certainly, the specialty is no place for charisma and youthful dynamism. It is no place for arid manipulators of the status quo. Its practitioners should know that gross abnormalities of fluid, electrolytes, and blood count can become

almost physiologic for a particular person. The marantologist could be curious without satisfying his curiosity. Brain scans and barium enemas are of little use unless they influence the management of the patient. The emphasis is on peace and comfort rather than on diagnostic activism (10).

Given data and information available on senile dementia and the helpless aged, it is difficult to assess the impact of a moonshot type of strategy. It is beyond my knowledge to predict possible breakthroughs in etiological research, where I have doubts about outcomes in the immediate future. So, there has to be action along several fronts simultaneously—Could we expand home care and housekeeping services, meals on wheels, and daycare centers? Perhaps the well-aged could help the helpless aged more. Are we as anomistic and individualistic as we seem to be? Can we turn ourselves around to each other rather than from each other? Funding agencies, private and public, must be satisfied with proposed programs for which specific goals and their attainment cannot be promised given the current state of knowledge. They must accept proposals that are aimed in a general direction.

We need to keep on testing the market with risk capital for sometime to come with what few funding services we want to risk.

Perhaps the foregoing cannot be called a strategy, but I feel that an attitude forms the matrix for a strategy. I am by no means sanguine that we are capable—not to mention willing—as a society—to manage the increasing pressure of the sick aged gracefully. The social system and the family unit are, in my opinion, being overloaded. Still, as compassionate human beings, we must try hard to prevent my prediction from becoming true.

ACKNOWLEDGMENT

The library research assistance of June Farrell Smith is gratefully acknowledged.

REFERENCES

1. Anderson, O. W. (1965): *Syphilis and Society—Problems of Control in the United States, 1912–1964.* RS#22, Center for Health Administration Studies, Chicago.
2. Birren, J. E. (1959): *Handbook of Aging and the Individual, Psychological and Biological Aspects.* University of Chicago Press, Chicago.
3. Birren, J. E. (1964): *The Psychology of Aging,* pp. 270–271. Prentice-Hall, Englewood Cliffs, N.J.
4. Busse, E. W. (1959): Psychopathology. In: *Handbook of Aging and the Indian,* Birren, J. E. (ed.), pp. 377–380. University of Chicago Press, Chicago.
5. Gordon, J. E. (1965): Control of communicable disease in man, golden anniversary of a book. *J. Am. Public Health Assoc.,* 55:4–11.
6. Gruenberg, E. (1977): The failure of success, Milbank Memorial Fund Quarterly, *Health Soc.,* 55(1):3–24.
7. Kane, R. L., and Kane, R. A. (1976): *Long Term Care in Six Countries: Implications for the United States,* pp. 76–1207. John E. Fogarty International Center for Advanced Study in the Health Sciences, DHEW Publications No. (NIH), Washington, D.C.

8. Muller, M. S., and Gibson, R. M. (1976): Age differences in health care spending, FY 1975. *Social Security Bull.*, 39:18–31.
8a. Muller, M. S., and Fisher, C. R. (1977): Age differences in health care spending, FY 1976. *Social Security Bull.*, 40:3–14.
9. Nandy, K. and Sherwin, I. (eds.) (1977): *The Aging Brain and Senile Dementia, Vol. 23, Advances in Behavioral Biology.* Plenum Press, New York.
10. *N. Engl. J. Med.,* (1972): 286:102–103.
11. Roth, M. (1978): Epidemiological studies, In: *Aging, Vol. 7 Alzheimer's Disease: Senile Dementia and Related Disorders,* pp. 337–339. Katsman, R., Terry, R. D., and Bick, K. L. (eds.) Raven Press, New York.
12. Shanas, E. (1961): *The Health of Older People: A Social Survey,* p. 76. Harvard University Press, Cambridge.
13. Shanas, E., Townsend, P., Wedderburn, D., Friis, H., Milhaj, P., and Stehouwer, J. (1968): *Old People in Three Industrial Societies,* p. 22. Atherton Press, New York.
14. Sherwin, I., and Seltzer, B. (1977): Senile and presenile dementia: A clinical overview, In: *Advances in Behavioral Biology, Vol. 23,* Nandy, X., and Sherwin, X. (eds.), pp. 285–294. Plenum Press, New York.
15. Strömgren, E. (1963): Epidemiology of old-age psychiatric disorders, In: *Processes of Aging, Vol. II, Social and Psychological Perspectives,* p. 141, Williams, R. H., Tibbetts, C., and Donahue, W. (eds.) Atherton Press, New York.
16. U.S. Bureau of Census (1973): *Some Demographic Aspects of Aging in the U.S.* Current Population Reports. Series P-23, No. 43. Government Printing Office, Washington, D.C.
17. U.S. Bureau of Census (1973): *Current Population Report Series No. 43, PT 23.* Government Printing Office, Washington, D.C.
18. U.S. Bureau of Census (1975): *Current Population Reports Series P-20, No. 287.* Government Printing Office, Washington, D.C.
19. U.S. Department of Commerce. Bureau of the Census. (1978): *Current Population Reports. Special Studies Services P-23, No. 69. Survey of Institutional Persons; A Study of Persons Receiving Long-Term Care,* p. 196. Prepared by Brown, R. F., and Stoudt, D. W., Government Printing Office, Washington, D.C.
20. U.S. National Center for Health Statistics. (1978): *Advance Data, No. 35.* Government Printing Office, Washington, D.C.
21. U.S. Statistical Abstract. (1977): p. 392. Government Printing Office, Washington, D.C.
22. Williamina, A., and Himwich, H. E. (1959): Neurochemistry of aging. In: *Handbook of Aging and the Individual,* Birren, J. E. (ed.), p. 189. University of Chicago Press, Chicago.

DISCUSSION

Dr. Pfeiffer: While we are all hopeful that research will solve the problem of dementia, our task here is concerned with what can be done now for patients with dementia, for the patients themselves as well as for their families.

The support structures defined in these papers were presented as (1) community organizations; (2) residential congregate living facilities; and (3) informal or family structures. There was little discussion about clinical manifestations of dementia. One of the striking aspects about dementia that has not received sufficient emphasis is the interesting discrepancy between level of cognitive performance and level of social skills. In many patients, cognitive skills can be severely impaired while social skills are well preserved. The retention of these social skills has a lot to do with being able to receive care and being maintained in the community.

What is involved in making the various support systems work is the maintenance or the reestablishment of social skills and the enlargement of whatever social network is there.

Another issue is particularly psychiatric in nature, i.e., the prevention of associated psychopathology, such as disability, anxiety, depression, paranoid delusions, etc., superimposed on the basic cognitive deficit. Whether a person can be adequately cared for depends not only on the severity of cognitive deficit, but also on whether associated psychopathology supervenes. Accordingly, the reduction of associated psychopathology, or its prevention in the context of a social support system, is an important issue.

Another issue emphasized in all the presentations on social support systems was the focus on "minimal intervention." I would modify that phrase slightly to say "minimal disruption" through intervention. I would not minimize the need for intervention, but rather suggest increased cognizance of the disruptive aspect of certain interventions.

In all three of these support settings, support can be most adequately provided if there is a fuller understanding of the nature of the disease process on the part of the caregivers—whether they are family or professional persons. This would include teaching the affected patient about the disease itself.

Finally, it is clear that very little data are available regarding pure senile dementia groups as they relate to various of these social support systems. Much more work is needed in this area.

Sir Martin Roth: I think I can best comment on points I have in mind by taking up the Sainsbury and Grad study that was described by Dr. Kahn. This experiment tackles so many important issues that it is worthwhile looking at it in retrospect.

The first point I would like to make about that important investigation is that it is not certain that they were necessarily achieving a higher degree of success in resettling or avoiding admission of individuals from the community, and providing community care for them. I think the data of the comparative study between Chichester and Salisbury showed that Chichester was successful in attracting a higher proportion of referrals and thereby also a higher proportion of individuals with a shorter duration, and a briefer history of illness.

Now, it is an admirable achievement to bring people to medical attention at the early stages of the development of senile dementia, and that alone would have justified the study. But the two groups, the Salisbury and the Chichester groups, were to that extent not strictly comparable, in that the individuals who had come with organic disorders to Chichester may not have been ill as long as those studied in Salisbury. I don't say that were a more strict comparison to be made, the result would not be upheld, but for the present it hasn't been made.

Far more important, it seems to me, are the respects in which the social scene has completely altered in the last 15 to 20 years. We must not assume that any success achieved 20 years ago in keeping people in the community can be wholly replicated at the present time. In the first place, we have a higher proportion of people above 80 years of age than there were, let us say, 15 years ago. And, I was very interested in Dr. Brody's story, which is very pertinent. One more terror to the prospect of growing old is the possibility of having children who are also candidates for geriatric care. This is a new prospect. It was not so much in evidence 15 to 20 years ago.

Second, fewer women are available—the many pairs of hands who were there to wash, to clean, to tend, to look after, to comfort, are not there anymore.

Third, in the idyllic situation described in the Bethnal Green studies by Peter Townsend, and in the studies by the international groups published by Shanas and her colleagues, you had a reciprocal exchange of services between the old and the younger generations, the elderly being helped in sickness to an astonishing degree.

Now, let me remind you of Peter Townsend's figure. He pointed out that if it hadn't been for the help of the members of the family, the burden on the health and welfare services would have been four to five times as great as it was. If only one-fifth of that care had been transferred to the health and welfare services, they would have burst the seams. He was describing a network of social supports with a mutual exchange of services, the younger generation gaining opportunities for participating in community activities in return for the support provided by the elderly.

Now there is evidence that this support system is being rapidly eroded. We do not know the rate at which this is occurring. And we certainly have done nothing to put something in its place. It is a matter of urgent and vital necessity that something be put in its place.

This brings me to the very important point regarding the means for bringing support to the aid of the family. For the present this is not being done. But it is important to undertake experiments to establish how far we can succeed in helping families and recreating networks to support the aged.

Another reason why we should not lean too much on these studies for guidance is that the burden on the family in terms of emotional strain, the interference with employment and daily life, the effects on children, which was described in the case of the Chichester studies, is considerable. There was a greater burden on the Chichester families and although there was willingness to accept the burden, one should not lightly generalize from that finding. The question of burden and the response to it needs to be reassessed in different types of social setting. It cannot be assumed that burdens are tolerated in the same manner everywhere or to the same extent that was the case more than a decade ago. We do not know, we cannot assume this is the case.

Now I shall consider perhaps the most important thing of all. Here I draw upon practical experience. That is, to press the tolerance, the endurance, the willingness to care, of families beyond certain points is misconceived policy because it is subject to the law of diminishing returns.

The success achieved in Newcastle was due in considerable measure to the trust by the community in the psychogeriatric services. There was trust that they would receive all possible support by domiciliary services. The day care would bring relief during working hours, admission would be arranged during holidays and for limited periods in the week. It was also recognized when their burdens were manifestly too much for them to bear, admission would be arranged.

Once this bond of trust between community and services is broken, there is a rapid downward spiral in confidence and the plausibility of community care with it. As soon as the possibility of chronic disease and long-term care begins to approach, admission may be demanded immediately.

So, one must strike a judicious balance between providing for community care that fosters the survival of old people in the community for longer periods, on the one hand, and keeping a sensitive eye on the community tolerance and welfare and its attitudes toward the service; for once that trust is impaired and tolerance weakened, the plans for community care are worth little more than the paper on which they are drawn.

I should like to pick up one further point, before we accept the view that giving more social work is more lethal than giving less, which is the conclusion that emerges from the Blenkner studies: one needs certain details. I suppose that if one didn't take great care in sampling, one could also show that more medical care is also lethal than less medical care.

I am reluctant to be persuaded without being shown good evidence that the groups investigated were comparable. Errors are so easily imported into such studies since those who utilize more care, differ in all sorts of imponderable ways, from those who receive less. They are likely to have fewer links with their families, less advantaged social circumstances, more physical as well as more psychiatric disability, both explicit and covert. So, before we assume that if you provide more care you will cause higher mortalities or cause them to be admitted into institutions more often, the relevant samples would have to be closely scrutinized.

Dr. Weinberg: In response to Sir Martin Roth, to the best of my knowledge, the Blanker studies were set up to ensure that there was a random assignment of subjects to each experimental group. Accordingly, I do not believe that his doubts, in this instance, can be justified.

Dr. Arie: We have done well to have a meeting devoted specifically to dementia, and to accept and recognize the responsibilities of psychiatry in relation to the elderly.

But, it is appropriate to remind ourselves that dementia, indeed the care of the elderly as a whole, is the monopoly of no group, and we must always be aware of the spectrum of care of which we are only one part.

I want briefly to explain what I mean. Dr. Kahn earlier gave us some examples of studies in Britain on which Sir Martin has commented very pertinently. One of these was a report by our colleague, Dr. Baker, a geriatric psychiatrist, on the extent to which he was able to reduce hospitalization of the elderly by extensive systems of day hospital care. This is an interesting claim, and I think Dr. Baker has much to support it. The trouble is that it illustrates the pitfalls of reporting on one sector of the spectrum of care without looking at the consequences in the other associated and interdependent sectors.

After Dr. Baker published that report, the next issues of the *British Journal of Psychiatry* had some very telling letters, including one from Klaus Bergmann, and letters from the geriatricians in the locality, who claimed that the patients whom Dr. Baker was not admitting were, in fact, being admitted by them.

In other words, any account of the operation of services for the elderly must not be particulate; it must be holistic. We must consider the whole interdependent care system all along the line, because changes in practice in any one sector are likely to have consequences for other sectors.

In Nottingham we are attempting to bring together in one university department the whole spectrum of services for the elderly. We have a department which we call Health Care of the Elderly, and we have abolished the term geriatrics.

The services for the elderly are under the rubric of Health Care of the Elderly, and Health Care of the Elderly is staffed by physicians, psychiatrists, social workers, nurses, physiotherapists, occupational therapists, research workers, and others. We attempt to provide a unified service and a unified educational experience, and to facilitate also monitoring of performance.

We are at an early stage and I can make no claims for this model except one, and that is that the job satisfaction of working and teaching in such a joint enterprise of colleagues within one department is striking. And feedback from our students is that they enjoy it too. So, we feel that we have got something interesting and good in Nottingham, and I hope there will be opportunities to come back and tell you whether it really proves to be good in the future.

Dr. Kahn: First, I appreciate Dr. Arie's comments amplifying on the material originally published in the British literature. This exchange illustrates one of the advantages of a meeting like this. Despite the limitations of any one facility, however, it is impressive that there have been numerous reports of programs in Britain in which day care has been described as a component of integrated mental health services for the elderly, effective in keeping substantial numbers out of institutions.

The other comments expressed earlier were concerned with those two classic evaluative studies, the Grad and Sainsbury study, and the research of Margaret Blenkner. Despite our repeated complaints about the dearth of evaluation, these must be considered among our finest examples of well-controlled studies, and the carry important implications for modes of mental health care. Sir Martin Roth has questioned the Chichester/Salisbury study on the grounds that patients in the two groups were not comparable, since those in Chichester had a shorter history of illness. He implies that this detracts from the value of the study, since the results could not be regarded as a "strict comparison" of the two programs on similar populations. It should be pointed out, first of all, that although ill for a shorter period, the Chichester patients were also more severely ill. But, more importantly, rather than being a complication, the differences in the character of the clinical populations referred to the two programs is, in itself, a major substantive finding demonstrating the advantages of the community program.

It has also been questioned whether or not the Chichester program is still appropriate today after the many changes in the social scene that have occurred. Obviously these social changes will have effects on mental health issues. Yet, the Chichester program continues to function. In a recent article, for example, Sainsbury indicated that the program was still as effective as it had been originally. From the description of British programs provided by Glasscote, it appears that new programs are continuing to be established along similar lines (1,2).

Some of the brief descriptions of their own current programs offered by the panelists here have emphasized the necessity for establishing the same attitudes of trust and dependability that were considered critical for the success of the Chichester program. The two major questions raised concerning the Blenkner study relate to the adequacy of sampling and the interpretation of the results. I would like to reiterate Dr. Weinberg's comment that Margaret Blenkner was a rigorous researcher who developed her study using very careful random sampling.

Her results cannot be literally interpreted as telling anything about good or bad social work. What she did point out was the often paradoxical effects of well-intentioned service to a severely impaired elderly population. Common practices, such as institutionalization, turned out to have the unfortunate side effect of being associated with increased mortality. To avoid the noxious effects of "over-dosing," she recommended minimal intervention. Dr. Pfeiffer has objected that the term should really be limited to "minimal disruption." But minimal intervention refers to other aspects in addition to disruption. It would mean, for example, that other potentially noxious effects would follow from services that infringe on the old person's ability to act as an autonomous, responsible, adult person.

Although some may feel discouraged by the results of the Blenkner study, it really has considerable positive importance, indicating, as it does, approaches for improving our services. This goal cannot be achieved by good intentions alone, however, but requires continued careful controlled study.

Mrs. Brody: I think we are making certain assumptions that we really have to look at, that fall into the area of value judgment. One of those assumptions is that it is always "bad" if a family puts an older person in an institution. That is an incorrect assumption. It can be just as neurotic and pathological, or whatever labels you may want to use, for a family to keep an older person in their home. I am thinking of a case record I read a couple of weeks ago, in which a women had not shared her bed with her husband for 5 years. She had shared it with her elderly brain-damaged mother so that she could supervise her at night and keep her from wandering. The husband was sleeping in the son's bedroom, and the son in turn was sleeping in the basement and was having school problems. Now, I submit that that is pathology, not health, and that sometimes health is in the direction of separating.

The other value judgment that we seem to be making is that we project our own feelings about going into an institution onto older people, who are at the point where they need it.

It is commonly said that most older people do not wish to go into an institution. You ask old people where they would like to live and they don't want an institution. That is understandable. But if people in this audience were asked whether they wanted to go into a hospital, they too would all say no. If you asked old people whether they wanted a visiting nurse they would say no, because that would mean that they would be sick. But, if older people—or any people—reach the point at which they need a certain kind of care, then attitudes change, and many, many people go into an institution voluntarily, feeling they need the security of the health care that is close by. Or, they want to relieve the family of a severe burden. So, we have to change our rigid mindsets about such situations.

With respect to the community services and family, the recent Social Security longitudinal study of retirement provided data to the effect that about 25% of all people in their late 50s and early 60s had a surviving very old parent; in about half of that group, both parents were alive.

In short, there are more and more very old people for the middle aged to take care of. What this means is that this whole business of the theoretical sociological life-stages that ended with the "empty nest" has to be rethought. What is happening for a subgroup of people who reach that empty nest phase—the romantic notion that they will then have plenty of time to enjoy their hobbies and peace and so on and so forth—for that subgroup of people those empty nests are being refilled with very old, very damaged people. Parent care of a very old, very damaged person—one who is incontinent, for example—is very different from care of an incontinent young child who will soon be trained. The stress can be enormous.

Now, what has happened in this country is that we have not developed supportive community care services. A question that was asked by the audience earlier was about what happens to the spouses and the adult children of people with senile dementia and the kind of services they need. We don't have all of those services. With the advent of Medicare, virtually overnight a medical care system was put in place in the United States, whatever its drawbacks. But the health services—the day care, the respite care, the home health services—all of those services are very scant and very uneven throughout the United States. In the vast majority of communities, it is impossible to mobilize a total package of needed services.

We are doing some research at the Philadelphia Geriatric Center in which we have identified triads of women: an elderly woman, her adult middle-aged daughter, and the middle-aged daughter's young adult daughter. We are asking questions of them in order to be able to project the kinds of services that successive generations will be willing to give to their elderly. We are eliciting their attitudes about parent care to determine effects of women's changing roles.

Our hypothesis is that what the families can and want to and will continue to give are the kinds of services such as emotional support, visiting, response in emergency, negotiation with the health system when necessary, keeping in contact and so on. Those services are what older people probably will continue to want from their families. Early data from the study indicate that the concrete instrumental kinds of services—the home health services, the maintenance of the immediate home environment, the bathing, and so on—are the sorts of services that the community must develop in the future if we are not going to put additional stress on the women who are already under severe stress.

It is for that reason that I do not think that the same kinds of programs will help all women. Some women may be willing to exchange money for working, but women who have an investment in career in terms of personal realization will not be willing to exchange their jobs for $50 or more paid to them for parent care.

Dr. Delise: Dr. Ringler remarked earlier that a new development in this field are the therapy groups for families of patients with Alzheimer's disease. He pointed out that one of these groups is already operational under the guidance of Dr. Eisdorfer. I am wondering if you could tell us about the origin of this group, how it was organized, and who is participating? Do you simply limit yourself to training family members to cope with the patient, or is there also an ongoing therapy group for individuals who have to cope with relatives with Alzheimers?

Dr. Eisdorfer: Let me try to answer all of your questions in substance, if not specifically. The group evolved out of a number of things. We have a Veteran's Administration Geriatric Research Educational and Clinical Center, which contains our Alzheimer's research ward, which has been run largely without the use of psychotropic medications. One of the things I discovered, partly in my clinical practice, was that I was spending approximately 5 hours or so with the family for every hour I was spending with the patient.

There are several issues involved. First of all, it is clear that you need to work with the family to help the patient and second, the family itself very often is in a state of severe crisis.

One of the things that became clear is that although many of the people who came to us were fairly well informed, upper middle class and so on, there was a lot of denial. The most common scenario is that the husband gets diagnosed as Alzheimer's disease and the wife refuses to accept the diagnosis. She takes him to a number of other diagnostic centers, until finally some exotic strategy is employed, which doesn't work, and she gets increasingly agitated and upset at the health system. I was getting the same story over and over again. Competent neurologists were telling his wife "your husband has Alzheimer's disease, and there is nothing you can do about it. In 3 to 6 months, he will be in a nursing home." Some of these families came to us after maintaining relatives in the community for 4 or 5 years. One of the other issues that may not have been raised is that some received surgical shunts, because of the interaction between the clinician and a very agitated, upset lady. The neurosurgeon figures, well, if it was my wife or husband, I would shunt him even if it was a one in a million shot. So they come to me then, sometimes a little toxic, usually on 15 to 20 mg of a potent antipsychotic drug and with a very disruptive family situation.

We also discovered that while the family was crucial in maintaining the patient in the community, economic considerations played a part. We never got paid for taking care of the family and the family was taking up the bulk of clinical time. For the clinician's practice, it is a most serious problem. I could see why physicians in group or private practice couldn't spend time with the family, despite their desire to do so, in caring for the patient.

When we opened up the Alzheimer's ward, these women, who had averaged over 5 years of working with their husbands in the community, who specifically didn't want their husbands in nursing homes, indicated that they really wanted to be involved in the ward.

The question was, do we ignore them, do we do what we usually do, which is to keep the relative out, or do we take an opposite strategy and incorporate them into the treatment process?

Having determined to involve them had obvious consequences. In my residency training program, I teach the residents, when in doubt, shut up and let the patient tell you. We were lucky enough to keep quiet and let the patients lead us to the fact that they were getting a lot of satisfaction from taking care of each other.

We found the patients who came to us quite demented were making friends with each other, and were apparently holding sustained conversations with each other even though I defy anybody to make sense out of the conversation. They walk up and down the hall as comrades and so on, and the wives became friendly seeing that the husbands were friendly. These kinds of pairings led to the creation of a weekly discussion group. It started with the ward and then gradually the word got out and it moved from Tacoma to Seattle. A lot of the women lived in Seattle, but their husbands were in Tacoma, and they would be there four and five days a week. Other people began to join it, and it had to be expanded beyond the VA group. We now have used a nurse and a clinical psychologist who work with the group in Seattle.

I have been working more recently with what evolved from this group, which is an incorporated group called Project Assist, which is designed to create a national consciousness about Alzheimer's disease. It is one of six groups nationally. Dr. Katzman told me about a similar group that is evolving in New York. I do know that there is a group that has evolved in Montreal, and one in San Francisco, and so I have been trying to help them to create a family self-help program. We are working not only with wives and husbands, but also with children. And, more and more the focus is on specific management techniques. At first families had no idea of what to expect. We are generating a number of videotapes with these families.

Our group is now mostly oriented to self-help, with a lot of internal communication, and a lot of help with psychological expectation. The majority of women with whom I spoke said that when they first were told their husbands had Alzheimer's disease, they were at least relieved. They thought, well, finally, now we have a disease we can cure, and it wasn't until it was explained to them that Alzheimer's disease was an incurable disease, and there was nothing they could do, that they began to recognize the profound consequences of what is going on. At this point, we take very little credit.

We have just been a catalyst in helping facilitate their goals.

REFERENCES

1. Glasscote, R. M., Gudeman, J. E., and Miles, D. G. (1977): *Creative Mental Health Services for the Elderly.* American Psychiatric Association, Washington, D.C.
2. Sainsbury, P. (1975): Evaluation of community mental health programs. In: M. Guttentag and E. L. Struening (eds.): *Handbook of Evaluation Research,* pp. 125–259. Beverly Hills.

Subject Index

Subject Index

A

Acetylcholine deficiency, 165
Acquisition process, 105–106, 110
ACTH$_{4-10}$, 170–171
Activities, daily, 2–6
Activities of Daily Living Scale, 133
Acute brain syndrome, 48–49, 98
Adaptation, 73–74, 98, 161, 211
Affective states; *see also specific state*
  pharmacological treatment of,
    161–179, 181–185
Age-integrated environment,
  250
Aged
  institutionalized, 305–309
  neglect of, 258, 261
  numbers of, 3, 13
Aggregrate networks, 289
Aggressiveness, 2–4, 203, 205
Aging
  and brain weight, 139, 148
  and cell number, 148
  and coping, 188–189
  and diagnosis of mental illness,
    181
  and MAO activity, 148, 175
  and mental functioning, 51–52,
    62, 63, 104, 124–125, 139–140
Agnosia, 92
Alertonic, 147
Aluminum intoxication, 71, 150
Alzheimer's disease
  age of onset of, 49–50, 85
  classification of, 49–50, 51–52
  components of, 88
  course of, 85
  etiology of, 86
  and excess mortality, 87–88
  and genetics, 51

and histopathological changes,
  47–48, 51
  intellectual impairment in, 51–52
  and longevity, 87
  and morphological changes, 51
  prevention of, 5, 13
  prognosis of, 87
American Indians, and natural
  support, 289
Amphetamines, 145, 147, 175
Amitriptyline, 174–175, 181
Amnesic syndrome, 44, 108, 109
Amsterdam, community mental
  health in, 255
Anabolic substances, 148–149
Anger, 203–204
Antacid gels, 178
Antianxiety agents, 173–174; *see*
    also specific agent
Anticholinergic side effects
  of antihistamines, 173, 181
  of antipsychotics, 177, 181
  of tricyclics, 175, 181, 183, 184
Anticoagulants, 149, 162–163
Antidepressants, 90, 174–176, 181,
    203; *see also specific type;*
    name
Antihistamines, 173, 181
Antipsychotic agents, 176–178, 181;
    see also specific agent
Anxiety, 188, 189, 193, 201–202, 226
Anxious-depressive type, 193
Apathy, 203
Aphasia, 90, 92, 110, 137
Apperception, 190
Apraxia, 91–92
Arecholine, 150
Arousal levels, 69–70, 75, 140
Asian-Americans, and natural
  support, 289